# THE PATH OF PRACTICE

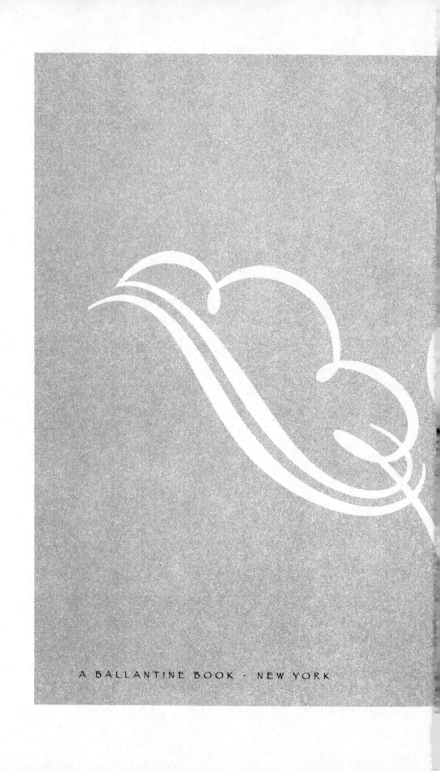

A BALLANTINE BOOK · NEW YORK

# THE
# PATH
# OF
# PRACTICE

*A Woman's Book of Healing
with Food, Breath, and Sound*

BRI. MAYA TIWARI

A Ballantine Book
The Ballantine Publishing Group

Copyright © 2000 by Bri. Maya Tiwari

Illustration © 2000 by Bri. Maya Tiwari and the Wise Earth School of Ayurveda Ltd.

Wise Earth *Sadhana* is a unique school of thought and practice developed by Bri. Maya Tiwari and based on Ayurvedic principles. The philosophy and practices set forth in this book are copyrighted by Bri. Maya Tiwari and the Wise Earth School of Ayurveda Ltd.

For information about Wise Earth *Sadhana* Training for Practitioners, you may write to: Wise Earth School of Ayurveda Ltd., 90 Davis Creek Road, Candler, North Carolina 28715

www.randomhouse.com/BB/

Library of Congress Cataloging-in-Publication Data
Tiwari, Maya.
The path of practice : a woman's book of healing with food, breath, and sound / Bri. Maya Tiwari.— 1st ed.
p.   cm.
ISBN 0-345-43030-1
1. Medicine, Ayurvedic.   I. Title.
R606.T594 2000
615.5'3—dc21                                                    00-062121

Text design by Debbie Glasserman

Manufactured in the United States of America

First Edition: November 2000

10  9  8  7  6  5  4  3  2  1

*To my Satguru,*
*His Holiness Swami Dayananda Saraswati,*
*and to the Great Rishis who*
*are the wellspring of wisdom in the universe.*

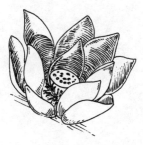

## OPENING PRAYER TO THE DIVINE MOTHER

*Sharanagata dinarta paritrana parayane*
*Sarvasyarti hare Devi Narayani namo'stu te*

Reverence onto You, O Goddess Narayani.
O You who are intent on protecting the distressed
and the dejected who seek refuge in You:
O You, Devi, who remove the sufferings of all.

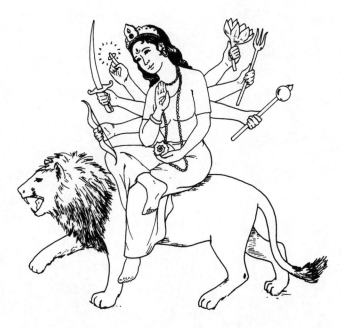

# CONTENTS

## ACKNOWLEDGMENTS

First and always, my gratitude to the Divine Mother, who guards and protects my journey and whose work it is I serve, and to Her spirited emissaries: my editor at Ballantine Books, Leslie Meredith—warrioress and spiritual visionary, whose uncompromising genius and skills make this book possible; and my agent, Janis Vallely, whose unflinching support and efforts have helped to bring this book to fruition.

My deep gratitude and appreciation to my remarkable editor, Deborah Chiel, whose insights, skills, and intuitive understanding of Vedic thought have helped to shape and hone my words into an exquisite work.

My gratitude to Dr. Christiane Northrup, Ilana Rubenfeld, and Sri. Deepak Chopra for their heartfelt comments on the book.

My deepest gratitude to Satguru Sivaya Subramuniyaswami and to the swamis and *sadhakas* of *Hinduism Today* for their support of my work.

Many thanks to my manager, Patricia Isa Peluso, who safeguards my work at large, and to the staff and students of the Wise Earth School of Ayurveda for helping to spread these teachings. My thanks to Pritha Singh, Karna Singh, Radha Singh, Bonnie Kirk, and Anu Priya for their *seva* to Mother Om Mission; and to Vic Insanally and Annette Arjoon, advocates of the Mother Om Mission work in Guyana, South America.

My thanks to Holly Hammond for her kind support and line editing of the work; Leslie Hawkins for manuscript support; and Marnie Mikell for her fine hand with the line drawings.

Finally, my gratitude and appreciation to my birth mother, Kalidevi, and my elder mother, Jayadevi, for their loving support; to my brother Chandra, whose sacrifice made it possible for me to walk my spiritual path; and to my brother Subhas, whose spiritual support helps me to sustain my spiritual path.

# INTRODUCTION

I am a Vedic monk—a *brahmacharini*. Since my initiation in 1992 by my teacher, Swami Dayananda Saraswati, I have dedicated my life to living in accordance with the natural rhythms of the universe; to teaching the wisdom and healing practices of the Vedas, the holy scriptures of India which date back to 1500 B.C.E.; and to helping others heal physically and emotionally. At my center, the Wise Earth School of Ayurveda, in the mountains near Asheville, North Carolina, I teach the knowledge and practice of *sadhana* and Ayurvedic healing.

Because of my experiences, I have a great deal of information—about breathwork, meditation, sound, yoga, and wholesome nutrition—that can help people, especially women, live healthy lives, cultivate healing communities, and help themselves and others heal from physical and emotional ailments. My students include doctors, nurses, yoga instructors, nutritionists, artists, social advocates, inner-city youth mentors, and interested laypeople.

Wise Earth *sadhana* teachings are intended for everyone—women, men, and children. Indeed, 35 percent of my students are men. However, this book has a strong focus on women, because they are the staff-holders of sacred life and nurturance. The aim of *The Path of Practice* is to evoke, inform, strengthen, and safeguard the memory of women as guardians of sacred healing. It is also meant to help men become awakened to the Mother's primordial healing energy that has existed within them from ancient times. Indeed, all but a few of the spiritual teachers whose work has informed my practice are men.

In addition, I conduct the Mother Om Mission, a charitable organization whose purpose is to educate at-risk communities about *sadhana* lifeways and to familiarize men and women with the primordial healing power that every human being possesses. I also travel all over the world conducting workshops for those interested in learning the path of practice, or *sadhana*.

*Sadhana* is a Sanskrit word whose root, *sadh*, means to reclaim that which is divine in us, our power to heal, serve, rejoice, and uplift the spirit. *Sadhana* practices encompass all our daily activities, from the simple to the sublime—from cooking a meal to exploring your inner self through meditation. The goal of *sadhana* is to enable you to recover your natural rhythms and realign your inner life and daily habits with the cycles of the universe. When you begin to live and move with the rhythms of nature, your mind becomes more lucid and more peaceful and your health improves. Your entire life becomes easier.

As you begin your journey along the path of practice, you must make the promise to yourself that you are willing to take a very clear look at yourself. Allow yourself to recognize the various disguises and false faces that you have assumed over the years. As you come to acknowledge and know each one, you will also come to see *beyond* them to your truest self. As you find out more about yourself and your strengths and weaknesses, you will also learn about your body, mind, and spirit, and their innate power. You will awaken to your own self-healing abilities. Whatever conventional, Western medical treatments you use, you will always be able to use your own natural abilities as well.

On the path of practice, we adopt the belief that disease happens from within, and so must any cure. We decide that any lack of peace or dis-ease or illness becomes an occasion to go deeper into ourselves, to examine where we must make changes in order to heal our bodies, feelings, or lives. We accept that our ailment is an assignment, and that to complete it satisfactorily, we must do research into it and into ourselves. Each of us is unique; no one else can complete our assignment for us. We can't even depend on the inherent beneficence of the universe to save us. The universe *will* support us, and *will* help us by revealing its sacred rhythms. It will help us see where we have gotten off balance and will always allow us to realign with it. But we have to do the work of self-reflection and healing that fits our individual inner life and outer life. On our individual path on the human journey, each of us is meant to learn the truths of our physical, mental, and spiritual lives that are particular to us and shared by others. These truths unite us to our families, our tribe, the entire human race, and the universe as a whole.

Early in life, I discovered for myself that serious illness can offer extraordinary opportunities for healing and self-knowledge. When I was twenty-three years old—at the height of my personal and professional success as a fashion designer in New York City—I was diagnosed with terminal ovarian cancer. Driven by my ambition, I had been keeping a fast-paced schedule of hard work and parties. I was also in flight from my traditional East Indian heritage and upbringing. My illness would eventually force me to realize that all pain is a reminder that we have strayed from the natural rhythms of life. Yet before I accepted this truth, I became exhausted from years of fighting the cancer with invasive treatments and surgeries. I gave up the struggle, left my life and friends in New York, and went deep into the snowy wilderness of Vermont to prepare to die. Instead, over the course of three solitary winter months, I was presented with the opportunity to face the changes I had to make in my life. I rested and fasted and dreamed, and I gradually saw where I had deceived myself; where I had allowed myself to become out of balance.

I also wept until it seemed as if I had no more tears to shed. I kept a journal, writing page after page about my personal and spiritual history. Having learned meditation as a child, I remembered how to do it again. In meditation, prayers, and dream states, I relived the anguish of my ancestors who had been uprooted from their native soil of India and transplanted in a foreign land, Guyana. I had spiritual visitations from my father, who lived far away, but convinced me that I must reclaim my life and fulfill my purpose. I also had visions of the Divine Mother, the infinitely beneficent feminine energy whom we can all call upon for help, guidance, and healing. I prayed to recover faith in myself and in the Divine.

When the snow began to melt outside my cabin, I reawakened to the sounds and beauty of nature. I heard deer foraging in the underbrush of the forest around my cabin. A bright-red cardinal was singing. The music of spring drew me out of my seclusion into the sun. It seemed to me at that moment, and in many moments since, that the cancer had knocked me down and stripped me of all my defenses so that I could get out of my own way. It forced me to reclaim my connection to my ancestors, to the natural rhythms of the universe, and to the infinitely loving, healing light of the Divine Mother.

When I emerged from my retreat and returned to the city, my doctors were astonished. They told me that they could find no signs of the cancer in my blood or lymph nodes. Determined to live a life of good health and serenity, I studied yoga, Eastern medicine, and natural farming. In the fall of 1986, I met my guru, His Holiness Swami Dayananda Saraswati, a South Indian monk and scholar. Under Swami

Dayananda's guidance, I made an intensive study of Sanskrit and Vedanta, that portion of the Vedas dealing with self-knowledge.

My purpose for writing this book, however, is not to convince you to become a Vedic monk or spiritual teacher like myself. Nor do I recommend that you renounce your present lifestyle or discontinue any medical treatments that you may be undergoing. What I want to share with you is my realization of some deep truths of the healing process that came to me through my own illness and subsequent life course. *The Path of Practice* is meant to be a guide for all people, especially women. It is a short course in healing and in living. Whether you are in good health but want to find a greater sense of balance and mindfulness, or whether you have been diagnosed with an illness—be it chronic or acute—this primer shows you how to make gradual changes in the way you conduct your daily life so that you will see profound changes both immediately *and* over time. You will be happier, healthier, calmer, and more resilient because of these practices. Indeed, you will notice that the effects of these practices spread far beyond your individual life. Because women have always been the guardians of life's wholesome practices, when we strengthen our health and spiritual power, we also strengthen the health and wisdom of the men, children, and communities around us.

## "THAT WHICH IS TO BE DONE"

To understand the philosophical basis of the path of practice, it's helpful to know something about Vedic history and culture. Vedic culture grew out of ancient *rishi* tradition, extending back to the Harappan civilization in India. Like the *rishis* before them, Vedic Yogis are adept at focusing their awareness and shifting their perceptual fields. In meditation, they enter elevated states to "see" the truth, retrieving information directly from the cosmos for the welfare of their community. The visions of the ancient Yogis created the healing arts of yoga, meditation, *japa* (the repetitive chanting of sacred Sanskrit words, or mantras), and breathwork, and informed the writing of the Vedas, the holy texts of the Hindu people of India.

Hinduism, the religion of my ancestors, sprang from the Vedic texts and traditions which promote harmony and unity among all peoples. The Vedic culture is not a set of religious or philosophical beliefs; rather, it is a universal and sacred way of life based on the idea that each one of us has the potential to attain the goal of *moksha*—liberation from the cycles of rebirth, the attainment of self-realization, and the recognition of the immortality of the spirit. The Vedic tradition does not seek converts from other traditions and religions. But it does teach all of us to discover our own true essence and our singular purpose in life. It also helps people find their own way back to the authentic traditions of their own ancestral and cultural heritage.

The Vedas consist of four parts—*Rig, Yajur, Sama,* and *Atharva*—and set out the sacred laws of the universe, as well as the mythology of gods and goddesses and the creative energies of the universe. They teach that health is a state of living in harmony with nature as a whole and with our own basic natures. Because we are formed from nature and have a sympathetic resonance with her, only nature can heal us when we become ill. When we eat when we are hungry, rest when we are tired, and create when inspiration comes, we live in sync with nature's tempos. Disease will not last in a body-mind that is flowing in harmony with the rhythms of the cosmos, which sustain the material world with energy.

According to the *Bhagavad Gita*, a great Indian spiritual

text, the only way to live in harmony with the cosmos is to "do what is to be done" in the present. This is the heart of *sadhana*—the practices that reflect and re-create within us the universe's energies and rhythms. In present-day India, the word *sadhana* is generally used to refer to rote, mechanical practices. Through my own teachings and life practice, however, I have redefined *sadhana*, restoring its original meaning of actions that reclaim the divine within. To practice *sadhana* is to act in ways that are derived from nature's intelligence and rhythms. *Sadhana* replicates the sacred in nature through everyday activities that bring us into harmony with the great cycles of the cosmos and that reconnect us to that which is divine in us: our power to heal, serve, rejoice, and uplift the spirit. In this book, *sadhana* practices revolve around breathing exercises and meditation, chanting and natural sounds, and natural food and nutrition. This path connects internal awareness to external rhythms and ultimately provides us with the gateway to our inner wisdom—the knowing that whatever is in us and outside us exists as a whole.

## THE HEALING JOURNEY

Each of us has the capacity to enter the vast universe within ourselves and become conscious of the Divine Spirit that is beyond the material reality we understand through our five senses. The practices of *sadhana* will help you learn to shift your perspective and enter a meditative state of mind many times throughout your day. You will come to see all obstacles and challenges in your everyday life as opportunities to learn more about yourself and your individual inner strengths. As you overcome each difficulty, you will become more focused and stronger in your purpose.

Each one of us has a unique purpose on this earth for

which we have been born. The Vedas call this our dharma, and by following the path of practice, you will be in harmony with this purpose. Harmony already exists at the core of every human life. Once we become conscious, we are able to recognize it. We become aware of the blessedness that surrounds us: the serenity in our living space after a long day's work; the beauty of dusk glimpsed through the windows; the sweetness of sparrows singing their songs; the warmth of the colors of autumn leaves.

When we are aware of our inner harmony, our power of intuition becomes active. We become more expressive, more fully alive, and more in tune with our bodies and all our healing energies. This intuition, together with our rational mind, will help us heal or get our lives more in balance. The rational mind is useful and has its place, but it cannot help us heal from within. Deep healing—healing at the inner source of the dis-ease or imbalance—is not a strictly rational process. Why illness arises, why bacteria or viruses sicken one person but not another, is a mystery that conventional, allopathic medicine has not been able to solve. While Western medicine can help you deal with physical symptoms and give you some time to pursue the deeper source of any illness or disease, it cannot help you see the meaning and opportunity in your imbalance. Your intuition, which you will discover as you follow the *sadhanas* I describe in *The Path of Practice*, can.

The path of practice described in this book is inspired by this wisdom and is the result of three milestones in my life. The first is my remembering, through my own painful experiences and through prayer and contemplation, the experiences of my exiled ancestors. Their experiences were important for me to realize because the energy of their spirits, disappointments, and traumas were passed on to me just as the form, color, and cellular makeup of my physical body were passed on to me. You, too, will need to explore your an-

cestral spiritual heritage as well as your physical inheritance
to find the best path of balance, peace, and healing for yourself. I will help you find ways to uncover what I call your ancestral memories—the ways in which the legacy of your
forebears affects your health and well-being.

The second milestone was my cancer journey, during
which I discovered that I could help heal my pain by living in
accord with the rhythms of the universe, awakening my intuition, and following practices that would heal me and keep
me healthy.

The third passage came when I began assisting women,
men, and children through their dark and fearful times, helping them restore faith in their intuition and rediscover their
natural rhythms and their birthright to harmony, healing,
and peace.

Nature expresses herself by providing food for every
species, by creating air and the means to breathe it, and by
moving in rhythms and cycles that keep all life in harmony.
Wise Earth *Sadhana's* practices of food, breath, and sound
enable us to sustain our health, realign ourselves with nature's cycles, and discover our rich inner realm of wisdom.
They help us to "sit in ourselves," to remain centered in our
consciousness with every action we take. By finding spiritual
accord in our daily routines, we can find this peace elsewhere
and everywhere. If we cannot find the harmony in our everyday actions, we will not find it anywhere else.

## FOOD, BREATH, AND SOUND

My own journey into health and wholeness began with the
*sadhana* of food. Remembering my mother's peaceful presence in the kitchen in Guyana where I was born, I undertook
cleaning and reclaiming my kitchen after I returned to my

New York City apartment from the woods of Vermont. There, I roasted grains and pounded them into flour; I combined aromatic spices and ground them into traditional Indian spice blends called *masalas*; I kneaded dough, rolled it, and baked chapatis over an open flame. But I wasn't just making a meal. Like my female ancestors before me, I strengthened my heartbeat with the sounds I made pounding grains; I balanced my inner breath with the circular movement of grinding spice seeds; I harmonized my senses and stilled my mind with the music I made by sifting beans in a basket.

In chapters 11 and 12, I will describe this process in greater detail, and discuss how you can transform your kitchen to reflect healthier, more organic approaches to food preparation and diet. Although you don't need to grind grain into flour, I will give you some grinding exercises to strengthen your own inner rhythms. I will also explain the Ayurvedic science of body types, or *doshas*, and which foods are most beneficial to the different types. Also provided are sample menus and easy-to-follow recipes that are appropriate for people of the particular *doshas* to eat in each of the six seasons. Unlike Western understanding of four seasons, the Ayurvedic calendar charts out six seasons involved reflecting the stages of the earth's yearly journey around the sun. (We will see more on the seasons in later chapters.)

Food *sadhana* is an inextricable part of a happy family life. Many cultures used these practices to bring family, friends, and community together. I recently heard a writer lovingly reminisce about the many hours she spent doing her homework at the kitchen table while her mother prepared dinner. Even the toughest algebra problems seemed easier to solve, she said, when the calculations were punctuated by the comforting, familiar sounds of her mother chopping vegetables, washing rice, or peeling potatoes.

I have no VCR, no movies on tape, no video games, no fast

foods, none of the things that children are supposed to enjoy. Yet my nieces and nephews—and my students' children, most of whom come from sophisticated urban households—love to visit me, because they can't wait to get their hands on my dough, spices, and grains. My seven-year-old niece begs me to let her knead the chapati dough, grind spices for the *masalas*, and shuck the corn. Another young friend of mine, who is all of two years old, was so enchanted with the process of kneading that we washed his feet, gave him a huge pan of dough, and let him at it. His face radiant with glee, he immediately began dancing on the dough. Together we create delicious meals that feed both body and spirit.

All physical life is composed of the same elements. The earth, water, fire, air, and space of our foods nurtures the earth, water, fire, air, and space of our bodies and minds. When you remain aware of this integral connection, every bite of food you take becomes a blessing from Mother Nature. With this simple awareness, you have begun performing *sadhana*, your path of practice. When we take care with our food, it nourishes and influences our life force, movement, and internal life—our personal rhythm or sound. Food, then, becomes our awareness manifested by thought and action. Each thought and action also becomes an expression of our unity with Mother Nature.

Sasha, an artist who is originally from South America, recently attended a beginner's Food *Sadhana* Practitioner Program at the Wise Earth School. Some twenty years earlier, her father had attempted suicide and suffered brain damage. Since then, he'd been confined to a long-term-care facility in South America. Sasha wept as she told me that although they spoke by phone from time to time, she missed him terribly. When I asked her when was the last time she'd gone to visit him, she described a collage of feelings—anger, guilt, fear, and a sense of abandonment—that had kept her from seeing him for many years.

I had noticed that Sasha particularly enjoyed drumming during our chanting classes, so I suggested that she send her father a recording of her chanting, singing, and drumming. She shook her head sadly as she explained that although her father loved music, the institution did not permit the residents to own any musical instruments or tapes. (I thought this was an extremely unfortunate policy, since research has shown that music has therapeutic value, as I will discuss later.)

"Why don't you bake your father a batch of cookies?" I suggested. "You can play your drum in between sifting and kneading and shaping the dough, so that you drum the sound into the cookies."

Sasha had reached the point where she could no longer tolerate the grief she felt over the long separation, and she liked the idea of nurturing her father in this small but meaningful way. When she returned home, she baked her father a batch of Ayurvedic oatmeal cookies, drumming and chanting throughout the process. She sent him the cookies, along with recent photographs of herself. Soon afterward, she called and spoke to him. His voice sounded more animated than usual, and his very first question was, "What did you do to those cookies? I've never tasted anything so delicious. They're so good, they make me want to burst out in song."

When we practice *sadhana* as Sasha chose to do, we exercise our divine choice to follow the path of practice in our everyday lives. The sense of well-being I gained from my food *sadhana* led me to the practice of conscious breath, the second foundation of Wise Earth *Sadhana*. Vedic thought teaches that breath is not just air but life force, *prana,* the organic energy that forms the currents of the subtle body. The subtle body is our nonphysical body that comprises the body's life force, intellect, mind, and ego. The subtle body is vital energy. *Prana* is generated within the chakras, the body's seven centers of energy, which are aligned along the central column of the spine.

According to ancient Indian folklore, the beautiful maiden Savitri was sitting by a lake playing her vina, a stringed instrument. As she played, the swans gliding past sang along to the tune. A passing hermit could not believe what he heard. "What powers have you that you can play and sing so divinely?" he inquired of Savitri and her swans. She smiled and responded, "My breath is full." The swans replied, "We eat the sacred grain." Divine breath animates and inspires us, and allows us to resonate with nature and communicate to and through nature's rhythms (the swans), as do the foods given by nature (the "sacred grain").

The life force of all creation, *prana* causes the earth to revolve around the sun, and the moon to orbit around the earth. *Prana* moves the air, water, nerves, memory cells, and the ocean tides. It is the basis of thought and consciousness within the body and in all creations. Conscious breathing helps to calm the mind so that our thoughts come into harmony with our intuition.

Later in these pages, we will learn about *pranayama*, the regulation and expansion of breath, which is one of the central practices of yoga. I will describe various breathing techniques specifically designed to control our physical and mental energies. Awareness of breath is the basis of meditation. When the breath is agitated or unsteady, our thoughts are scattered and our actions confused. When our breath is steady, so are the mind and body. As you will see, meditation is not an act of will or simply the practice of sitting and observing the breath as it flows in a calm, steady manner. The purpose of meditation is to quiet the mind, give a focused energy to the nervous system, and transcend visible, audible, tangible reality. The moment-to-moment awareness that you cultivate through *sadhana* practice is the ultimate aim of meditation.

One major obstacle we Westerners face in achieving harmony with the larger forces of nature is our reliance on the thinking mind. In the Vedic tradition, the mental plane is only one component of our intelligence which helps us to create, assimilate experience, analyze situations, and solve problems on the physical level of reality. Thought alone, however, cannot connect us to inner awareness and cosmic consciousness. In fact, the judgments and preconceptions of the rational mind often carry us away from the Divine Source. Meditation, contemplation, and everyday spiritual practices enable us to connect thought to consciousness and activate our intuition, or *buddhi*.

In the late 1960s Herbert Benson, M.D., conducted research at Harvard University that measured physiological responses in practitioners of meditation. To his amazement, Benson found that meditation slowed their heart rates, decreased their respiratory rates, and slowed their metabolisms. He named this state of diminished stress, with its many positive effects on the various systems of the body, the "relaxation response." Benson's experiments proved to the scientific and medical communities what Vedic seers have known for thousands of years: Meditation is good for our physical as well as our spiritual health.

The practice of sound is the third foundation of Wise Earth *Sadhana*. The yogis use sound to awaken consciousness. According to the Vedas, sound is the source of all life. Although we perceive our bodies to be solid matter, every cell is formed from vibrations and interactions of energy. We are made of living sounds, and our individual rhythms are dependent on the greater vibrations of the universe to sustain them. We carry the universe's primordial sound internally in our energy centers, or chakras, also referred to as our vibrating cores of consciousness.

The Vedic seers tell us that the universe's most sacred sound, Om, resonates within the space of the sixth chakra, located midbrow, between the eyes, in the area known as the "third eye." "The essence of thought, word, and sound is *Om*," says the *Chandogya Upanishad*. Om represents pure consciousness. Through practice of Vedic chants and sacred Sanskrit words, known as mantras, each one beginning and ending with "Om," we may harness our inner power of our intuition.

Through the intonation of sounds, the practitioner evokes tremendous power within, strengthening the breath force, energizing the mind, and immunizing the body. The Vedic seers defined mantra as both the medium of sound meditation and the means to invoke the divine energy of the deities. I am not alone in believing sound therapy to be one of our greatest medicines. Indeed, a wealth of scientific evidence points to the healing power of sound.

At the Wise Earth School, we use many different forms of sound and chanting to enhance our *sadhana*, as I will explain in chapters 9 and 10. One dramatic example of how the sound energy of the universe functions through vibrations was demonstrated by Joey, the three-year-old son of Marian, one of my students. Joey was born profoundly deaf. After many rounds of rigorous medical testing, the doctors declared that his condition was irreversible and he would never be able to respond to sound. But one morning, as Marian was drumming and chanting along with one of my recordings of Vedic chants, Joey came into the room and suddenly began dancing in perfect time to the chant. Stunned by his reaction, Marian called out his name. Joey gave no sign of hearing her, but continued to cavort about the room. As soon as she turned off the music, he stopped dancing. When she turned the tape back on, he began again to move to the beat.

Of course, Joey could not hear the music, but he could feel the vibrations of the drums, and he was responding to the rhythm of the chant. The grin on his face was proof of his excitement over having found a way to "hear." Healing sounds thus can have a far deeper effect than their audibility. Just as the earth moves in harmony with the vibrations of celestial music, we, too, can become aware of these rhythms and move in harmony with all. Basavanna, a spiritual poet who lived in Karnataka, India, around 1200 C.E., declared: "Make of my body the beam of a lute. Of my head, the sounding gourd. Of my nerves, the strings. Of my fingers, the plucking sticks. Embrace me close and play, play your song, O Lord of the meeting rivers."

## FOLLOWING YOUR OWN PATH

Any wholesome practice from any tradition, when performed with a sense of awareness, can be considered *sadhana*, whether that means the dance of the Sufis, the study of the Talmud, an African initiation ritual, fasting at Ramadan, or counting rosary beads. The eighteenth-century Japanese Zen master Hakuin Zenji said, "Everyday mind is the Way." By everyday mind, Hakuin meant our capacity to dwell continuously in the present moment. When we engage every moment without the fears of past or future, each action we perform is filled with consciousness.

If you know and enjoy the wholesome foods and music of your own ethnic culture, I urge you to incorporate them into the *sadhanas* that I will describe in the pages that follow. Keep in mind that your innate spiritual rhythms include the memories of food, breath, and sound from your childhood; specifically, the foods your parents or grandparents prepared and served you, and the music they played. Keep them in your awareness as you read *The Path of Practice*, because they could become the keys to helping you remember and resolve your ancestral memories.

A life of *sadhana* flows easily and gently, not because it follows a set of rules or strictures, but because we learn to move within the currents of sound and energy that surround us. We rise with the sun, lie down with the moon, partake of the food that each season brings us. We breathe in accord with the daily lunar and solar rhythms. We give voice to our inner sound with healing chants and prayers and, even more important, through silence, the basis and origin of all sound. When we live in this simple way, peace pervades our days.

This book presents many ways to practice *sadhana*, but I invite you simply to begin with a recognition of the life force in your breath, the joy in the sound of your voice, and the blessing in a morsel of food. Do those exercises to which you feel drawn. You can return later to the exercises that initially do not call to you. The *sadhanas* are meant to be a lifelong practice incorporated little by little into your daily routine until your thoughts and rhythms are realigned with Mother Nature. As you will learn, there are also practices meant to be done only at particular times of the year or in certain circumstances.

I have been doing these practices for more than twenty years now, and I have students who have been doing them for nearly a decade. As we began our conscious practices of food, breath, and sound, our health improved and happiness increased, and as we continued we became more awakened to our inner wisdom. We would no more forsake them than we could stop eating or breathing.

One final word on the prayers and invocations in this book: As a Vedic monk, I am naturally inclined to present prayers from my own tradition, and to invoke the names of the deities that I have learned to call on in my meditations. These are also universal sounds in Sanskrit, a language derived directly from the cosmic sound. Whatever your religion, these are the sounds of inner freedom and you may call upon them to heal and be made whole, without feeling that you are betraying your own core beliefs. The names of Shiva, Shakti, Durga, Kali, Vishnu, Lakshmi, Brahma, and Saraswati have meaning for me both as a Hindu and a universal being. All the names of Spirit are sacred, whether we speak of Jesus, Buddha, Yahweh, Allah, or Tara. If you feel more comfortable substituting a name from your own religion or culture, by all means, do so. As in all things, I encourage you to explore and derive strength from your own heritage and traditions, and to understand Vedic ways and wisdom as a universal gift belonging to every person and creature in the universe.

Start small. Spend a few minutes attuning your breath in the morning and evening, as described in the exercise that follows. Cook one meal a week according to Ayurvedic principles. Listen to music when you prepare your food; it doesn't matter whether you choose Vedic chants, Chopin, or Coltrane, as long as the music speaks to your heart. Chant the simple, one-syllable primordial sounds of *om* and *ham* and others from chapter 10. You will come to see that your practice of food, breath, and sound are all three aspects of an indivisible whole, three different manifestations of spiritual nourishment. Eventually, they will feed your desire to extend your practice.

As you read *The Path of Practice*, remember that *sadhana* is a journey. Start where and when you are able, with whatever practice calls out to you. You can move as as slowly as you like. You might choose to spend a month working with each *sadhana* separately and then combine all three, or you may prefer to begin practicing them all at the same time. Open your heart and mind, and see what grows. You may discover that the path of practice connects you to a rich and ancient past, and to an entirely new life of joy and radiant health.

*Part One*

# FINDING
# THE PATH
# OF HEALING

# Chapter 1

## MIGRANT SPIRIT:
## MY HEALING JOURNEYS

*In my dreams, I visualize your dark eyes*
*Peering to penetrate the misty haze*
*Veiling the coast of Guyana . . .*
*Per Ajie,*
*I can see how in stature*
*You stood shoulder up*
*Head held high*
*The challenge in your eye.*
*Yet none dared tell Sahib*
*Whipped in fields*
*Lest on kith and kin*
*Of outraged woman*
*Descend vengeance.*

—From *Per Ajie*, by Guyanese poet Rajkumari Singh

According to Vedic tradition, each person is born to a purpose, a destiny formed from our ancestry. My family name, Tiwari, means "three Vedas" in the Brahmin tradition of India. This implies that my ancestors were versed in three of the four primary Vedas, which are the *Rig, Yajur, Sama,* and *Atharva* Vedas. My destiny is in my name, one carried by a long line of sages, monks, and priests.

Like many people, however, I took a long journey away from my roots and then a circuitous route to return to them. My story is an example of how someone can become alienated from her truest self, but rediscover her identity, strengths, and gifts by becoming attuned to the rhythms of her family and cultural heritage.

I will describe my childhood and lifesaving odyssey from

estrangement to reconciliation in the belief that my story may motivate you as you embark on your own healing journey. My hope is that my example, extraordinary though it may seem, might serve as an inspiration and a model, whether the healing you seek is physical or spiritual, or both. In chapter 2, I talk about how keeping a journal helped me endure the darkest episode of my life, and in chapter 8, I discuss specific journaling techniques to help you recover ancestral memories. For now, I recommend that as you read my story, you begin recording whatever thoughts, feelings, or insights arise about recurring themes from your own past, as well as reactions to experiences in the present. Pay particular attention to memories of food and sound.

I come from a migrant people. During the late 1700s, the British, in their continued quest to expand their already vast empire, confiscated lands from the native people of the Caribbean islands, then traveled to Africa and brought people back as slaves. Later, they lured impoverished souls from their homeland in India with the promise of good fortune in the far-off West as indentured laborers.

My great-grandparents were exported from India, as if they were bales of cotton. Along with thousands of their countrymen, they endured a terrifying passage that lasted three to four months over turbulent seas. En route to the West Indies, many Indian women were raped by British soldiers; their husbands were beaten and cast out to sea or left stranded on isolated shores. The spirits of those who survived were broken for the rest of their lives, and the violations they suffered remained indelibly stamped into the psyches of generations that followed.

The fabric of my life, and of my illness, was woven with

threads that extend back to my childhood, and even further back to the lives of my ancestors. In order to find my way out of the confusion that my cancer represented, I had to untangle the knots in those threads and look closely at their colors and textures, their twists and frays.

In less than 200 years of colonial rule in Guyana, the British had succeeded in usurping the native Amerindian land and crippling the native ways of life. They fractured the culture of the African men and women whom they had forced into slavery so that virtually no evidence remained of their traditional practices, except for some traces in food and language. Slavery had only recently been abolished in Guyana when the first of my Indian ancestors arrived in 1875. They were given the chance to work the land and, in time, the opportunity to own it, a privilege much more generous than anything afforded the Africans. In the face of what appeared to be a systematic campaign to obliterate their ancient, rich Vedic culture, they managed to maintain their spiritual practices in the privacy of their homes and temples, although in a substantially reduced form.

My own great-grandparents survived the brutal ocean voyage from India and disembarked in Guyana with few resources, except for their determination to create a better life for themselves. Nineteenth-century Indians rarely traveled beyond their villages, let alone across the ocean. Like the people of all ancient cultures, they were rooted deeply in the land and in the dharmas, the values and laws set down for them by their forebears. Most of India, however, was mired in poverty. So, along with thousands of others, my people set out to find a more prosperous life in a new land. Their passage from India was itself against the sacred laws of the Vedas, which counsel people not to leave the land of their birth to cross the oceans. Because they challenged this long-standing tradition, my migrant ancestors were resented by those they left behind, and so were further alienated from their roots, isolated in a new land.

My great-grandparents brought with them the seeds of their native foods, and they turned to the bountiful land for survival and sustenance, and to heal their devastated spirits. By the time I was growing up in Guyana in the late 1950s, my grandparents and their compatriots had re-created the lush landscape of India. They had also kept alive traditional Indian practices of weaving baskets and fishing nets; carving stone mortars, pestles, and grinding stones; and constructing their houses in time-honored ways.

Although as a child I was not fully aware of my great-grandparents', grandparents', and parents' experiences, I had an intuitive sense of their emotional pain. By the age of six or seven, I had a strong impression that my own innocence had been violated, even though my people never spoke of their past. Somewhere within me, I carried an unconscious memory of the atrocities endured by my elders. Only later would I learn that these intuitions were indeed historical fact. These feelings were my first brush with apprehension of a larger consciousness to which I would later connect, and from which I would derive insight, healing, and my life's mission.

My parents' generation had inherited the aggrieved memories of the sexual violation endured by their parents. The men whose wives had been sexually abused often blamed the women for these violations. Many men rejected their wives, and this legacy was passed down to their sons and sons' sons. Wife-beating was prevalent among the Indians in Guyana.

I loved my elders wholeheartedly, and tried in little ways to heal the unspoken anguish I sensed. I served my aunts concoctions of brews and teas, anointed their feet with herbal balms, and combed their long hair. But the sorrow remained etched on their faces, and I could smell it on their sun-parched skin.

The women were allowed to express their grief only at elaborate funeral ceremonies, where they wailed and keened, pouring out their pain in haunting cries. At weddings and other festivities, they sang native songs, unearthing rich and passionate incantations in a mixture of Hindi, Urdu, and Guyanese English. They chanted long and fervently, until their agony was temporarily appeased. Afterward, a joyous vibration would flood the air, like a bright ray of light piercing through dense clouds. Their bodies would sway in sensual folk dances, their suffering forgotten for the moment.

Although I don't believe most of the elders of my family were ever able to heal their spirits from the pain endured over history, I would learn later in life that a devastated spirit can become whole again; broken hearts can heal. I inherited my family's wounded spirit, and then caused more pain to myself and our collective spirits, which I believe led to my developing cancer. Yet my own healing from that cancer attests to the possibility of redemption and wholeness. In the words of the contemporary poetess Rashani:

> There is a brokenness out of which comes the unbroken. There is a shatteredness out of which blooms the unshatterable. There is a sorrow beyond all grief, which leads to joy. And a fragility out of whose depths emerges strength. There is a hollow space too vast for words through which we pass with each loss, out of whose darkness we are sanctioned into being.

## IN MY FATHER'S HOUSE

My paternal great-grandfather came to Guyana in 1889 not only because he wanted to improve his family's economic circumstances, but also because he was a *pujari*, a Hindu priest. The British had agreed to bring over a handful of *pujaris*, in response to the Hindu immigrants' belief that the priests could end the severe drought of 1889 by performing the *Chandi Homa*, the Vedic ritual intended to bring the rains. Although the priests fasted for two months and performed various religious rituals deemed necessary to summon the rains, the skies remained dry.

My great-grandfather persisted, however. Newly arrived in Port Mourant, he entered a pit that had been dug for Vedic fire rituals, and he fasted alone for two more months, until the heavens finally opened up. The villagers lifted his emaciated body from the pit and later placed there a Shiva lingam, the ancient Hindu "mark of Shiva." The first *mandir*, or temple, in Guyana was built on that spot. My great-grandfather served as head priest of Shivala Temple, as it was named, until his death, soon after the drought ended.

My father, Bhagwan Rampersaud Tiwari, was the youngest child of a large family and grew to be a great teacher. His golden skin, black mane of hair, and muscular build exuded the beauty and brilliance of Surya, the Vedic sun god. When he was eighteen, his mother became terminally ill. His father had died some years earlier, so my father nursed his mother during the last days of her life. This experience had a profound effect on him and imbued him with great compassion.

My father was a bit of a renegade, however, and eventually took two wives, which, although an ancient Indian tradition, is not generally accepted among modern Indians. He often needed to soothe the sensibilities of these two proud women, Jayadevi, whom I called my "older mother," and Kalideva, my birth mother.

After the birth of his first child, my father became less rebellious and began to reclaim his connection to the culture of his homeland. He studied Hindu scriptures and practiced the *pujas*, or ritual sacrifices, which are observed in every orthodox Hindu home. An omnivorous reader and a great intellectual, he took correspondence courses from universities in several different countries, and earned a degree as a dental technician from a major dental school in the United States. He even crafted his own dental tools. Diplomats came from all the nearby islands, including Trinidad and Jamaica, to have my father work on their teeth. He was also the local marriage and family counselor, astrologer, and an avid mandolin player, whose favorite Western tune was "Red River Valley."

In his spare time, my father built a Hindu temple in our village. He was proficient not only in Sanskrit but also in Urdu and Hindi. After he mastered the Hindu scriptures, he undertook to study the Bible and the Koran. As a result of his understanding of these religions, he was able to counsel the clerics in our area, and helped mend the differences between Hindus and Muslims, Africans and Indians, by quoting their scriptures and showing the sameness of Spirit that underlies our apparent differences. While remaining stalwart and devout within the Hindu tradition, he was careful to direct his children's education so we would grow up open-minded and tolerant of other cultures, and live as friends with our African neighbors.

My father almost single-handedly built our wood-frame house, with its generous verandas, all according to sacred Vedic architecture. The traditional earthen stove, for instance, was on the east wall. I always think of my mother,

her face bathed in the golden morning light as she stood there cooking the *dhal*, or mung beans, for breakfast. Our day started early, with the roosters crowing at four A.M. (Today, roosters crow all day long, sad evidence that they've lost their alignment with nature's rhythms.) After my mothers had awakened us, they would perform their early morning rituals, while Father led us in chanting our prayers. Breakfast was prepared over a wood-burning fireplace, with a sample of the meal always offered to the fire (representing sacrifice to the Divine) before we were served. Then, we changed from our Indian-style pajamas into our uncomfortably stiff school uniforms—navy blue pleated skirts, starched white shirts, and striped ties. Our bare feet encased in black patent-leather shoes, off we went for a thoroughly English school day. Only after returning home did we regain our Indian identities, with hours of Hindu language and scripture lessons taught by my father or older mother.

My father sought to prepare his children (eleven in all, including my cousin Mahendra, who was raised in our household as a brother) for life in Guyana and in the world outside our small community. He moored our British education with anchors of our tradition, realizing that only through education might we break the bonds of grief we had inherited from previous generations.

Some afternoons, exhausted from school and play, I would lay my head in my mother's lap as she playfully pulled at my hair looking for lice, a recurring problem in our rural school. The village women, comfortably seated on their verandas, cleaned and sifted grains and *dhals* in their handmade baskets. *Shee, shee, shee* was the comforting whisper of the afternoon slipping away. These were the sounds of life, nature's harmonies and rhythms that brought us together.

The communal atmosphere extended to cooking and all the kitchen activities such as pounding grains and spices, and all the other preparations that were part of our daily life. The whole community was tied to the earth in ways that today may be hard for many city dwellers and suburbanites to imagine. Just outside our homes lay vast marshlands of tall grasses, where cranes and other wildlife thrived. I can still conjure the smell of the mud in Guyana, which is different from the smell of mud elsewhere in the world. It was rich and black and silky, and when the rain fell on it, the sound it made was full and round and musical, like that of tadpoles plopping into a pond. I became acutely aware of the variety of sounds in Guyana, and although I have visited and lived in rural areas of many different lands, I have yet to hear the sorts of sounds you can hear in that jungle-ocean terrain. Guyana was a mysterious land, layered with Indian harmonics, African rhythms, and British hierarchies.

This way of life, tied to the rhythms and wisdom of the earth, sowed in me the seeds of my rediscovery of *sadhana* many years later. Despite my parents', grandparents', and great-grandparents' suffering and estrangement from their motherland, and the brutal realities of living in a colonial society, they preserved the ancient ways that were being lost throughout India and the rest of the world even then. They spun together the rhythms of planting, harvesting, singing, and dancing and wove them into a life that revolved around the home. Although the women were traditionally the healers and instructors in these ancient ways, my father insisted that his daughters also be well educated—which was unconventional then—and always gave our schoolwork priority over kitchen chores.

After our country gained independence from the British in 1966, civil war broke out between the Guyanese of African and Indian descent. Sixty-five percent of the Indian population fled the country. History repeated itself for my family. My father skillfully planned the exodus of his five elder children, including me, to three different countries—Britain, the

United States, and Canada—where he intended for us to continue our education. His love for people regardless of race and color saved his and his family's lives. When the civil war worsened and the black militia government began murdering Indians, the Africans in my father's community helped him to flee to Canada.

My emigration to New York City in 1968 was the beginning of my escape from the sorrow permeating my family and country. I was sad to leave my family, yet exhilarated at the thought of the great adventure that lay ahead. Driven by a deep desire to build a new and independent life for myself, I turned my back on my past. I avoided the growing Guyanese enclave in the borough of Queens, preferring to live in Greenwich Village, where I found an apartment on Horatio Street. Lancaster Village, where I had grown up, was a community of perhaps 500 people. My new village had a thousand times more inhabitants, yet I felt comfortable there from the very first day.

## CRAFTING THE MASK

At the age of sixteen, I plunged headlong into a love affair with New York. Although I had never seen abject urban poverty before, and I was stunned by the dirty streets and littered subways, the city smelled of freedom—the freedom to express myself.

I attended business school for one month while I applied for admission to New York University. I planned to study law, as my father had wanted. But while I was waiting for a response from NYU, I met Stella Adler, the renowned drama teacher. After attending a few of her classes, my academic plans were derailed; I had fallen in love with the theater. Stella unfolded European and Russian plays with the flawless methodology she had gleaned from Stanislavsky, the great Russian guru of the theater, adding her own peculiarly American insights. Although I was too young to qualify for her courses, she bent the rules and, in 1969, allowed me to enroll in the Stella Adler Conservatory, from which I graduated in 1973.

The theater was the perfect training ground for my new life, since I was deliberately crafting a role for myself as a successful, modern young woman. By role-playing, I learned to function in a world that was unimaginably different from the one in which I had been raised.

As I worked with Stella, she became my friend, my greatest guide, the angel on my shoulder. She groomed me, brought out my intrinsic strengths, and sent me for voice training with Helena Monbo, a highly respected vocal coach. Through Stella's genius, Helena's wisdom, and my natural penchant for the dramatic arts, I was becoming a disciplined actress. In the early 1970s, however, when more consideration was given to the color of an actor's skin than it is today, roles for women of color were hard to find, especially in classical plays. Stella sent me to Joseph Papp, the founder of the famed New York Public Theater, to audition for the role of Lady Macbeth. But even this great theater visionary, who would soon rattle the dramatic community with his race-neutral casting, felt the time was not yet right. He instead encouraged me to get into costume designing. Although the idea didn't appeal to me at first, Stella helped to persuade me to try to make my way in the fashion industry.

I had had no special training for this new direction, yet somehow I convinced myself that I could become the fashion director of a high-profile retail organization. I scheduled meetings with any industry top gun who would see me, but after my fortieth interview I still had no offer. I eventually encountered the fashion director at Bergdorf Goodman, who helped me land my first job in 1972, at Gimbels. I learned the ropes quickly there and, within the first year, I had completely restructured the fashion department and upgraded the image of Gimbels' main branch. Profits tripled in the areas I worked, lending me the clout I needed to carve out my own niche. Oblivious to the reality that I wasn't qualified for the job, I never questioned my abilities.

All the while that my confidence was growing, I was unconsciously tormented by the awareness that I was turning my back on my family and my past. I was relieved to find a culture in New York in which my people's sorrow, as well as my own inner conflict as an Anglo-Indian, could be put aside. I did not feel alone or scared, but liberated. Rabindranath Tagore's words echoed in my heart: "Freedom is all I want, but to hope for it I feel ashamed." I was ashamed to disregard my father's wishes, and this shame would be a stepping stone in the road leading me away from him. I felt guilty for leaving my family to face the atrocities of war without me. I felt guilty for seizing my individual freedom, far away from the grief of my people.

My career flourished. By 1974, at the age of twenty-two, I had opened my own exclusive Madison Avenue boutique, featuring my original designs and selling to celebrities such as Jackie Onassis and Rudolf Nureyev. Within a year, I had launched boutiques, which I called "Maya," in some of the highest-profile fashion stores in America: Bloomingdale's, Saks Fifth Avenue, I. Magnin, and Neiman Marcus, among others.

I was among the first fashion designers to create clothing from stretch fabrics. Inspired by my father's crafting of his own equipment and machinery, I directed technicians to retool the production machinery to allow me to work in new ways with Spandex as well as with natural fabrics such as cotton, wool, and linen. Soon the fashion magazines were referring to me in the most glowing terms. Mary Reinholtz, a fashion editor at *Women's Wear Daily*, dubbed me "the high priestess of stretch clothing" and Sally Kirkland, a fashion doyenne who was also an editor at *Life* magazine, declared that thanks to my designs, America finally had its own fashion image.

Although the name of my line was simply my given name, it could not have been more appropriate. Often mistranslated as "illusion," the Sanskrit word "maya" also means the manifestation of the one God as the multiplicity of forms in the material universe, the ignorance that draws a veil over the face of the One Reality so that all we see is diversity, and the wisdom that ultimately leads us to pierce the veil and see the One beneath the many. Although I have experienced the fullness of maya at different stages in my life, I was heavily veiled in my fashion career.

My glossy lipstick, fashionable clothes, and platform shoes distracted me from the health problems that were developing in my body. My spirit was becoming more and more exhausted, yet I responded by keeping frantically busy, suppressing any awareness that something could be wrong with my life. Long workdays often lasted into the early morning hours, followed by partying with other successful, similarly veiled and deluded revelers.

I even participated in that defining moment in American popular culture, the 1969 Woodstock festival. Immersed in the chaotic atmosphere, I caught a glimpse of Swami Satchidananda, dressed in his brilliant orange robes, as he blessed the thousands gathered to celebrate rock music with an opening prayer. Was it not a sign of divine synchronicity that the most revolutionary cultural event of the decade should send me a message from my roots?

At this time, my dreams were haunted. The fires and blood of the racial wars in Guyana invaded my sleep. Living in New York, I ignored all news of Guyana, estranged myself from my family, and tried desperately to rewrite my past by creating a present that utterly shut it out. I should have known that I could not sever the connections to my ancestral roots or ignore my inner anxiety and lack of grounding. As civil war tore through my country, cancer began to wage war within me.

## JOURNEY WITH CANCER

By March 1975, at the age of twenty-three, I had been suspecting for months that my spiritual dis-ease had taken on a physical form inside my body. Something was terribly wrong. My dreams were becoming ever more disturbed, my conscious thoughts erratic. A great gray cloud had descended and enveloped me. My energy was low and my appetite scant, which was unusual for me. My abdomen was distended. I made an appointment to see my gynecologist.

On the way there, I walked past Jackson Square Park across from my apartment, as I had done countless times before. Every day I saw a flock of pigeons there, foraging in the dirt for crumbs. Normally they ignored me, but on that day, as I neared them, the birds abruptly flew away. I understood their odd behavior as confirmation that I was harboring some fearful illness. Later that day, I again deliberately walked toward the pigeons. Once more they hastily took flight.

When the gynecologist probed the tumor in my uterus, the pain I felt was so intense that I fainted on the examination table. The diagnosis based on the biopsy revealed an unusual strain of ovarian cancer that had invaded my uterus, but one deemed not fatal if prompt action were taken. In one sense, I felt inexplicably relieved, for the diagnosis validated my psychological and spiritual exhaustion.

I returned home from the doctor's office after receiving the diagnosis, and slept for almost two days. Although the doctors had emphasized that my cancer was probably not terminal, I felt that it might be. I remained buried in my bed with the lights out, and I stopped eating and contemplated the possibility of death at an early age. Now I realize that my fear was not a fear of death, but a fear of the changes I sensed I needed to make in my life. I probably would not have had the courage to change direction had I not contracted such a serious disease.

Except for telling three dear friends, I kept the burden of my secret to myself. I knew that my illness, and the steps I had to take to heal, would be even more painful under the scrutiny and concern of others. I understood that I was about to begin on the deepest and dearest relationship of my life— my engagement with cancer.

The cancer had moved from my ovaries into my womb, the most sacred core of my womanhood. It had robbed me of my essential female prerogative, the ability to bear children. But the cancer also made me aware of the presence of the Divine in my life, of something beyond my everyday routines of work and friends.

One morning, during my darkest despair, as the iridescent glow of Manhattan's predawn streaked through the slats of my window shades, I suddenly sat up in bed. The room was filled with light, as bright and pure as the full moon. The Divine Mother, draped in white, appeared in the window, surrounded by a crystalline light. At home in Guyana, I had grown up surrounded by many images of the Divine Mother in her various manifestations, and we had offered daily rituals and prayers in her honor. Now, I recognized her as soon as she appeared. Her arms were outstretched in a gesture of invitation, her palms facing me. I felt my spirit freed, my heart released from its depression. Then, she was gone.

Some years later, when I studied the Vedic texts, I learned of the infinite, all-encompassing nature of the Divine Mother's spirit. Her feminine energy and healing spirit are transmitted to everyone, and she bequeaths to each of us the power to nurture and protect. The *Devi Mahatmya*, the classic fifth-century text in praise of the Divine Mother, describes her as "the power who is Consciousness in all beings."

At the time of my illness, however, I knew only that she had given me the gift of lightness and serenity. I opened the blinds to let in the daylight and fresh air. I began to eat again. The next morning, I had a vision of a small bluebird, perched in midair before the same window where the Mother had appeared the previous morning. The bird beckoned me to fly skyward with it. Afraid of falling, I hesitated, but the bird gave me the understanding that I would be safe, and that I must obey. As I approached the window, the bird was transformed into a vast field of white light, in which I hung suspended. Only then did I realize that the bluebird was another manifestation of the Divine Mother. The bluebird has always symbolized for me the attainment of happiness, so she had appeared to me in that form.

The Divine Mother's two visits in as many days marked a turning point in my life. I decided to reclaim my life and seek help. Little by little, I grew to feel her presence through everything that followed.

Buoyed by the Mother's visitations, I returned to the doctor who had diagnosed me. Together, we mapped out a plan of treatment that included a complete hysterectomy in June 1975, followed by six months of localized radiation treatments. Despite these radical therapies, X rays taken soon after I completed the radiation revealed three tumors attached to one lung and both kidneys and hinted at others. Perhaps most disturbing of all, the radiologist told me he suspected that the rapid eruption of these tumors had been stimulated by a slip of the surgeon's knife during the hysterectomy. This might have caused a tumor the size of a tennis ball to burst open and spew cancer cells into the surrounding tissue.

During the radiation treatment, he said, these renegade cancer cells had grown into the six or seven more tumors that had attached themselves to my kidneys, lungs, and other vital organs. To determine the nature and size of these unseen tumors, I submitted to three exploratory surgeries over five months. Then, during the next year and a half, I underwent eight more operations, including two eight-hour procedures, to excise the tumors they had seen on the X rays, as well as others they found attached to my stomach and small intestine.

In October 1977, I lay on a cold gurney awaiting what was to be my final surgery. The raw, antiseptic odor and the cacophonous clatter of stainless-steel equipment almost made me despair once again. Even though I was then estranged from my father, I tried to envision his image and drew deeply on my memory of his energy for solace. Slipping back to when I was two years old, I recalled how Father had cared for me through a bout of diphtheria. Then, I heard his rich voice calling me, keeping me alive with his love.

As memories flooded through my mind, the attendants pushed me brusquely under the glaring lights. I had been wearing a nonremovable partial dental bridge, attached to the other teeth with gold bands.

Just as I was about to go completely under the gas, the bridge slipped. In the split second before I blacked out from the anesthesia, I felt it obstructing my windpipe. I was unable to say or do anything to get the surgical team's attention. I fleetingly thought how ironic it would be for me to die during surgery, not from my disease but because I had choked on my partial bridge.

A short time later, I awoke to find myself serenely floating above the heads of the surgical team in their green scrubs. From my perch near the ceiling, I saw myself on the operating table. I noticed the wound in my belly, the skin neatly pulled back like the flap of a leather briefcase. The surgeon's hand probed in the aperture while two attendants swabbed the leakage. Then I became aware of the concern in the room: my vital signs were not good. The team of baffled doctors and nurses was anxiously trying to restore them to normal.

I had become the witness to my own operation in a classic near-death, out-of-body experience. As I circled overhead, a nurse pried open my mouth to discover that I was choking on something. Three attendants rapidly moved closer to my face, and one of them reached into my throat to retrieve the partial bridge. While my physical body lay on the table within the clasp of death, my subtle body (the vehicle in which the soul encases itself) had already begun its ascension. Only when the bridge had been removed from my throat was the subtle body drawn back into the physical body.

As I regained consciousness in the morgue-like cold of the recovery room, I saw my oncologist smiling down at me. I was embarrassed to face him, but he quietly slipped my bridge into my hand and whispered, "This will be our little secret." Even though my misguided decision could have cost me my life and untold grief to those who had attended me during surgery, he never chastised me in any way.

In all, I endured twelve major surgical operations and many devastating rounds of radiation therapy over two and a half years. By November of 1977, my doctors had determined that my cancer was, in fact, fatal. As I lay in my hospital bed, after yet another X ray to assess the effects of the most recent course of radiation, they admitted that they had run out of options. I had, at most, two months to live. Their strongest, most compassionate recommendation was that I remain in their care while they administered heavy doses of morphine to relieve my pain and wait for the inevitable moment that I would draw my last breath.

## THE SOLACE OF DEEP SNOW

An hour after receiving what amounted to a death sentence, I left the hospital without telling anyone. I was overwhelmed with sadness, not because of my disease or even the prospect of death, but because of the dismal mode of death they were envisioning. I traveled as fast and as far from the hospital as I could, seeking refuge in a friend's ski cabin in Sugarbush, Vermont. The thought of dying with a drugged spirit filled me with dread. The offer of morphine had shaken me back to reality. I wanted to live long enough to discover my true spirit. Determined to meet my maker with whatever dignity I could muster, I prepared to spend my last days alone, without medical intervention, in a desperate plea to the gods and goddesses to set my soul free.

It was December, so I kept the fire burning day and night in the cabin's huge fireplace with wood provided by my host. I fasted and wept and poured out the most closely guarded secrets of my heart in a journal. In vivid dreams and visions, I saw my people's tumultuous passage to the New World and felt the quiet sorrow that we descendants still carry. I had tried to run from that grief as if it were not my own, but the cancer had come to re-create it in my life. This unresolved sorrow, I now understood, had been handed down to me in the form of impaired energy within my vital tissues, giving rise to illness and emotional suffering. Had I faced the pain earlier on, the energy would have flowed through me unimpeded. The self-knowledge would have

made me strong rather than sick. Because I ignored and sup-
pressed it, however, it became blocked in my body, in the
part of the body that connects one generation to another.
Every person's reproductive cells are direct links to their ancestors. By cutting myself off from my family, I had caused
my regenerative energy to derail, to become stagnant and
diseased. Thankfully, the energy of the Divine Mother drove
me to seek help and sustained me through my operations.

My father's love and wisdom would also come to my aid.
One night as I sat staring at the fire, his face suddenly appeared within the flames. Glancing out the window, I saw
him there, dressed in white. Was he really there, or was I hal-
lucinating his presence? I wasn't sure, and remained frozen
in my seat. An instant later, my body seemed to dissolve into
a sense of lightness. I felt comforted, no longer lonely. A few
nights later he appeared again. I wept as I shared with him
my loneliness and anguish, and asked his forgiveness for
abandoning the family and my spiritual roots. He spoke to
me gently but firmly, reminding me that if I deliberately
thwarted my life force by inviting death, my next life would
be even more difficult. He pointed out that I had allowed my
present-day pain to block my remembrance of my connection to the Divine.

He read me scriptural passages from the *Bhagavad Gita* on
the true nature of karma and dharma. Karma, he explained,
holds both positive and negative consequences for us. The
universal law of cause and effect impels us into countless rebirths to address and undo the negative results of previous
actions.

In the traditional Hindu belief system, all of our actions—
including our words, thoughts, and deeds—plant seeds that
ultimately will bear fruit, whether in this life or the next. We
can modify the results of our karma through conscious ac-

tions today, but we cannot do so if we ignore our responsibility for our personal or ancestral past. The results of all actions, however, are in accordance with the Divine, and all should be seen as blessings. We should not become attached to the fruits of our actions or our individual identities, as none is entirely due to our own effort, cleverness, or ancestry, but stem from our interconnections with universal energies and with the Divine. As Gandhi put it, "We must renounce the possessor."

In recognizing our ultimate connection to the Divine, we also recognize the ancient truths that we must live by as well as the unique role each of us is destined to fulfill—our dharma. When we shirk that responsibility, the *Gita* tells us, we plant more unfortunate karmic seeds that will be reaped in this life and future lives.

My father's teachings shook me to my stubborn core. His words were a clarion call to awaken more fully to my true identity. He showed me that I had been killing myself spiritually, shutting out the nourishing energy of my people by cutting myself off from my roots. I had also shirked my spiritual duty and nature by caving in to death, and I had to change my mind and my mode of existence in this very lifetime. Before his apparition departed, he told me that my body still possessed sufficient *prana*, or vital breath, to sustain my life. This was a shock, since I had completely accepted the doctors' prognosis that my life was almost over.

With the hope of re-creating my connection to the Divine, I prayed fervently to recover faith in myself, even if I could not regain my life. Faith in ourselves is invariably faith in the Divine. I asked to be forgiven for all the trespasses in my life. I acknowledged my insecurities and lack of self-esteem, which had led me to live behind a mask, dishonoring my culture and family. I wept for weeks following my father's appearance, until the fears, grief, anger, hurt, humiliation, and guilt were lifted from my spirit. After four months of reconciling these inner conflicts, my emotional and physical pain dissipated.

When the worst of winter had finally passed, I was drawn outdoors and beyond my grief. The sun high in the sky brilliantly illuminated the ice on the trees. My being felt permeated with prismatic colors. The gray cloud around me lifted, and a deep peace dawned within me. I marveled at having reached such a profound tranquility, feeling as if I were suspended in air, floating like a ribbon in the bright skies.

At first, I thought these feelings were the peace that the Divine Mother gives us just before death. But one afternoon, as I walked outside, the crunch of dried brambles beneath the melting snow was precisely the invigorating sound my body needed. (I would later use that same sound for moving energy when counseling patients who feel sluggish or stuck.) That was the day I awakened, the day I came alive again. In waiting for death to come, I had found new life. I had no doubt that my cancer had finally begun to retreat.

Two months later, I returned to my apartment in Manhattan. Soon afterward, I visited my friend and teacher Stella Adler. We spent several days together during which I described my experiences in the winter woods. Although I had been reduced to skin and bones, partly because of my illness and partly because of my fast, she agreed that I seemed to have gained new life.

I was twenty-eight years old and weighed only ninety pounds, with barely enough fat and muscle to buffer me from the frenzied pace of life in Manhattan. My hands and head shook involuntarily, and a fierce coldness permeated every vein and limb. The ends of my nerves were frayed. I felt raw and vulnerable and shuddered at any loud noise. I had frequent lapses of short-term memory, and my dream state was still troubled. It would be difficult to maintain the center of peace I had discovered during my sojourn in Vermont, but the sense of wholeness remained. My mission, then, was to rebuild my life around the healing presence of the Divine Mother. As I began my journey back to health, I had no idea where my path would lead me. But I was sure that if I remained committed to opening my heart to the Mother's nurturing energy, I would discover the road She meant for me to follow.

# Chapter 2

# THE MANY FACES OF
# THE DIVINE MOTHER

*Aditi, mighty Mother of just rulers and queen
of those who follow Cosmic Order, great
protectress with a far-extending reach
untouched by time, gracious guide, to you
we cry.*
—*Yajur Veda* (21.5)

When I returned to New York, the Divine Mother paved my
way back into a life gentler than the one I had left, positioning herself at my every turn. For instance, a few short months
after I resumed my life at Horatio Street, the annual Vedic celebration of the Mother, *Navaratri,* with its nine-day pageantry
of fire rituals, music, songs, prayers, and meditations, took
place. A hundred or so devout celebrants had gathered at the
Integral Yoga Center, across the street from my apartment, so
it was an easy walk for my weak body and a synchronistic
event for my soul. *Navaratri* honors the Mother in her three
primary forms: Lakshmi, the creator who grants prosperity;
Saraswati, giver of wisdom and creativity; and Durga or Kali,
governess who upholds cosmic law and universal reverence.

Although you may want to involve yourself in the energy
of the Divine in whichever form is familiar to you, I invite
you to explore further the Divine Mother to understand the
feminine power and potential that is available to you for
your life and your healing.

As the Mother herself says in a medieval text called *Shakta
Advaita,* "Who and what I really am—cosmic awareness so
vast I effortlessly hold trillions of universes in the palm of my

hand—is beyond the capacity of human minds to understand. Therefore, imagine me in whatever form appeals to you, and I promise in that very form I will come to you."

After the *Navaratri* celebration, I had a dream of the Mother in her form of Kali, which means darkness: the dark void of the cosmic womb. Kali is honored in India as the form of the Mother from whom the universe emerged and to whom it must return. To her devotees, she is the Great Mother who nurtures and cares for them. She is also the force who insists on retooling our thoughts and actions which run counter to her laws and rhythms, and who dissolves the universe when the appointed time comes.

When the delicate balance of the life force is disturbed and the ecosystem shifts out of kilter, when creatures turn on one other, the Mother takes the shape of Kali, a fierce and powerful warrioress, who defends the individual and universal order. The song *"Devi Stotram"* praises the power of Kali:

> Reverence to the three-eyed Durga [a name for Kali], whose luster is like lightning, who is seated on the lion [lord of animals], who is fierce and who is waited on by maidens carrying weapons and clubs. Reverence to the eight-armed Durga, who holds in her hands the discus, conch, trident, club, sword, bow with its string drawn, and lotus and whose eighth hand demonstrates the mudra of peace.

The protective warrioress energy is a primal part of every woman's maternal instinct. Many stories have been told about mothers who perform extraordinary feats of physical strength to save their children from danger. This feminine strength is in all females of all species. A few years ago in India, for instance, I witnessed a mother elephant demolish the engine of a train after it ran over and killed her calf. My mother's people came from Chennai in South India, where the Warrior Goddess is devoutly worshiped. They attribute their inordinate strength and well-being to her. My mother continues to uphold spiritual practices that ensure Kali's protection—and I see how this grace has been passed on to protect me. Once invoked, Kali's protection will last for generations to come.

## THE SPIRIT OF PROTECTION

As Kali, the Mother redirects her universe, creating natural phenomena such as hurricanes, tornadoes, and earthquakes. She is also the source of emotional upheaval in the form of illness, disappointment, and failure, all of which tend to block us from moving forward. These negative and destructive forces, whether manifested as external or internal turbulence, may be perceived as spiritual opportunities to make constructive changes in our lives. They mark the time for us to pause, examine ourselves and our motivations, and reorient ourselves. We must all strive to create meaning for ourselves out of so-called disasters, which, although it may be difficult to see at first, are expressions of the Mother's great love and nurturing spirit. When we veer away from the divine path, the Mother responds with tough love, strength, and action. Just as she sends us situations and disasters that terrify us, she also gives us the courage to conquer our fears.

Some years ago, I got a frantic phone call from Gloria, a British-born student of mine who was on her way back to the United States after spending several weeks in England. Although she had a perfectly valid visa to reenter the United States, the American immigration authorities at Heathrow Airport, outside London, had refused to let her board her plane. Desperate for help, she called me from the immigration offices seeking counsel.

"There is a reason why this is happening," I told her. "What do you still need to accomplish in England?"

Gloria burst into tears and for about a minute, all I heard were her sobs. Finally, she collected herself enough to tell me that she had lost touch with her family seven years ago. Her father had been an alcoholic all through her childhood, and although he was sober now, she still carried the psychic scars of his drunken rages. She had promised herself that during this trip she would be in contact with her family. But as the days passed, her resolve had weakened, and she had never gotten around to calling them.

The solution seemed obvious to me. "The Divine Mother will not let you leave England until you've reconnected with your family," I told her. "I think that you have no choice but to return to London and give them a call."

Gloria reluctantly agreed to follow my suggestion. When I heard from her next, she was back in San Francisco, and her voice sounded light and ebullient. "I not only rang up my parents, I actually spent a few days with them," she said. "They were so happy to see me, and I was able to work through a lot of negative feelings from the past. It was such a joy to spend time with my dad without having to worry that he was going to turn angry and ugly. You must have been right about the Divine Mother, because when I showed up at Heathrow a week later, I had absolutely no problem clearing immigration."

I have turned to Mother Kali to help me move past the pain of recovery and overcome the obstacles in my spiritual life. Twenty years ago, I sought out a Vedic astrologer who gave me a Kali mantra, which I still use today, to invite the Divine Mother's healing energy into my life. Time and again,

Mother Kali has helped me to overcome many of my fears and limitations.

To avail yourself of this feminine power, envision yourself as a female warrior, and take a few minutes every day to bring Kali's presence into your life. Find a quiet place where you will not be disturbed and repeat the Kali mantra as many times as you feel is appropriate. (One young student of mine, a real estate broker, often chants the Kali mantra while driving the forty-minute trip between her home and office. She says that the mantra prepares her to cope with the various crises that regularly come her way at work.)

OM SRI KALYAI NAMAHA
[ohm shree kahl-yi nah-mah-ha]

OM is the cosmic sound, the mystic name of God. SRI invokes the Divine Mother, in all of her aspects. KALYAI invokes the Divine Mother in her aspect as destroyer of negative forces and remover of obstacles. NAMAHA means "to that Divine Name" and is a form of closure to Vedic mantras.

**The Practice: Contemplating the Warrior Goddess**

When you need spiritual guidance or the courage to deal with a particularly painful situation, you may want to visualize the five different aspects of Kali, each of which teaches us a significant life lesson. (See box on page 51.) After your visualization, recite the Durga mantra to seal the Warrior Goddess's lessons and protection within yourself. You may even want to find a poster of the Warrioress Kali and hang it in a place where you can sit in quiet contemplation of her striking features. As you meditate, invoke within yourself her five aspects in order to remove whatever barriers you encounter on your physical, emotional, and spiritual path.

## THE FIVE ASPECTS OF KALI

1. I am Beauty—passionate protector of life

* Kali is young, beautiful, and dark-skinned. Her crowned hair is long, red, and streaming with vitality.

2. I am the Dancer—bestower of creation and restorer of equanimity

* Kali dances on Shiva and Shakti, the cosmic couple whose union brings about the creation.

3. I am Wisdom—dispassion that cuts through ignorance

* In her hands, Kali wields the sword of knowledge, which cuts through ignorance; scissors, which cut attachment; a severed head, which symbolizes the letting go of rational mind and ego; and the lotus, which represents the fulfillment of spiritual life.

4. I am Shakti—primordial energy of creation

* The coiled snake around Kali's body shows her transformative powers of Shakti.

5. I am Rebirth—cosmic memory of all that exists

* Kali wears a garland of heads around her neck, strung with the umbilical cord of the soul, which represents the cumulative wisdom and memory of human existence.

**The Practice: Reciting the Durga Mantra**

The Durga mantra is a means to seal the protection and healing energy of the Great Warrioress within you. Take a few quiet minutes every day to recite the Durga mantra. (The number eighteen and its multiples have strong significance in Vedic numerology. The number one represents the process of evolution toward nonduality—the Infinite Whole. The number eight, maya, represents the Divine Manifestation through which the soul evolves. Therefore, you may want to repeat the mantra at least eighteen times.)

OM SRI DURGAYAI NAMAHA
[ohm shree dur-gah-yee nah-mah-ha]

DURGAYAI invokes the Divine Mother in her aspect as destroyer of negative forces and remover of obstacles in the maternal, material, and spiritual fields.

## HEALING CURVES AND RECOVERY

After returning to New York, I fortified my spirit through the repeated recitation of my mantra, and reentered the world of fashion to make a living. At the same time, I started to study the classical Tantric texts, and discovered a number of beautiful teachings in them about the Divine Mother. These were great comforts to me, not only because of the intense physical pain I had endured from the cancer and my alienation from my family and heritage, but also because I had suffered terrible sorrow and anguish from my hysterectomy. Being a young woman, I had fully expected someday to become a mother, so the removal of my uterus was a great loss. It was only after the Mother entered my life that the void that replaced my womb became filled with Her light. A verse from the *Devi Upanishad* describes my feeling toward Her: "I salute you, Mother, who dispels great fear, averts great difficulties, and is the essence of great compassion."

My growing awareness of the Mother's presence in my life led me through many passages of faith. On New Year's Day, 1979, I met Sundari, a beautiful classical Indian dancer, who taught me to do the classical dance of Devi. (Devi means "shining one," referring to the Divine Mother conceived in her manifold aspects.) Soon afterward, I felt the life force, or *prana*, moving through my empty womb-space. During the next year of studying dance under Sundari's compassionate instruction, I began to heal that pain. Dancing helped my breath to move harmoniously up my spinal column and through my body, strengthening my life force. Dancing drew me closer to the Mother's presence. I came to realize that every gesture we make can flow in accord with the Divine Mother's energies and invoke those energies, when we are conscious of Her immense presence in our lives.

During my early recovery, I also sought comfort in reading "Song of the Lord," in the *Bhagavad Gita*, composed 2,500 years ago. The *Gita* opened other pathways for me and led me to discover India's later generations of spiritual mystics, such as the Alvars and Bauls, who composed the *Bhagavata-Purana* and *Gita-Govinda*, works about redemption through love and devotion to God. In the *Bhagavata-Purana*, the Lord is looked at as a lover: "Just as fire that is ablaze with flames reduces wood to ashes, so devotion in Me removes all sins." The *Gita-Govinda* uses sensual metaphors to demonstrate the physical passion that a devotee experiences when he or she contemplates the Divine: "He laid me down on a bed of chutes. For a long time he rested on my breast, while I caressed and kissed him. Embracing me, he drank from my lower lip."

With the Mother as my guide, I began to experience profound passion, a sense of purpose, and prayer. I also began to reconnect with my people and their reverence for Mother Nature through traditional practices of spiritual dance, poetry, and song; yoga postures; and natural food preparation. Through such acts of devotion to the Mother, the rawness of my body and spirit began to heal. Through this early practice of *sadhana*, I began to understand that I would never again be lonely, because the Primordial Mother was now within me.

As my faith in the Mother grew, I began to understand that I had to acknowledge my vulnerabilities—those moments when I was feeling most wounded and defenseless. I learned that I could turn to the Mother to help me gain new strength and insights—in short, I had to allow a rebirth to take place. This was my earliest premonition of the significance of my womanhood—an energy the Vedic masters call *shakti*—the primordial feminine energy within each of us that can emerge to nourish and heal all things.

According to the Vedic seers, a woman's femininity cannot exist apart from her *shakti*—the one energy that gave birth to everything. *Shakti* is the Mother's power behind creation, and signifies the sacred mysteries of creation, regeneration, and destruction—a metaphor for womanhood. At the beginning of Creation, as it is written in the *Shakta Advaita*, the Divine Mother took form and set in motion the wheel of manifestation. She bestowed her healing spirit into the womb and regenerative energy of every female of every species in the universe. We receive the *shakti* energy, which has been passed down through our female lineage as part of our ancestral memory, through our mother's womb. The sacred scriptures of Tantra inform us that this primeval energy remains in its potential form within men, while it is active within women. To grow spiritually, to evolve into consciousness, both sexes must revere and refine the *shakti* energy within themselves.

The Divine Mother endowed all females with two gifts: the power to nurture and the power to protect. *Shakti* is more than the energy of reproduction. It is the spirit of protecting the sacred, gathering food, worshiping the Divine, and giving birth to children, to inspiration, to ideas, and to art. The *Atharva Veda* speaks of the spirit of nurturance: "The Goddess whose name is 'Nurturance' dwells by Her cosmic order. It is by reason of Her color that these trees are green, and green their garlands of flowers."

As Aditi, the Mother fed the gods her milk and taught them the healing secrets that are carried in the seed-memory of plants, herbs, and minerals. In Ayurveda, herbs represent the Goddess. From the dawn of time, the healing efforts that upheld life came from the feminine. She restored joy and health and wisdom to the body with her herbs, teas, ointments, foods, and rituals. Every woman carries Aditi's memory of nurturance in her maternal memory, intuition, and spirit.

You can begin the process of nurturing yourself and, therefore, your men, children, and all other creatures by recalling your *shakti* power. Vandana Shiva tells a riveting story that illustrates this truth in *Non-violence in Animals*. A woman in India protested against the digging of a quarry, even when she was beaten and pelted with stones. "What is it that gives you all this *shakti*?" she was asked. "Do you see this grass growing?" she replied. "We come to cut this grass, and every year it grows back. The power in the grass is the power in me. Do you see the trees growing? They are two hundred years old. Every year we cut these trees to feed the cattle and to keep our children alive so that the children have milk, and still the trees keep growing and that *shakti* is in me. Can you see this stream of clear sparkling water? This water gives me life and that gives me my *shakti*."

The first step in recalling your *shakti* is to allow yourself to accept that you already have it. Recognize it within you. Acknowledge it in your feelings and actions. Become attentive to the Mother. Start to notice her presence in everything around you. A good way to get started in recalling your *shakti* is to find an image or aspect of the Mother that speaks to you—Aditi, Gaia, Ishtar, Aphrodite, the Blessed Virgin Mary, Avilokiteshvara, or any form of the Divine Mother—and keep it close to your heart. You may see her in your dreams, or you may turn a corner and find her in a stranger's act of kindness, in a remarkable teaching or teacher, in the partner of your dreams. Her image may pop up where you least expect it, to guard, comfort, or redirect you to a new depth of fulfillment.

Yesterday I picked up a fallen branch in my garden and saw, etched naturally in the pattern of the wood, a clear depiction of the goddess Saraswati, seated with the vina, an ancient stringed instrument, in her lap. Some weeks earlier, I sat submerged in the warm sulfur springs near my home in the Smoky Mountains. I leaned back, entered a deep silence, and gazed up at the clear, autumn sky. Suddenly, a butterfly alighted on my face. I could feel it almost imperceptibly nibbling at the drops of water on my cheeks. It stayed there for many moments before it flew away. The butterfly was the Mother's sign, an acknowledgment and reminder that all was peaceful in my life and within me.

We must recognize the Mother in all her aspects. To the sages, the streams and rivers that flow in the Himalayas are the divinity of Dhari Devi, "Goddess of the Current." Himalayan peaks such as Badrinath and Kadarnath are also adored as her manifestation. The next time you stand in an open meadow, notice your mind shift as you watch the wind sweep through the grass. When you are in a rainstorm, listen to your heart pound with the pulse of the drops and rhythms of the water. This alignment with the forces of nature is a function of our *shakti-prana*, the breath of the Mother moving within you.

A powerful way to cultivate the *shakti-prana* of the Divine Mother is to practice the goddess pose, *shakti asana*.

### The Practice: Goddess Pose

With your head pointing east, lie on your back and stretch out your legs, hip-width apart. Let your arms fall to your sides, palms up. Bring the soles of your feet together so that your knees fall to either side, extending the stretch without straining. Feel the stretch in your pelvis, and visualize the intake of breath coming in through your vulva. Let this energy flow

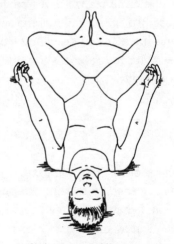

Shakti asana, *goddess pose*

up into your belly. Then slowly release it downward and out through your vulva. With each intake of breath imagine Shakti in the form of white light flooding your belly. Experience the splendor of her being within you. Hold the posture for approximately five minutes, unless you feel any discomfort. Gradually increase the time as you practice this pose and become more comfortable in it.

It's important to remember that *shakti-prana* is not exclusive to women; it is experienced by men, children, and all life-forms.

Your body is the temple of your spirit. It encompasses a subtle body and a physical body. The subtle body is a complex network of energy within us that is composed of breath and memory, mind and intuition, and the capacity for consciousness. Our joy and well-being do not depend on our physical body, but on learning more about the spirit within us and the greater life force of the universe. This knowledge of spirit will actually help you take better care of your body and yourself as a whole. After my cancer, learning about the subtle energies made me realize that I could never again return to a life based solely on the material world. Although I still spent several hours a day designing clothes, I no longer identified myself with my career. My work was now merely a means to pay the bills.

## CREATING A SACRED SPACE

As the inner space of my body and mind became clearer, I recognized that I needed to reclaim the physical space that was within me and that surrounded me. A serene environment cultivates a serene mind and helps to heal us. Because we are created from the primordial space, re-creating that space around ourselves, in our homes or at work, is necessary to reclaim our vastness of spirit, the freedom of the soul. The *Rig Veda* says: "The Primordial Vastness is the sky; the Primordial Vastness is the space. . . . The Primordial Vastness is all that was born and shall be born."

After cleaning my apartment thoroughly, I would be able to breathe more easily, and thus achieve a greater sense of emotional and mental calm. I began by cleaning out my files. I made a ceremonial fire in the fireplace and burned most of my correspondence and early journals and poetry, all laden with the sorrows of my cancer ordeal. I dispensed with most of my possessions, which had become unimportant to me. The process of weeding through my belongings also gave me the opportunity to review my past, which assisted my recovery. Old psychic burdens started to ease. Speaking my heart's clearest intentions, I made a silent vow never again to sever my ties with the Mother's rhythms.

Next, I established an altar, placing statues of Hindu gods and goddesses on my prayer stand as a daily reminder of my devotional duties. Each day I offered fresh flowers in a simple bowl and burned sandalwood incense to reflect the purity of being I sought. I prayed for clarity, for my family and teachers, and for all who had helped me through my battle with cancer. I prayed out of gratitude, and in acknowledgment of the Divine Spirit in myself. My spirit was starting to become stronger, and I was gaining a new modicum of peace.

I then went to work on my kitchen, giving away appliances and foods that no longer fit with my desire to prepare and eat healthy, nourishing food. Memories of my family's simple kitchen in Guyana flooded my mind, but since I couldn't daub the walls of my New York apartment with mud or replace the gas range with a wood-burning stove, I settled for acquiring several earthen and wooden bowls, straw baskets and a sieve, and a large mortar and pestle. To the extent that I could, I replicated the environment of the *sadhana* kitchen of my childhood. Just as my people had turned to the timeless *sadhanas* of Mother Nature to heal their ruptured spirits in the New World, I, too, found great solace and healing by following the wisdom of the seasons in the sacred food that nature provided.

I turned my attention next to my bedroom. I could not live with the memories that had seeped into the bed during the hours I had spent weeping there at the time of my illness. I asked a carpenter to build me a wooden bed frame, constructed low to the ground, because the ancient seers tell us that we must touch base with the earth as often as we can each day. This enables us to commune with the earth's magnetic energies, which in turn helps to revitalize our vital tissue energy and memory. My friend Aveline Kushi gave me a gift of a futon she had brought with her from Japan.

Finally, I sorted through and reorganized my closets, converting one into an office where I could put my mail, pay bills, and deal with life's worldly details. I also cleaned out the area around my bed and set up a small nook for reading and writing, separated from the rest of the room by a set of panels made from wood and rice paper.

Later, I would study Vedic architecture, a discipline where structures are specifically positioned in keeping with the Earth's astrological energies. Over the years, I've continued to refine the rhythms of my living and working space. My bed is now out of the direct line of the bedroom door, positioned so that my head points south so I can absorb the energies of the moon, as well as the powerful energies of Shiva, who is said to sit in the south. (The Vedic seers believe that pointing the head of the bed toward the east is also auspicious because we are thus able to replenish the body's solar energies from Surya, the Sun.)

I was surprised by the sense of joy and lightness I experienced from ridding the closets of clothes, accessories, and memorabilia. I felt as if I had released a huge amount of stuckness within me. Later on, I came to see that storing possessions and papers, then forgetting what has been packed away, is a metaphor for our unresolved ancestral memories. When our closets are stuffed and crowded, we forget what's there. When our space is organized and in constant use, we know what we have to work with.

Once I cleaned out and redesigned my living space, I found I had both greater mental clarity and more time to engage in life's wholesome practices. I began doing yoga at the Integral Yoga Center. New friends steered me to the Kushi Institute in Boston. I traveled there for two weeks of every month to study the fundamental principles of Oriental healing, based largely on Zen Buddhist principles, which I gradually adapted to my own Vedic tradition.

Remembering the beauty of my grandfather's fertile fields and gardens in Guyana, I learned natural, organic ways of planting, harvesting, and preparing foods. I surrounded myself with harmonious sounds from outings in the wooded parks of Boston and New York, and from my large music collection. As a result, my entire being began to resonate with renewed joy and vigor.

As I divested myself of my possessions and my old work-identity, my family and ancestral traditions took their places in my life. I located and reunited with my parents and siblings, who had emigrated four years earlier from Guyana to Canada. Twelve years had passed since I had last seen them, but they embraced me warmly without reprimand or harsh words. The reunion with my father was especially warm and emotional. We wept for several days and celebrated for many more. Although we had been rudely uprooted from two countries, we had all regained our lives; I from my struggles with cancer over the past five years, and they from the political war that had ravaged Guyana.

After catching up with one another's activities in the years since we had last been together, I took my leave and returned to New York, refreshed by their love. By acknowledging and embracing my family, I was finally able to heal from the deepest place in my soul and begin to become who I was truly meant to be.

The day I arrived back home in Greenwich Village, I walked over to Jackson Square Park. As I neared my favorite bench, a flock of pigeons swooped down to hunt for food. I watched them closely, wondering if they would confirm my sense of wellness. Indeed, as I sat down, they clustered at my feet, pecking at the ground and eyeing me for a handout. I felt embraced and welcomed by these emissaries of the Mother.

Birds have been perceived for thousands of years as messengers of the Divine Mother. The Inuit people of the Arctic believe that shamans take the spirits of birds during their journeys into trance. Twice-born, first from the mother and then from the egg, birds symbolize a spiritual rebirth within one's own lifetime. This, then, was the day of my spiritual rebirth.

I knew that it would be only a matter of time before I left the fashion industry. As my interest waned in worldly affairs, my desire increased to pursue the health of the spirit. I began to visit and share my newfound nutritional secrets with cancer patients. Even at that very early stage in my long journey of holistic learning, these patients became a sort of *sadhana* community, a harbinger of my future work and mission. My mind reclaimed its natural joy as I dedicated myself to service and living according to nature's rhythms.

A GIFT FROM MY FATHER

Almost seven years after I was first diagnosed with cancer, I started to lose my grounding and began to revert to my formerly frantic lifestyle. Although I had been phasing myself out of the fashion industry, I was now offered the chance to develop an international franchise for my design business, and I was once again gripped by the desire to make my mark as a designer. During a phone conversation with my father, I admitted that I was tempted by the prospect of expanding my business overseas. Sensing that I was in danger of slipping back into my old ways of being, my father came to visit me. He helped me see that I was succumbing to the forces that had pulled me under before and reminded me of the pain I had endured to relearn the truths of my soul. He also warned me that I would be wounded irreparably in this life if I were to forfeit the wisdom and insights I had gained in order to pursue worldly goals.

Father's stay lengthened from several weeks to several months as he undertook to deepen my knowledge of a holistic life by teaching me the Vedic Scriptures and ways of nutrition. Every day after I returned from work, we would go to shop at the Chinese markets and natural-food stores. Although both my mothers and their mothers were good cooks, I really learned to cook from these months with my father. He taught me how to use ancient Ayurvedic principles of cosmic balance within a meal. My hours at work shrank to a minimum as I hurried home each day to my lessons in Ayurveda and the sublime philosophy of Vedanta—the teachings of mother India that had developed over several millennia. Often, I found my beloved father, his face bathed in the pink glow of the Manhattan dusk, preparing dinner or poring over his cherished scriptures. Just as he had done during the visions

I'd had of him while I was in Vermont, he elucidated the *Bhagavad Gita* and Upanishads, expanding on his explanations of the deeper meanings of karma and dharma.

We had wonderful conversations about the knowledge he had transmitted to me in that cabin in Vermont. Like excited tourists returned from a trip to a fascinating country, we compared notes on our visionary journeys. Through visions he had had of me at that time, he had known all about my struggle with cancer, and told me that at the very time I was receiving his guidance, I had also appeared to him on the astral plane—that inner and higher plane that our consciousness and spirit can visit—and confided my pain and guilt. The dates, times, and content of our mutual visions coincided closely. My father even knew the exact moment that I had finally become free of cancer. He had been in his garden in Lancaster, Guyana, when a large seagull—another emissary of the Divine Mother—came to sit with him. At that moment he knew, and rejoiced in my healing.

Now, Father pointed out, my life was again becoming too deeply immersed in ceaseless activity, especially of the mind. He set about to replant the seeds of Vedic tradition deep in my soul. He told me many stories about his mother, who was a great devotee of the Divine Mother. One story, in particular, made quite an impression on me.

As I mentioned earlier, my father was sixteen years old when his mother became ill. His many brothers and sisters were married by then, so he was living alone with her and caring for her as her condition deteriorated. For the two years before she died, he bathed, dressed, and fed her. "All the good fortune I received in my life is due to my mother's blessings," he repeatedly told me. His generosity and devotion to his mother did, indeed, bring him immeasurable grace and drew him close to the Divine Mother.

In between spiritual teachings, Father kept me busy performing wholesome activities: grinding grains, rolling chapati, pounding spice seeds, kneading dough, and stirring *dhals*. When I became impatient, he would remind me of the great legacy of *sadhana* I had inherited from both sides of my ancestry.

One afternoon he announced that we were going over to Jackson Square Park, across the street from my apartment, to bake bread. My building was home to many stars of the fashion and acting communities, and my first thought was, *What if one of my friends comes by and sees Dad and me crouched in front of a fire?*

"Dad, it's a public park," I protested weakly. "All the better," he replied as he picked up the bag of ingredients and walked out the door and into the park. But my embarrassment soon vanished as he squatted on the earth to demonstrate this ancient art of baking. I saw a man who would not censor his expression of personal freedom or compromise his reverence for Mother Earth. People began to draw close and watch with obvious fascination as we dug a pit, gathered brambles, and lit a fire in it. (My doorman, normally a rather prickly sort, went down to the basement of our building, removed the legs from some broken chairs that had been piled in a corner, and brought them over for us to use as kindling.) We rolled the dough and put it on some pieces of kindling, which we placed in the earth. Then my father took a big rock and covered the pit, leaving a small hole for ventilation. While the bread baked, he sat and happily answered questions about this *sadhana* from the people who had gathered to watch. When it was ready, we shared the bread with the crowd and also fed our beloved pigeons.

Father had come into my life again with a definite purpose: to reunite me with my ancestral past. He explained that our ancestral memories are like a river, flowing continuously from generation to generation. Although we can manipulate the river, we cannot alter its ultimate destination. He explained that we stand on the shoulders of our ancestors, but if we're not aligned with their rhythms, we have to carry them on our backs. If we take up their traditions of *sadhana*, however, their energies give us strength. He reminded me that I was born on an auspicious day, Lord Rama's birthday, and that my path in life was a highly spiritual one that could be traced back thousands of years to my ancestors.

I will always remember his last words to me before he left New York: "You are blessed, Maya, and you must never forget Devi's—the Divine Mother's—presence in your everyday life. She has saved you in order to help the distressed in the world and has brought you back to your rightful path." Long after he had returned home, my father's teachings continued to occupy my mind. Whatever I have achieved since then has been informed by his nurturing words, and his profound love for the Mother and the migrant spirit of my ancestors. He enabled me to reclaim my true purpose and put to rest a life of material desires.

While he was in New York, my father foresaw his impending death, which came at the age of seventy, just a few months after we parted. United by a common bond of sorrow, my mothers, siblings, and I all grew closer, relearning who we were for one another. My father's death was a great blow to me, and I felt the urge to throw myself onto his cremation fire. He had touched me at the deepest core of my soul, and now he was gone. I had just found my spiritual legs and wondered how I was going to carry on without his guidance. Two pillars had been taken from me—the motherhood in the form of my womb, and now my father was gone, too.

## THE GURU'S LIGHT

I prayed to the Mother to show me the way, and she responded a week after my father's death. I had a dream in which Father sat with his back to me, wearing his white priest's robes, performing a fire ritual. I was overjoyed to see him, but as I approached him, I chastised myself for clinging to his form and holding him back from his journey. Just then, he turned around, and the fire painted his robe orange. I saw that the person seated there was not my father, but someone I had never seen before, a stoic man who looked me straight in the eye.

Two weeks later, a friend gave me a tape of Vedic chanting, saying, "You'll hear your own voice in this voice." I was captivated by the beauty of the tape. And when I looked at the photograph on the box, I was astonished to see the face from my dream! The person chanting was Swami Dayananda Saraswati, who would become my beloved guru.

I still miss my father, but I continue to feel his energy. I am most grateful for having had him as my first and greatest teacher in this life. When he was taken from me, the Divine Mother brought me Swami Dayananda, who has been both father and mother to me. The *Shiva-Samhita* explains the merits of a spiritual teacher, or guru, in this way: "There is no doubt that the guru is father; the guru is mother; the guru is God. Therefore, he [she] should be served in deed, speech, and thought."

After my father's death, I left New York and the business world to devote myself totally to Vedic studies under the tutelage of Swami Dayananda, whom I had met in the autumn of 1986. I became the first of my people in one hundred eleven years to return to India, where Swamiji gave me an elemental introduction to the motherland. As we drove that first day to his ashram in Rishikesh, he asked the driver to stop the car. He took me down to the banks of the river Ganges, filled his hands with water, and splashed it over me. "Welcome back to your Mother," he said.

Five years later, I returned to the sacred river with my teacher to receive his initiation into the life of a *brahmacharini*. This term means literally "one whose conduct is of Brahman"; one whose behavior springs from consciousness. On the eve of my initiation, while I was observing a silent vigil, a storm raged through the night. Great gusts of wind sent clouds of dust swirling up from the riverbank, creating magnificent images of my ancestors' faces against the dark sky. It was as though the storm had uprooted all the unsettled karmas of my people's past and brought their spirits to bear witness to this life-changing event. Whatever separation of the spirit they had endured could now be melded into wholeness, healed into sanctity. I understood that they had always been with me to help me cross the valley of ancestral pain, and that they had led me to this moment. A journey spanning three generations had now come full circle.

# Chapter 3

## THE ORIGINS AND PRACTICE OF *SADHANA*

*As oil in sesame seeds, as butter in cream, as water in the riverbeds, as fire in the parched kindling, so is the Indwelling Spirit grasped in one's own self when one is dedicated to seek out Consciousness.*
—*Svetasvatara Upanishad* (1.1)

In the beginning, there was absolute stillness. Nothing existed—neither time nor space, gods nor goddesses. Not food, breath, or sound; only the dimensionless force of consciousness was there. Shiva, the primordial force that upholds the universe, awakened. Filled with immortal love, Kameshvara, another name for Shiva, created the moon and constellations, the stars and celestial lights of the sky, setting the rhythms of love and procreation. The universe began.

The creator Brahma hibernated in the lotus-womb of Mother Universe. The lotus blossomed and Brahma awoke. Inspired by Ardhanaranari, Shiva in the form of half-man, half-woman—the unified symbol of creation and the entire cosmos as One within itself—Brahma created the beings.

First, he created Prajapatis, the founding father of creation, and then the exquisite Ushas, the first woman, whose name means "the light of dawn that illuminated the world." So beautiful was Ushas that Brahma himself was consumed with love for her. To escape his fierce obsession, Ushas ran from him, shape-shifting herself into various animal forms. Shiva was unable to withstand the weakness of Brahma, so he took the form of the wrathful Rudra and unfurled himself from the brow of Brahma to save Ushas from his reckless pursuit. He shot at Brahma with his blazing arrow, and fastened him to the sky. The gods bowed before Shiva, acknowledging him as the Mind of the Cosmos, in the words of the *rishis*, Shiva's students, "As a symbol of our devotion to you, O mighty Shiva, we heretofore call you Pashupati, the protector of the animals and the one who controls our beastly passion."

Thoroughly transformed by Shiva's fiery arrow, Brahma appealed to Ushas to let him be her partner, and not her master. Ushas reinvented herself as Saraswati, accepted Brahma's offer, and gave him the wisdom and creativity necessary to create the universe and its beings. Together, they created the celestial beings, and the ghosts, ghouls, and goblins of the spirit world.

Saraswati became the Mother of all animate beings. But soon the people and animals became hungry, restless, and violent. They turned to their protector, Pashupati, for help. Shiva moved his energy into the womb of Mother Earth, producing such immense heat that she became fertile, bringing forth a vast abundance of trees, plants, herbs, grasses, shrubs, and creepers. The hungry birds and beasts feasted on the bountiful vegetation and celebrated their master Shiva, resounding the name Vriksha-Natha, lord of vegetation.

Then, Shiva created the elements: earth, water, fire, air, and space. "Without death, there is no continuance to life," he mused, and thus he created death—not as a finite end, but as a gateway to new life. Rebirth ensured the harmonic cycles of life necessary for the development of consciousness. Shiva saw the beings as birthless and deathless, each enduring the process of rebirth, the ever-generating wheel of karma necessary to refine individual and collective consciousness.

Soon afterward, the creatures became discontented and restless, fighting among themselves. Shiva could not bear the chaos and disharmony he witnessed, so he called upon his consort, Shakti, and enfolded her within himself, drawing the two polarities of manifestation back into its source. We derive from the unity of these two energies the symbol for cultivating consciousness and the purpose behind the practice of yoga. Moving as one, they ascended together to the very summit of consciousness to discover the cosmic mind, which Shiva himself had created. Shiva realized that human beings were caught in the smoke screen of disillusionment, turning away from the true reality of existence—unified harmony.

Merged into Shakti, Shiva projected his thought into the center of the cosmos within himself. He explored the extensive realms of the universe's mind and realized that Brahma had created not only the world of matter, but the world of mind. Shiva saw that the minds of the beings were vulnerable, susceptible to the perceptions of the senses and ensnared by the tantalizing display of the external world that pulls them away from the rhythms of universal law. Shiva recognized that the minds of the beings must be nourished and decreed the universal laws of dharma, to protect and nurture the beings.

Shiva knew that the beings could cultivate health-giving and spiritual serenity and therefore gain consciousness only through the observance of the sacred laws of nature, dharma. He understood that consciousness continually and simultaneously expresses itself in a multitude of dimensions and forms. Dharma is the cohesive factor in this dynamic process which governs and brings into balance the natural laws of the universe.

Thus came Manu, the first lawgiver of humanity, who set out to uphold dharma and ordained that human beings must observe it by repaying special obligations to the universe. These eternal obligations are: *Pitri Rina*—debt to the ancestors; *Rishi Rina*—debt to the gurus, both ancient and contemporary spiritual teachers; and *Deva Rina*—debt to the celestials, to the deities, and to nature. Among the three human obligations, the third is paramount. "Reverence to the

Divine, reverence to Nature—to the earth, river, wind, fire, and space, to the animals, plants, and every blade of grass, every speck of dust," declare the Vedas. The path of practice shapes this vision.

Shiva's work was not yet finished. He knew that the cosmic laws could be upheld only if the minds of the beings were illumined so that they understood dharma, the spiritual focus of life. As he sat again in contemplation, he pondered this question: "How do I steer the mind of creation toward enlightenment?"

Creation stood still until Shiva awakened at last from his inner journey, having found the way to enlightenment: He recognized that he must demonstrate to the beings that all forms of destruction, decay, and disease are caused by conflict that begins in the mind. The beings perceived themselves only in the visible, audible, and tangible form of embodiment, rather than as the source of enlightenment. He had to find the way to make them see that the body/mind is a source of illumination.

So it was that Shiva assumed the role of the cosmic teacher, and through his power of *darshana*, the principle of spiritual transmission, he communicated the truth of enlightenment into the minds of the celestials, seers, and sages. He had discovered the path of harmony wherein the minds of celestials and humans alike can flow in accord with dharma. The ultimate goal of dharma is the integration of the individual with the cosmos through the development of consciousness. Yoga, the inner pathway that merges the mind with cyclical rhythms of the cosmos, is the means to this end. Perfecting the practice of yoga, Shiva showed the seers how to transcend the fields of perception and find the hidden reality of the self and universe behind the apparent mirage, Maya.

As Dakshinamurti, the benevolent teacher who sits in silence facing south, Shiva is the first guru of self-wisdom.

Gods, sages, and celestials hastened to be in Shiva's presence and receive his *darshana* of cosmic truth. With his inexhaustible compassion, Shiva drove out the darkness of ignorance from the minds of his students, the celestials and sages, so that they were released from *samsara*, the resulting misery caused by the mind's separation from consciousness. They attained *moksha*, liberation from the relentless cycles of rebirth.

The Vedic seers described this momentous occasion in cosmic history as follows: "This Great Lord, through the power of His compassion, transmitted the knowledge *'Tat Tvam Asi'* (the ultimate vision of being One with the Whole). With His hand gesture, *jnana mudra,* or 'wisdom seal,' Shiva banished delusions from our mind, demonstrating that all reality secedes to One, Infinite Consciousness, the ineffable truth of the Self."

The sages' hymn of praise for Shiva also gave recognition to Shakti, the power behind Shiva. They knew that the consciousness they had experienced sprang from the integration of the two primordial energies, Shiva and Shakti. The great sage Adi Shankara in his poem *"Saundarya-lahari"* puts it this way: "United with Shakti, Shiva is endowed with the power to create the universe. Otherwise, He is incapable even of movement." Shiva's experience of yoga arose from the integration of Shakti's powers within him.

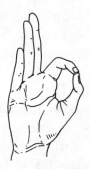

Jnana *mudra*

## THE VEDIC VISION

This ancient, traditional Vedic creation story shows a deep intuition of the interplay of physical and subtle matter and energy, body and mind, individual spirit and cosmic consciousness. It is a beautiful depiction of essential truths in forms that help us remember our human and spiritual origins and our spiritual obligations to ourselves, to the human beings who brought us into this lifetime, and to the universal energies that nourish and sustain us. It brings home the universal importance of daily *sadhana* in its epic drama of the origins of *sadhana*.

Although it is a rich, complex story that has been interpreted in many ways for centuries, the main theme I would like you to remember as a context for your practice of *sadhana* is that there is one underlying force that upholds life. The Vedic masters call this force Brahman, infinite, dimensionless consciousness, the highest teachings of the Upanishads and nondualism to be found in the end portion of the Vedas, called Advaita Vedanta, the wellspring from which the Wise Earth tradition of Ayurveda comes.

In the vision of Advaita Vedanta, physical and subtle matter and energy, each form of creation, all things known and unknown, visible and invisible, the individual and the universe, each separately and together is essentially the whole—complete unto itself. Everything in the universe is represented by two basic categories—*aham* (literally "I"), the subject; and *idam* (literally "this"), the object—into one or the other of which everything exists. The subject is never independent of the object. Indeed, the individual and the universe each separately and together are the infinite, dimensionless whole. To practice *sadhana* is to discover interconnectedness between *aham* and *idam*—the individual self and the material world, our thoughts and our actions—and to transcend our manifold experiences into awareness.

Each of us has the capacity to engage our power of awareness and to be released from the tethers of identifying the conscious, whole Self with any of its parts—body, mind, memory, ego, will, thought, and action. In the *Sama Veda*, it is said, "The Self resides in the lotus of the heart. Knowing this, consecrated to the Self, the seer enters daily that sacred sanctuary. Absorbed in the Self, the seer is freed from identity with the body and emerges in pure consciousness." *Sadhana* is about awakening to our true Self by living in the wholesome practice and recognizing every speck of life to be the whole. Through *sadhana* and rituals, we can consciously integrate the universe's diverse energies within ourselves and in our world, and move ourselves and others toward healing and wholeness.

Now we will undertake to illuminate our understanding further by exploring the Vedic vision of integrating our primordial energies. Let your spirit stretch back to the dawn of the universe. We will journey together to the most ancient womb of the Divine Mother who gave birth to the cosmos and learn about the inseparable, unified cosmic force of the universe, Shiva and Shakti. We will discover inner harmony through the age-old practice of yoga—the unification of body, mind, and spirit.

To prepare ourselves for the next stage of spiritual practice, we use a mantra to evoke the spirits of Shiva and Shakti. You may spend a few minutes every morning reciting this Shiva-Shakti mantra:

*Mangalam Dishatu Me Maheshwari*
*Mangalam Dishatu Me Sada Shiva*
(man-gah-lam dish-atoo may mah-haysh-wah-ree
man-gah-lam dish-atoo may sada shee-vah)

May Goddess Maheshwari be auspicious within me
May God Shiva be auspicious within me

The Vedas tell us that Shiva is the unmanifest conscious-ness—an energy that surrounds all creation but is not seen with the naked eye. Without Shiva creation could not occur. In the final days of my recovery from cancer, when I was blessed to spend time with my father, I came to see through his guidance that all of our fathers partake of Shiva's primor-dial male energy. When fathers and other benevolently pater-nal men use this energy wisely, they build solid foundations from which we all can grow into a Oneness with conscious-ness. My father's instruction helped me to strengthen my faith in my spiritual traditions, which led to my devotion to the Di-vine Mother. The father-mother energies work together.

Shakti represents consciousness in the form of expression—the cosmic energy through which manifestation occurs. Shiva, having seen the truth of the universe, represents cosmic in-telligence, and Shakti, who created the rhythm for the cos-mic laws that would guide the universe, represents earthly, earthy influences. Shakti is a dynamic force—a yang force. Shiva is a universal energy—a yin force. As all-pervasive forces of consciousness, Shiva is called Parashiva, and Shakti is called Parashakti. They are the pillar and platform of cre-ation, the most significant metaphor for inner harmony. We all carry within ourselves these two intersecting powers.

*Yoga Chudamani Upanishad* informs us: "The purpose of yoga is to unite these two principles so that Shiva and Shakti become one within the self." The word "yoga" is derived from the Sanskrit word *yuj*, meaning to join or unite. It refers to union with the Divine, the inner pathway that merges the mind with cyclical rhythms of the cosmos. Yoga, which encompasses far more than physical poses, includes a wide range of spiritual practices: *dhyana* (meditation), *pranayama* (breathing practices), hatha yoga (yoga postures), mantra (rhythmic sounds), mudra (sacred gestures), *sruti* (prayers, chants, and invocations), and *yajna* (rituals), to name a few.

As you begin the practices of yoga that I teach in this book, please recognize that the energies of both Shiva and Shakti are manifest within you: the *ha* and *tha* principle, representing the lunar and solar life force. The fundamental goal of yoga is the union of these two primordial energies and the integration of all life forces. The cultivation of yoga is the way of *sadhana*, and the way to good health and higher consciousness.

## INTEGRATING PRIMORDIAL ENERGIES

To begin this process of integration, let's explore the two aspects of the primordial force that continually overlap to maintain all of creation. Shiva is the primordial masculine force, and Shakti is the primordial feminine force. We each carry these sacred energies within us and connect with them in visible and invisible, imaginable and unimaginable, conscious and unconscious ways. Full consciousness involves a vision of both Shiva and Shakti.

## MUDRA: A YOGA PRACTICE OF INTEGRATION FOR EVERYONE

A very simple yoga practice with which you can start the process of integrating your innate feminine (lunar) and masculine (solar) energies is the ancient and powerful mudra. The word "mudra" is derived from the Sanskrit root *mud* ("to bring joy"). It is a sacred hand gesture that we use to merge the two primary energies of Shakti and Shiva, and seal them within our body.

Mudra as a spiritual practice may be traced back to the most ancient Vedic rituals for the Goddess. The gods and goddesses of the Hindu pantheon are depicted with their hands in various mudra positions evoking tremendous powers. The mudra positions connect us with our inner divinities and bring awareness to the subtle body—the personal energy field that surrounds us; our energetic body double or vibrational field. They also make us aware of our hands as sacred limbs reaching into the universe and conducting energy inward and outward.

Like the practice of mantra, mudra is used as a meditation tool to redirect the energy of the breath *(prana)*, strengthen the life force, and stabilize the body's energy.

## SHIVA LINGA MUDRA

The practice of the Shiva linga mudra, which merges our Shakti and Shiva energies, brings the nervous system and breath into a state of balance. It calms our mind, expands our intuition, and improves our health. Linga literally means "attribute," or "sign of Shiva." The sages conceived of this and other sacred symbols as necessary forms of worship, since most people need a visible, tangible form to gain access to the intangible, invisible, infinite Spirit.

Numerous legends exist about the Shiva linga. According to the *Padma Purana*, the sage Bhrigu arrived at Mount Kailas to find Shiva and Shakti so absorbed in their love for each other that they refused to acknowledge his presence. Angered by this rejection, Bhrigu cursed Shiva and wished him to be remembered as a linga, a phallic-shaped stone, caught in Shakti's vulva. In other words, the linga cannot stand without Shakti at its base—the male energy emerges from and is supported by the feminine force. The *Linga Purana* tells us that the linga is Shiva's cosmic pillar, which emerges from the base of the earth, Shakti, and stretches forever into the sky. This pillar of infinity emanates the Cosmic Sound, om.

The Shiva linga mudra is a vital practice for strengthening your *prana*, or breath-energy, which will, in turn, make you aware of the rhythms of your subtle body. This practice brings about a deep state of calm within the body and harmony within yourself and your relationships.

### The Practice: Shiva Linga Mudra

Find a quiet place and sit in a comfortable cross-legged position on a pillow or upright in a straight-backed chair. Bring your left hand close to the chest with the palm facing upward. Keep the fingers together. Make a fist with your right hand and place it securely on the left palm. Extend the right thumb upward. The right hand is a metaphor for your solar breath and the left hand for your lunar breath. The configuration of this mudra integrates the energies of Shiva and Shakti within you.

Close your eyes and meditate on God Shiva, the Exquisite One. Visualize him in the form of a linga, sitting firmly on the base of Shakti. Now, visualize Shakti as the Formidable One. Hold the mudra for five minutes or so, then release it. Continue your meditation by visualizing Shakti's energy supporting Shiva within you.

To enhance your visualization of God Shiva, you may want to find a representation of Him in a painting or small statue.

### The Seven Cosmic Aspects of Shiva

- Shiva is sky blue in color. (Symbol of the All-Pervasive.)
- He has four arms and carries the trident. (His arms represent the four directions; the trident represents the three cosmic forces of activity, equilibrium, and inertia.)

• He wears the crescent moon in his long knotted hair. The river Ganges flows from the top of his head. (The crescent represents primordial masculine energy and the Ganges River symbolizes the flow of consciousness and means of purification.)

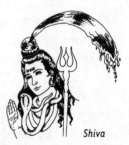
Shiva

• He is smeared with holy ashes and wears a garland of skulls. (Symbols of complete renunciation.)

• He has three eyes. (These represent the sun, moon, and fire. His "third" eye represents the primordial fire.)

• He wears the serpent around his neck. (Sign of *kundalini-shakti*.)

• He sits on a tiger skin. (The skin represents Shakti's power.)

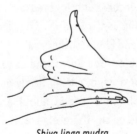
Shiva linga mudra

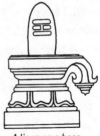
A linga on a base

If you regularly cultivate this simple practice, you will begin to acquire insights into your natural rhythms which are aligned with nature's rhythms. Your practice will evolve over time and should not be rushed. Gradually, you will find yourself stronger and more at peace, and wanting and able to express a spirit of unity and harmony with all things.

Visualizing Shiva in his seven aspects is a significant practice for me. It restores vitality and clarity of mind and evokes the spirit of oneness within me. Men will find that the confidence they gain from this beginning exercise will pave the way for further practice.

As you go through each of your daily routines—waking, breathing, bathing, praying, cooking, eating, walking, chanting, working, shopping, meditating, sleeping—strive to be conscious of your thoughts, actions, and speech. Your daily *sadhanas*, by their very nature, participate in both the male and female, solar and lunar cosmic energies. According to the Vedas, everything in the universe exists as a result of bringing these two energies into balance through awareness and spiritual practice, the heart of which is *sadhana*. Throughout the book, I will describe specific *sadhana* practices and ceremonies, all of them grounded in Vedic thought, that promote the merger of our Shiva and Shakti energies within each one of us, and thus facilitate our union with the cosmos.

## THE SIMPLE WISDOM OF *SADHANA*

After my father died, I returned to the homeland of our ancestors in an attempt to unearth and revive the ancient practices of *sadhana* that had been the heritage of my people in Guyana. The India to which I traveled, however, was not the India of my childhood fantasy, or the one my great-grandparents had left decades before.

I arrived in the motherland to find that the wholesome practices of the earth had been greatly diminished, especially in the urban centers. Although those practices can still be found today in some of the rural villages, they had largely been abandoned. Yet I had to climb high into the Himalayas to find practices that satisfied my deepest intuition of how *sadhana* should truly be practiced, and the Earth and the Divine Mother honored. I visited my paternal great-grandparents' village, which happens to be in the vicinity of my teacher's ashram. There I found the ancient Krishna temple where my great-grandfather had served as a *pujari*. I was told that I bore a striking resemblance to him.

As I traveled in India, I realized that, in a sense, I was fortunate to have been born not in India, but in a place that had kept the Earth *sadhanas* alive. Because Guyana was a hundred years or so behind the technological world, we had been able to safeguard our ancestral memories.

There, my grandparents and their courageous fellow travelers had preserved the life-sustaining practices by their tireless stewarding of the rich rice fields, plantations, forests, rivers, and animals. The land was the hearth of my people's practice. Through *sadhana*, they cultivated an alliance with nature's rhythms. The Vedic rituals they performed were not the rote repetitions of actions and syllables that these ceremonies had become in India, but rather a living re-creation of the sacred, tied to the bounty of the good Earth and the sweat of the people.

By preserving the cherished memories of their homeland, my parents and grandparents reclaimed the sacred within themselves and began the process of healing their broken spirits. Whatever love, redemption, and healing they created in their lives, it was through their devotion to *sadhana*. My maternal grandfather, for example, was a devoted farmer who spent most of his time on his vast plantation. He seldom went home, preferring instead to live beneath the shade of the banana leaves that shielded him from the relentless sun of the tropical skies.

My grandfather spent most of his time in silence. When my siblings and I visited him on his farm, he served us fresh foods from his fields that had been cooked on an open fire. He cured many by his touch and was known to fix a sprain or a broken limb by holding it firmly in his weathered hands. My mother performed the same magic, gently massaging our heads to cure our headaches and healing our stomachaches by touching various energy spots on our bodies. She washed our feet at night to ensure a sound sleep, and, before exams, she held my head in her lap, which seemed to enable me to retain great amounts of facts and information. All these comforting acts of love encouraged the energy of *sadhana*, which had been passed on to her by her father, to blossom in the hearts of us children.

Later, when the civil war chased much of the Indian population from Guyana, it seemed part of the Divine Plan to spread these seeds of *sadhana* to people throughout the world.

The Buddha taught that there is no such thing as an enlightened person, only mindful and conscious actions that lead us to enlightenment. In the words of Swami Dayananda, "Sit in yourself every moment and you will find the way." For a mind that dwells continuously in consciousness, with full awareness of the present moment, every thought is a reflection of consciousness.

When we engage every moment without the cares and fears of the beyond, we are able to harness the spirit of *sadhana*, and every moment is filled with divinity. *Sadhana* can be practiced simply by breathing, having a compassionate thought, saying a kind word, reaching for a blade of grass, plucking a fruit from its vine, sitting in the sun and feeling its warmth, touching the earth with bare feet. In short, *sadhana* is being aware of the integral connection that keeps us forever dancing in rhythmic measure with the cosmic pulse. Our moment-to-moment awareness of this connection is the heart of *sadhana*.

A Vedic story illustrates the courage and beauty of human life when we recognize the spirit within. A deer went searching for the source of the exquisite aroma of musk that permeated the air. The deer roamed far and wide through the forest, never realizing that the scent, in fact, emanated from its own belly. Unlike the deer searching for the source of its own scent, we have the ability to recognize our "musk"—the consciousness that is within us. Once we develop this awareness, we become attentive to our activities and to every moment of our being. As we move closer to our inner spirit, we move toward living in the present and stop the constant fretting about what will come next.

When we remain mindful in every moment of the day, filling each second to the brim with nourishing practices that regenerate body, mind, and spirit, we heal ourselves and help others to heal themselves. The path of practice helps us to find our inner voice and walk our own true path. Only then can we live a life of simplicity—one that flows in harmony with the cosmic rhythms.

Nature provides a broad foundation for spiritual practice. You can begin your practice of *sadhana* by noticing the obvious: the sound of raindrops falling on a pond, the smell of fresh air on an early spring morning, the taste of summer's first peach, the chill from an early winter's wind. The sound, smell, taste, and feel of nature immediately arouse your consciousness. You can replicate this experience of nature in your own kitchen by smelling the rich aroma of ghee as you prepare it (see recipe on page 329) or cutting vegetables along their lifelines (the lines of the life force etched in every food through which it receives its energy and vitality from Mother Earth). When we train the mind to observe the simplest and most obvious details, such as the "lifeline" of a food, we are living in the spiritually nonharmful way. The Tamil scripture *Tirukural* advises, "What is the good way? It is the path that reflects on how it may avoid hurting, harming any living thing." As you engage in these practices, you will find your breath moving with ease, your mind becoming gentle and peaceful, and your inspiration coming alive.

*Sadhana* is the practice of meditation in motion, and this practice is like a lotus. Deeply rooted in the mud, the lotus expresses its essence in an exquisitely beautiful flower. Like the unfolding of the lotus petals, the application of *sadhana* must be both gradual and continual in your life, abiding within the cyclical rhythms of nature. These practices hold the promise of making every moment a meditation. As a result, you become awakened to your purpose and your individual memory, inviting full recognition of the self as sacred.

Practice *sadhana* as divine action. Engage in it for the sake of refining the action and not for its apparent results. Plant a seed for the joy of planting it. Living in *sadhana* brings alive your alliance with the cosmos. When you practice according to the cosmic rhythms and relinquish an expectation of control over your own life and nature, your sense of separation from the boundless presence of the Divine Mother evaporates, as do your personal grief and strife.

Finish every activity you begin. The rhythms of nature decree that each occurrence has its own completion. By bringing each action to closure, you signal the universe to grant you time to replenish your natural energies. With each completion comes a feeling of exuberance—the swell of joy after planting the fields for the season, finishing a painting, or washing dishes after a delicious, health-giving meal. The heart becomes light and resolved, and the *prana* flows gently through it. The spirit of grace that brings gratitude to the universe for her bountiful gifts is kindled.

Whenever I complete a project, I set aside a few days to sit in silence or find some other way to refresh my spirit and renew my energies. Recently I finished teaching two intensive weeklong practitioner training programs. Rather than plunge headlong into yet another obligation, I decided to go visit my mother, who lives several hours away from me. She was in the process of moving to a new home, and I felt blessed to be able to spend time with her, helping her pack and get ready for the move.

As we sat together sorting through her belongings, separating what she wanted to keep and what she wanted to give away, we shared a stream of memories. We laughed and cried as we recalled various incidents from my childhood in Guyana, and I truly felt the spirit of the Divine Mother in my own mother's presence. The simple tasks we shared—making porridge in the morning, doing the laundry, filling up boxes with clothing and household items—helped to rest my mind and revive my *prana*, so that I returned home eager to embark on my next project.

A task completed with thanks becomes an invocation to the Divine Mother. But *you* have to set aside the time to mark that completion, just as you find time to accomplish the task. The first step is to reorder and recover the path of *sadhana* in your daily life so that you can reclaim the cosmic patterns and rhythms necessary for health and consciousness. Although a great lapse in the traditions of *sadhana* has occurred over the past two centuries, you can be a catalyst for a greater consciousness through your individual efforts and example. As Robert Muller writes in *Birth of a Global Civilization*, "The human species is engaged in a major transformation. Through the human species, the universe is becoming conscious of itself."

You can begin your journey on the path of practice by embracing the integration of body, mind, and spirit through the three principal *sadhanas* of breath, sound, and food. Each of these is essential to our existence: we cannot function without breath; we are immersed in the sound of our mother's heartbeat and biological rhythms from the moment of conception; we are dependent on the bounty of nature's foods for sustenance and growth.

# THREE STATES OF NATURE'S SADHANA: OJAS, PRANA, AND TEJAS

According to the Vedas, three states are responsible for the birth of creation: *ojas, prana,* and *tejas.* To quote the *Svetasvatara Upanishad,* "The never-created creator of all is Pure Consciousness, the creator of time, all powerful, all knowing. He is the Lord of the Spirit and of the three conditions of nature." Just as breath, sound, and food are integrally connected, so are these three cosmic essences from which they derive. In a sense, they can be thought of as the body's immunological factors, because we cannot sustain life without them.

Just as we cannot separate body, mind, and soul, we cannot separate *ojas, prana,* and *tejas.* All three are intertwined; if *prana* becomes unbalanced, so, too, do *tejas* and *ojas.* They function as an inseparable unit and prepare our consciousness to come alive. We may look at *ojas* as our soul-nourishment, *prana* as our soul-breath, and *tejas* as our soul-vibration. From the universal perspective, *ojas* is the container in which *prana* and *tejas* are carried, infusing life into manifestation.

*Ojas* brings cosmic memory to earth through nature's foods. *Prana* brings the life force energy to earth through nature's movements. *Tejas* brings the cosmic vibration to earth through nature's harmonious sound. We glean the essential nourishment of our three essences through the *sadhanas* of breath, sound, and food.

*Ojas,* which maintains our physical body, rhythms, and impulses, is responsible for safeguarding our internal bodily functions. *Ojas,* which means the glow of health from which we derive a strong, vibrant immune system, is the force of water; it enables us to sustain wholesome activity in our lives.

*Prana* maintains breath, intuition, and memory (or our astral body) and animates our life force. The most pervasive force of our lives, it is formed from the element of air which brought forth the astral body, the source of our life force, as well as the emotions of enthusiasm, courage, and joy.

*Tejas,* our mind's subtle fire, makes cosmic sound audible and produces our inner powers of transformation, our inner voice, and intuition. *Tejas* gives life to cosmic sound and brings forth our ability to change. It is responsible for sustaining the most subtle component of our body, the causal body.

The cosmic overlays of food, breath, and sound are similarly inseparable. When we engage in one form of *sadhana,* we inevitably come to embrace the other two. I found this to be the case, for example, with Jody, a journalist who attended a weekend workshop I gave for cancer patients several years ago in New York City. Jody had been diagnosed some months earlier with cancer of the liver, and had already undergone surgery to remove the malignant tumor. Her doctor believed that with chemotherapy, she could probably beat the cancer. Despite the positive prognosis, Jody felt hopeless and depressed about her situation. She later told me that she had decided to attend the *satsanga* (gathering with the spiritual teacher) because she thought I might be able to offer her some spiritual advice and solace.

Jody listened attentively, even jotting down notes as I talked about Vedic lifeways, but I could see from the expression on her face that she shut down as soon as I began to describe the food practices that had helped me so much in my own recovery. During one of the breaks, I asked her whether she planned to try out any of the food preparation *sadhanas* and recipes that I had discussed. "No way," she said flatly.

"I'm too busy with my work, and besides, I've always hated cooking."

I was struck by the vehemence of Jody's response, so I asked her to tell me about herself. She talked about the demands of her work, how much of her life had been taken over by deadlines and the pressure of chasing down the next great story. Then, almost as an afterthought, she mentioned that she had had a whole other career as a pianist. "But I couldn't make enough money as a musician, and I'd always been a pretty good writer, so I went into journalism," she said. "I haven't touched a piano in years. These days, I don't even have time to *listen* to music."

In separating herself from her instrument and the practice of creative expression through music, Jody had severed her connection to cosmic vibrations, to *tejas*. The joy she had once derived from playing the piano had been replaced by anger and resentment. "Would you be interested in taking up the piano again?" I asked. She shook her head, no; that part of her life was a closed book. But she did agree to my proposal that as part of her healing process she set aside time each day to listen to some of her favorite recordings of classical music.

A month later, Jody sent me a letter, saying how happy she was to have rediscovered the pleasures of music. She had even begun regularly visiting a friend who owned a baby-grand piano so she could resume playing. "My technique is very rusty," she wrote. "But as soon as I put my fingers to the keys, I felt a deep, familiar happiness that I've been missing for a very long while."

I wrote back and suggested that she add to her practice several of the chants that I had taught at the workshop. Soon after that, I received a package from Jody—a tape of her chanting as she accompanied herself on the piano. She had also enclosed a brief note: "I'm feeling much better, more hopeful about my recovery. I've cut back a bit on work, and I'm trying to incorporate into my life more of the practices I learned at the workshop. But I still haven't made peace with the food *sadhanas*."

My next suggestion to Jody was that she buy a *suribachi*, a round Japanese mortar and pestle used for grinding spices. Musicians tend to like the *suribachi* because when they use it, they create a pattern of continuous, rhythmic sound. "I know you don't want to cook, Jody, but loving sound as you do, you might enjoy the music you can make in your own kitchen," I wrote.

I was not the least bit surprised when Jody informed me in her next letter that she had found her way into the kitchen and made several of the *masalas* that she had tasted at our workshop (see recipes on pages 317–319). Soon after that, she reported that she had started preparing complete dishes, combining chanting with her cooking. The last time I heard from her, she was feeling very fit and optimistic, and had moved on to doing yoga, meditation, and other practices that involved strengthening her breath.

In Jody's case, the activity of one *sadhana*—sound—attracted the other *sadhanas* and energies into her life so that they all became aligned. You may want to start your practices with food or breathwork, knowing that no matter where you begin, you, too, will start to bring all of these energies into harmony. In later sections of this book, I offer practical instructions for how to recover the *sadhanas* of breath, sound, and foods, so that you can journey safely and successfully into the manifold realms of your being and explore the immense world of energy, memory, and spirit.

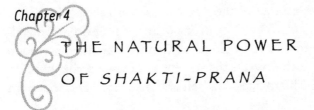

# Chapter 4

# THE NATURAL POWER
# OF *SHAKTI-PRANA*

*The power who is Consciousness in all being*
*Reverence to Her, Reverence to Her, Reverence*
*to Her*
*The force who exists as Shakti in all beings*
*Reverence to her, Reverence to Her, Reverence*
*to Her. . . .*
—Devi Mahatmya

My Vedic spiritual heritage goes even farther back than the *Shakta* tradition in India where the Goddess religion still thrives and the Mother of the cosmos is a living reality in the hearts and minds of millions of devotees. The more we nourish the seed of the Mother's presence within us, the more we participate in her extraordinary energy. As the Mother's presence fully awakened within me during my recovery, for instance, I gained many insights into the workings of my subtle, spiritual body. *Shakti* is the Mother's most powerful force within us and in the universe.

## THE POWER OF *KUNDALINI-SHAKTI*

As the active force of manifestation, the Divine Mother is often depicted as *kundalini-shakti* by the symbol of a serpent. The Sanskrit word *kundal* in fact means "one who is coiled." The serpent energy also represents the Mother's breath and rhythms within us. The serpent is associated with the goddesses of many cultures throughout the world.

Coatique, mother of the Aztec deities, is called "She of the Serpent Skirt." The Minoan Snake Priestess of Crete is a goddess. In the Mayan culture of Central America, the moon goddess, Ixchel, wears the serpent as a crown on her head. In Egypt, the hieroglyph for "serpent" also represents the word "goddess."

The energy of *kundalini-shakti* "sleeps" in the root chakra, the energy center at the base of the spine, where she is depicted as coiled three and a half times around the lingam, the symbol of Shiva. *Kundalini-shakti's* potent energy influences and controls the rhythms of body, mind, and spirit. Both women and men can evoke kundalini experiencies; it is by no means a phenomenon that is exclusive to women. Ancient stone-images show Shakti with the kundalini serpent emerging from her yoni, or vulva, a powerful symbol for a woman's energy and potential for spiritual transformation. The serpent's movement up the spine results in enlightenment.

I have had several firsthand encounters with kundalini's movement after years of practicing *sadhana*, meditation, and silence. When *sukshma-prana*—the subtle breath—began to gather force traveling through my chakras, my *kundalini-shakti* was awakened and started its numinous ascent up the central pathway of my spine, a process that persisted for three years. During that time, all my senses were heightened, most particularly my intuition, and in many situations I could "see" a person's condition before he or she gave me any information about the nature of the problem.

One day, when I walked to the road to pick up my mail, my feet suddenly rose several feet off the ground so that I floated to the mailbox. One of my neighbors, who happened to be passing by, greeted me with a wave, and seemed not to notice that anything out of the ordinary was taking place. I realized that my subtle body had elevated itself, but my

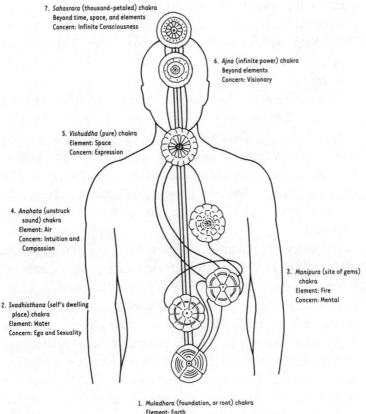

7. *Sahasrara* (thousand-petaled) chakra
Beyond time, space, and elements
Concern: Infinite Consciousness

6. *Ajna* (infinite power) chakra
Beyond elements
Concern: Visionary

5. *Vishuddha* (pure) chakra
Element: Space
Concern: Expression

4. *Anahata* (unstruck
sound) chakra
Element: Air
Concern: Intuition and
Compassion

3. *Manipura* (site of gems)
chakra
Element: Fire
Concern: Mental

2. *Svadhisthana* (self's dwelling
place) chakra
Element: Water
Concern: Ego and Sexuality

1. *Muladhara* (foundation, or root) chakra
Element: Earth
Concern: Survival

*Seven chakras: unfolding kundalini energy in the projectile movement of the chakras'*
*energies. Each chakra, rooted in the* sushumna, *the column of energy up the spine,*
*emanates its own energy and flows into the energy of the other chakras.*

physical body remained on the ground. This phenomenon recurred often during my meditations; I would feel my body rising from the ground while *prana* throbbed in my right temple.

As kundalini arose within me, for many weeks my internal body blazed with fire: the Mother's fire cleansing my body's impurities. I would often feel her brushing against my temples like clouds drifting by my face, or the caress of soft down feathers. I lived in the blissful state where everything I saw within and without was golden. I recognized this light to be the Mother and her celestial offspring, Surya, the sun.

I heard exquisite Vedic melodies in my mind, which I later identified as songs from the *Atharva Veda* and *Chandogya Upanishad*. One such song says: "Now, that golden image seen within the sun has a golden beard and golden hair. He is exquisitely luminous, even to his fingertips. His eyes are like the lotus of Kapyasa. His name is High. He is lifted above all ills. Verily, the one who knows this rises high."

Once the kundalini energies subsided, I realized that my spiritual intuition had increased as my *shakti* had increased. *Shakti* is the spirit of our primordial feminine energies within and its activity promotes the union of body, mind, and spirit. Goddess Shakti's rhythms move within every man, woman, child, and creature through *shakti-prana*, or Mother's breath, which pervades the two lower chakras located around the perineum and sacrum. *Shakti-prana*, the body's inherent life force, protects the reproductive organs and especially the primordial feminine energy of Shakti within our genitals, womb, and belly. It also gives us tremendous power to bring forth life, to move energy, and to heal ourselves. Working with women all over the world, I have witnessed great miracles as they learn about their inherent *shakti* power. If we are to become conscious again, we must reclaim the sacred feminine within each and every one of us, so that we can evoke and influence the healing energy in men and children, as well, by supporting the path of *sadhana*.

The power of your *shakti* goes beyond the space of

the womb and its magic of bringing new life into the world. Your womb also has a divine function, which is the cultivation of nurturing and healing powers of the Mother within. In working with your *shakti*, you will discover profound physical and spiritual health. In so doing, you as a woman also affect and influence the well-being of all living things.

## MOON ENERGY

The Vedic seers teach that a woman's *shakti*—her power, fertility, and nurturing spirit—is linked to the lunar cycle and the sacred substance of Mother Moon. The ancients called the dark days of the moon "woman's moon" or "resting moon," linking a woman's physical, emotional, and spiritual state to the lu-

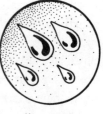

Moon energy

nar wheel. Many other cultures similarly revered a woman's sacred connection to the moon. German peasants called menstrual blood, *die Mond,* the moon. The French called it *le moment de la lune,* the movement of the moon. In India, a particular blood vessel in the vulva is called *chandra-mauli,* moon-crested, and the vagina itself is known as *chandra-mukha,* moon-faced.

In olden times, the first sighting of the rising moon from below the depths of the western horizon was hailed with joy and celebration. The rising moon represented the Mother's act of resurrection—a metaphor for a woman's menstrual cycle. A Gabon pygmy song echoes a woman's intimate relation to the moon: "Moon, O Mother Moon, O Mother Moon, Mother of living things, hear our voice, O Mother Moon. Keep away the spirits of the dead. Hear our voice, O Mother Moon, O Mother Moon, O Mother Moon."

The moon gives its nourishing essence to nature's foods and the vital tissues of the body, and it controls the musical note of the heartbeat and the curvatures of our breath. She sustains the ultimate essence of life and procreation carried in a woman's womb. Just as the ocean tides are affected by the movement of the moon, so, too, are the waters of the womb.

Women's natural feminine rhythms are supported by monthly menstrual cycles. Our earliest female ancestors innately appreciated this wisdom on a cellular level; deeply attuned to nature's cycles, they menstruated with the new moon, when the moon's *ojas* energy (which protects our physical bodies) is at its lowest ebb, and the sun's absorbing energies are at their peak. As their menstrual blood began to flow, they set themselves apart from the men and children to observe the *sadhana* of rest and replenishment. The new moon was a time when women temporarily shed the burden of their responsibilities to focus on self-renewal and self-nurturing in a spirit of sisterhood and community.

In our postindustrial era, the use of contraceptive pills and devices, hormonal therapies and antibiotics, and the chemical alteration of the world's food sources have disrupted our inner rhythms, causing our menstrual cycles to shift out of sequence with the cycle of the moon. This misalignment impairs the flow of *shakti-prana*, a primary subtle *prana* in women, and this impairment triggers hormonal imbalances and disease.

The *shakti* energy provides a broad foundation for healing physical and emotional wounds. Every cell, tissue, and memory of a woman's body is permeated with the billions of years of memory and energy inherited from the Divine Mother's *shakti*. Her milk flows through our breasts, and in the fullness of her moon, her nectar courses through our wombs, thus determining the time of ovulation. During pregnancy, as our bellies swell with life, we emulate Mother Shakti growing into plumpness, from the silver of her crescent moon into the roundness of her full moon. The Mother who surrounds us is also within us in the form of *shakti-prana*.

Our *shakti-prana* circulates through and around the womb, a woman's area of greatest vulnerability. This is a lesson I learned firsthand. Too often, we do not recognize the sanctity of the womb, and the sacred *prana* that governs it. Herein lies the paradox of the *shakti-prana*: this profound source of feminine power also makes us extremely susceptible to disease. When you care for your womb, and thus honor your *shakti-prana*, you heal your feminine life force and protect yourself from illness.

Since my recovery from ovarian cancer, I have undertaken to educate and inform women of their *shakti* energy and its workings with the lunar wheel. Menstruating with the new moon is the central practice for recovering your womanly health. Each year, I help almost a thousand women realign their menstrual cycles with the new moon. Many women are able to shift their cycles within the first three months of conscious practice, while others take up to six months or longer. Most women report a dramatic improvement in health as soon as their menstrual cycle starts to flow in accord with the new moon.

## A WOMAN'S MOON CYCLE

The first step in strengthening *shakti-prana* is to familiarize yourself with your inner rhythms. Every creature bows to the cadence of nature. Males of all species move with the rhythms of the sun. Females of all species move with the rhythms of the moon. Native women chart the passing of the years by the number of children to whom they give birth, and mark the passing of the months by their monthly cycles. To help you keep track of your cycle, I would like you to use a calendar that marks the cycles of the moon. Just knowing whether the moon is waxing or waning helps you become more attuned to nature's rhythms. I also suggest that you note in your lunar calendar when to perform certain *sadhanas* that I will describe later.

Our menses greatly affect our *shakti-prana* because the monthly cycle is the primary means through which this *prana* is revitalized, cleansed, and restored. Based on my experience and intuitive sense, I believe that Vedic culture honors the *shakti-prana* by recognizing that a woman's blood preserves her *shakti*, and that this blood carries the Divine Mother's potential for bringing new life and rebirth. The seers attributed this phenomenon to the workings of the red *bindu*, the cosmic seed of Goddess Shakti, located in the root chakra, where kundalini lies. When *shakti-prana* is strong, the *bindu* acts as magnetic lodestone, drawing the energy of the moon in to revitalize the womb. The rhythm of the red *bindu* also causes us to discharge our uterine lining at the appropriate time during the new-moon phase, so that our hormone levels are naturally reset.

Unbalanced hormonal levels, along with poor nutrition, stress, excessive exercise, and a general disregard for nature's rhythms, are the key causes of menstrual disorders such as amenorrhea (lack of menstrual period) or menorrhagia (abnormally heavy menstrual bleeding). As disruptive as these disorders can be to one's health and life, it can sometimes be a fairly simple process to heal them in natural ways that restore *shakti-prana*. Jennifer, a personable young woman who lives not far from my school in North Carolina, came to me for advice because she hadn't menstruated in six months. She was not pregnant, and at thirty-one, she was much too young for menopause. Aside from not having a regular period, Jennifer also felt bloated and lethargic, complained of insomnia, and was often heavily congested.

My first question, as always, was, "What's going on in your life right now?"

"I'm upset because I just lost my job," she said. "For the past eight months, I've been working in the marketing department for a company that sells organic foods. Then they decided to move their headquarters to another state. They wanted me to go with them, but my husband's doing research at the university here and he can't leave his lab."

"Did you enjoy your work?" I asked her.

"I loved it," she said emphatically. "Before that, I was a chef for seven years, which meant I was working five nights a week until midnight. Then I'd be so keyed up that I couldn't go to bed until two or three in the morning. I'd spend most of the day sleeping, and I never got to see my husband. Of course, now that I'm unemployed, I've reverted to being a night owl. I stay up way too late, watching TV, then sleep until eleven."

The reason for her missed periods had nothing to do with the stress of losing her job. By sleeping with the sun and waking up with the moon, she had disrupted her body's natural rhythms. My first advice was that she return to a more normal sleep schedule by getting up at six or seven, and going for a walk, though I cautioned her to avoid too much exercise at this point. I counseled her to cook wholesome foods, which I knew would not be a hardship since she loved to cook. I also told her that during the dark moon-cycle (a week before and after the new moon), she should take twice-daily doses of *trikatu*, a combination of *pippali* (a type of pepper), black pepper, and ginger, which are meant to give fire to the body. Finally, I suggested warm baths and a lower-back scrub of fresh, grated ginger, wrapped in a washcloth or handkerchief.

Jennifer began menstruating again the very next month at the new-moon phase. Her *shakti-prana*, which had become stagnant, was revived, so that her lethargy rapidly diminished and her spirits improved considerably. When I last spoke to her, four months later, she still hadn't found work, but she was having regular periods at the new moon and she was feeling optimistic about her job search.

## SADHANAS FOR WOMEN

According to Ayurveda, all disorders relating to the womb—premature puberty; irregular, scanty, or excess menstrual flow; premenstrual syndrome; infertility; vaginal infections; venereal disease; osteoporosis; uterine, ovarian, and breast cancers; and birth defects, to name a few—are linked to the monthly cycle. It is not surprising, then, that women are particularly vulnerable to mind-body imbalance and disorders when they are menstruating. As much as possible, during your menstrual flow, you should slow your pace and reduce your activities to the bare essentials so that your body experiences the least degree of stress. Refrain from bathing, and limit yourself to quick, cool showers or sponge baths. Abstain from sexual activities. Refrain, as well, from all cooking *sadhanas* in order to prevent the powerful energies from the menstrual blood from pervading the foods. Maintain a light wholesome diet of salads, fresh juices, light grains (basmati rice, millet, couscous, amaranth), pasta, tofu, leafy greens, and fresh fruits. Herbal teas such as raspberry, organic rose flower, peppermint, ginger, lemon balm, hops, and chamomile are also revitalizing during this time, as are any healthy ancestral foods that lighten your spirit.

Even if your cycles no longer coincide with the moon's rhythms, you may observe the *sadhanas* set out below, which will help you restore your natural cycles. If you have entered menopause, you should continue to practice these *sadhanas* for a few days during the new-moon cycle until you are sixty years of age. This practice will help you maintain healthy hormonal levels, and recall the natural rhythms of your *shakti-prana* and the vitality of your womanly spirit.

The full moon is the natural time for you to enjoy and celebrate your womanhood. When the moon is full, you are under the influence of its cooling, *ojas*-producing essence, which inspires ovulation and heightens your sexual impulses and vitality. This is a natural time for having sex, and for practicing *sadhanas* such as aromatherapy; warm, fragrant baths; and oil massages. Hearty *ojas*-producing foods are recommended: organic milk, pancakes, crepes, homemade breads, soups, casseroles, risotto, pilaf, polenta, a variety of whole and cracked grains (bulgur, couscous, brown rice, basmati rice, arborio rice), beans, pasta, fresh vegetables, salads, and desserts such as custards, puddings, fruit pies and tarts, and strudels. Wholesome ancestral foods that reinforce your spirit of abundance and celebration are also appropriate at this time.

## SADHANAS FOR THE NEW MOON

The practices set out below will help you strengthen *shakti-prana*, rebalance your hormonal system, and rejuvenate your womb and womanly spirit.

**The Practice: Activating Solar Breath to Strengthen *shakti-prana***

You can start to shift your menstrual cycle to the new moon by activating your solar (right) breath a few days before your period begins, regardless of which phase of the moon your cycle occurs.

Lie on your left side, close the left nostril, and slowly inhale and exhale through the open right nostril. Do this practice for a few minutes every day on the three days before your period begins. The solar, or *ha*, breath invokes the power of the red *bindu*, the *shakti* in your root chakra, and helps it gather its forces so that it thoroughly collects the menstrual waste before ejecting it from the body.

*Yoni Mudra—Womb Seal*

The next practice is called yoni mudra (womb seal). It is the most powerful mudra to draw Shakti's power into our bodies, into our womb or belly, strengthening and enhancing her *prana* within us. Because mudras enhance the breath, they bring awareness to the subtle body. This mudra strengthens *shakti-prana* and directs the menstrual blood so that the flow begins at the time of the new moon.

The yoni mudra is especially sacred to women. Among other benefits, it locks the opening to the womb, so that the circulation of *shakti-prana* in this region stays within and intensifies. As you practice this meditation, you will feel the subtle movement of this breath in the root chakra area. The breath may appear as a light, thready, serpentine movement along the spine or as a pulsating pressure in the womb region. This healing practice is good for you even if you are no longer menstruating or sexually active.

You should practice yoni mudra, in addition to solar breathing, for three days directly before the new moon and the full moon. You can also use it whenever you feel the need to revitalize *shakti-prana, except* during your menstrual cycle. As a reminder to do this practice every month, circle these dates in your lunar calendar.

### The Practice: Yoni Mudra—Strengthening *Shakti-Prana*

Sit in a meditative posture and cup your hands together, palms facing up. Cross your right pinkie finger over the left and fully extend the middle fingers to meet at the tips to form a pyramid shape. Cross the ring fingers behind the extended middle fingers and hold them down with the index fingers. Tuck in your thumbs to touch the bases of the middle fingers. Hold this hand gesture for five minutes.

If your fingers are stiff, you may initially have some trouble with this rather complicated mudra but over time your fingers will become more flexible. Within the first week of doing the practice, your fingers will begin to bend more easily, and within a month, as the *prana* improves in the womb, you will find this mudra quite simple and satisfying.

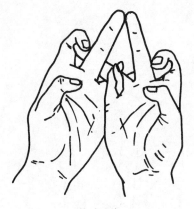

Yoni mudra

## The Observance: Taking a Womanly Reprieve

Your primary *sadhana* during your menstrual period is to allow the richness of your blood to flow back to the earth. In ancient times, women would gather in an area that their men had specifically prepared and set aside for them to squat on the ground so that their blood could nourish the *shakti* energy of the earth. Traditional Vedic practice encourages women to take turns helping to care for, and feed, the families of menstruating women. You can also encourage your spouse and older children to participate in the food *sadhanas* and managing the family kitchen during these times.

## Sadhanas *for the Full Moon*

In the early evening, during the first three days of the full moon, begin to evoke and strengthen your abundant, fertile, feminine moon spirit with the three practices that

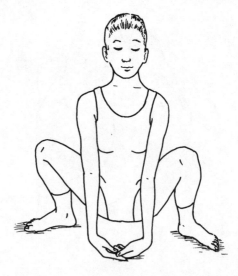

*Squatting posture*

follow: the squatting posture, *kapalabhati* (fire breath), and basking in the full moon. Circle these days in your moon calendar so that you remember to do your full moon practice.

### The Practice: Squatting Posture—Opening Feminine Spirit

In ancient times, women squatted during their menstrual cycle in order to return the blood to the earth. Our female ancestors could control their menstrual flow because they were aligned with their *shakti* power. The *shakti-prana* of women today is weaker, however, because we do not use it properly, so you should avoid putting pressure on the uterus or creating an unnaturally strong flow of blood by squatting during pregnancy or the menstrual cycle. Squatting is especially beneficial in treating diseases or disorders such as cancer of the uterus, ovaries, or breast; sciatica; infertility; sexual dysfunction; menstrual disorders; infections; headaches; hemorrhoids; constipation; excessive dryness of skin; and for general maintenance of a mother's health after childbirth. Assume a squatting posture by positioning your feet hip-width apart and parallel, and bending your knees. If you can't bring your heels flat to the floor, place a small pillow beneath your heels for support. Bend slightly forward, and rest the palms of your hands on the floor. Exhale vigorously through both nostrils. After you've emptied your lungs, begin a series of gentle inhalations and exhalations while holding the squatting posture. Continue for five minutes. Then move on to the next practice.

### The Practice: *Kapalabhati*—Fire Breath

The breath is a purification exercise for everyone but it is especially beneficial to women. The abdomen acts as a bellows that fans the fire within. To recharge *shakti-prana* and sexually regenerative energy, sit on the floor in a comfortable cross-legged posture. Exhale by repeatedly forcing the breath out through both nostrils eighteen times in quick, rhythmic succession. To make sure you are exhaling fully, place your right hand over your belly and feel the pumping motion of your diaphragm. Afterward, take a slow, deep inhalation, then commence another round of the rapid exhalations.

*Kapalabhati* breath is a powerful practice that activates the magnetic power of the *bindu*, the *shakti* in the root chakra. It draws the essence of the full moon into your womb and aligns your female energies with the rhythms of the moon. You can practice this breath throughout the two-week period of the full moon, but should refrain from practicing it during the new-moon cycle.

### The Observance: Basking in the Full Moon

In Vedic practice, women convene on the third evening of every full moon to bathe or walk in the moonlight, or to sit together in meditation beneath the full moon. The village women on the Corentyne coast where I grew up would come together to drum and sing songs to Mother Moon. They would chant, *"Chandra ma ma, Ayiye, ayiye, ayiye"*—an invocation inviting Mother Moon to draw closer. Indian women today still gather on the first three evenings of the full moon to anoint one another with fragrant oils and sing songs to the Divine Mother. I regularly invite students to observe the ritual of the Third-Night Moon with me. We sit in a circle where the full moon can be clearly seen, drum the *dholak* (a traditional North Indian barrel-shaped drum), and sing Vedic songs to the Divine Mother. Afterward, we observe silence. I encourage the women to continue this practice in my absence, and many of my female students convene in small groups all over the country to pay homage to Mother Moon with the Third-Night Moon ritual.

## LEGACY OF OUR MOTHERS

You can deepen the process of healing *shakti-prana* by exploring and refashioning your relationship with your maternal forebears, beginning with your own mother. The bond we share with our mothers is profound: We carry their joy (and their pain) in our spirit, their patterns of breath and cellular memory in our *shakti-prana*.

I had taken so much about my birth mother for granted, but after my father's death, I started to cultivate a warmer, more intimate relationship with her, as well as with my "older" mother. Today, I dearly love and am close to both women. We often sit together for traditional ceremonies, sing songs, and play the *dholak* and harmonica. Their energies and experiences are built into the foundation of my intuition and strength.

Each mother played a distinct role in my early life: My older mother wielded more authority in the home. She had more formal education than my birth mother, so she helped me with my homework and with my various hobbies, including designing clothes and painting with watercolors. My birth mother guided my spiritual development and taught me the daily prayers and rituals. She frequently bathed and massaged me, and she taught me to plant, harvest, and care for the garden.

I would have been a much healthier and gentler person had I been closer to her in my early years. When we talked about my experience with ovarian cancer, I discovered that she, too, had endured difficulties with her womb. She was only seventeen years old when I was born, after a long and painful labor. She subsequently had a miscarriage, two Caesarian births, and then a hysterectomy.

I have noted repeatedly that women who have troubled relationships with their mothers also have deficiencies in their *shakti-prana* and cannot connect with the Divine Mother's purifying energy. The feeling of separation from the Mother can give way to anger and frustration—both of which are debilitating. These emotions block your ability to communicate and move forward with your life. You can take your first step toward dissolving these emotional impediments by recognizing that much of the anger and frustration is from your own unrealized dreams and desires, about choices left unmade, or the need to fulfill somebody else's vision of how you should live your life. For instance, I had tried to ignore my spiritual calling by hiding behind my intellect and a demanding career. I had kept distant from my mother—the one person who had always known my true purpose—because I had avoided my path. After my recovery, I came to understand that I had resented my mother's unrelenting honesty—the same honesty that is now the wellspring of my spirit and purpose.

Before you can begin to turn your course toward the light, you must first *want* to move beyond your anger or resentment toward your mother and other female forebears. To start the process of recovering your maternal trust and love, I recommend a simple breathing exercise called *sitali*, or serpent's breath, for cooling the breath and dissipating anger.

### The Practice: Serpent's Breath Exercise

Curl your tongue so that it forms the shape of a U and draw an intake of breath through it, which will make a hissing sound as you inhale. Hold your breath for twenty seconds or longer, and then exhale through your nostrils. *Sitali* breath is excellent for beginning to heal a difficult relationship with your mother and for reducing fiery conditions of body and mind.

Another simple method for dissolving anger is to say to yourself, "Do not go there. An angry thought is a toxic thought." After enough years of practice, the mind begins to check itself so that it becomes difficult to register an angry thought.

Before we can heal the hurts of our maternal wounds, we must begin to appreciate all things feminine. Nature offers constant reminders of how feminine energy pervades every-thing around us. In the woods near my home, I observed a doe plucking mouthfuls of fresh, dew-laden grass and gently feed-ing her young. I also watched with delight as a mother finch built a nest on my windowsill for her four eggs. After the chicks hatched, she steadfastly kept watch over them, leaving the nest only occasionally to forage for food. Ten days later, she led the young birds on their maiden flights. They returned to their nest that evening for the last time. The next morning, at dawn, they were gone. These creatures showed me the natural strength and vitality of Shakti.

All mothers, of all species, instinctively know when their young are in need of help. Recently, I slipped and fell down a muddy hillside. The phone rang the moment I entered my hut. It was my mother, who said, "I just had an impulse to call and make sure you were all right." Perhaps you have similar stories of your encounters with the Divine Mother in nature or with your own mother.

Although some women can be more harmed than nurtured by maintaining contact with their mothers, such cases are the exceptions. In all but the rarest instances, the conflict can be resolved and the relationship repaired by observing spiritual practices that keep the heart open and energy unimpeded. Try to put aside your expectations of who you think your mother should be, and "see" her for who she really is. This sacred act of simply "seeing" her will dissolve the negativity between you. You can cultivate compassion for your female ancestors and acknowledge their travails if you envision them as the beautiful spirits that they are.

You would be surprised how simple gestures can mean so much to the recipient. Every fall, for instance, I make herbal bouquets from my garden and distribute them to the women who are most precious to me. Sometimes I dry the herbs and create potpourris, and sprinkle them with essential oils. I also make natural facial scrubs from ground mung *dhal* and Aegean Sea salt, put them in little brown paper bags, and tie them with tall, dried grasses from my garden. A gift need not be expensive, so long as your intention is to convey thoughtfulness, love, and caring.

You may also choose to recite this invocation in praise of Mother Earth, our greatest nurturer, or you may offer prayers to whichever deity with whom you feel an affinity, to evoke a spirit of appreciation for the feminine force that surrounds us.

*O Mother Earth, provider of nurturance, health, and wisdom*
*Guardian of the magical secrets of the Earth—*
*May I celebrate your beauty, wisdom, and grace.*
*May I find your wholeness within me.*
*Fill me with your divinity and vision to appreciate*
*The sacred feminine in all things.*

## CONNECTING THE LINKS
## IN THE CHAIN OF HEALTH

Besides the emotional and spiritual links to our mothers, we also inherit the physical rhythms of our mothers' health. As a spiritual counselor to hundreds of women with cysts, tumors, and cancer, I have noted that their diseases can often be related to the condition of the maternal uterus during pregnancy. Women, in particular, can benefit from knowing the links between their health issues and those of the women in their family, going back as many generations as they can trace.

Claire's story is an illustration of this principle. I met Claire seven years ago when she attended my women's workshop at the New York Open Center. She was just thirty years old. Six months earlier, she had discovered a fibroid the size of a large grapefruit growing rapidly in her uterus. She was one of the first to approach me when we broke for lunch. "I'm determined to avoid surgery," she said, after describing the size and location of her fibroid. "What Ayurvedic therapies can you recommend to help me?"

I asked her whether anything unusual or difficult had happened to her during the past two years. Her eyes immediately filled up with tears. "I was living with someone for four years. We split up a year ago. The breakup was his idea."

Next I asked her, as I always do when diagnosing the origins of a woman's health condition, about her relationship with her mother. "We get along well," she told me. "But sometimes she can be difficult. She's been a nervous wreck ever since she was divorced from my father five years ago, so she takes medication for depression."

As part of a noninvasive regimen to help her reduce the tumor, I suggested that Claire spend some time talking to her mother about the last three generations of women in her family, and the difficulties they may have had giving birth. I also gave her a Wise Earth nutritional regimen that included organic vegetables and herbs, such as arugula, endive, radicchio, and mustard; whole grains, particularly barley and millet; and beans, such as mung, aduki, soya, chickpeas, and black beans, all of which are especially beneficial in the treatment of fibroids. I suggested she take hip baths in warm water with *triphala* powder and aloe vera gel, and that she drink raspberry, rose petal, and red clover teas.

A month later, Claire wrote me a letter documenting her discoveries. Her great-grandmother had had a hysterectomy after giving birth to her second child, and her grandmother had undergone a Caesarian section to give birth to Claire's mother. Claire herself was a "preemie," born five weeks early.

Like her maternal ancestry, Claire carried a weakness in her uterus. Although she hadn't said that she was lonely, it seemed obvious to me that she was still mourning the loss of her partner. She had also alluded to wanting to be in a new relationship, but hadn't met anyone with whom she could connect. This grief was further fueled by her mother's unfulfilled longings and depression. Over the years of talking to women who have fibroid conditions I've noticed that they all share a deep sense of loneliness, whether they admit to it or not. Claire also had deeply etched lines that ran from the corners of her nose down past the corners of her lips, which according to Ayurvedic diagnosis is a classic indication of ancestral grief and loneliness. Thus, she had filled the void in her womb with a fibroid.

Claire was able to connect her maternal ancestral memories with the condition of her own uterus. In combination with the Wise Earth *sadhana* practices she had adopted, she turned the corner in her healing process and within a year was free of the fibroid. When I saw her next, she radiated good health and the lines on her face were considerably less pronounced. She sounded cheerful and vibrant as she talked about the drawing class in which she had enrolled. She was no longer brooding over finding the next "Mr. Right," but rather, was looking within to express herself.

Claire influenced her mother's healing as well, once they were both aware of the loss and loneliness that had made them vulnerable to illness. She shared with her mother the Wise Earth regimen and taught her the women's healing poses she had learned at my workshop, as well as the Ayurvedic diet. By addressing their shared vulnerabilities, they have been able to redirect their relationship to one that cultivates love and creative fulfillment.

## REKINDLING YOUR INNER FIRE

To recapture your *shakti-prana*, you must nurture a larger vision of who you are. You are not only an earthly mother, wife, daughter, sister, friend, or career woman. You also live on the subtle plane of the spirit. From earliest times, rituals have been used to invoke our consciousness of the subtle plane and our connection to it. *Yajna,* the ancient practice of worshiping the deities and their subtle energies through fire ritual, is observed in millions of Hindu homes. Indeed, fire is the elemental energy of all Vedic rituals devoted to appeasing the gods and goddesses. The *Rig Veda* tells us, "The devout performers of solemn ceremonies are led to the doors of the inner sanctum of the Divine. At the fire sacrifice, ladles placed to the East are plying the fire with melted butter, like the mother cow licks her calf, or the rivers caress the fields."

Fire rituals, combined with meditation, generate heat within the body to burn away physical impurities, illumine the mind, and facilitate our communion with the celestials. The Devi fire ritual described below is a powerful Vedic women's rite that will deepen your awareness of both the Divine Mother and your earthly mother in everyday life. It will also help restore maternal ancestral memory and health. Devi is another name for the Universal Mother, but for the ritual you may contemplate any image or aspect of the Mother with which you feel comfortable, be it Devi, Blessed Virgin Mary, Gaia, Gwan Yin, Avilokiteshvara, Nammu, Hahai'i Wuhti, Au Sept, Mawu, Ishtar, Akua'ba, or any other.

My earliest memory of my two mothers is of their lovely

faces lit by the fire of their early morning rituals. The Devi fire ritual is for every woman, no matter what your relationship is with your mother. Men and children may also participate, but take care to keep the children a safe distance from the fire pot. There may be times when you will want to invoke the Mother's *shakti* energy without performing the actual fire ceremony. You may do this by keeping your chosen image of the Mother in mind while you recite the prayer of your choice, or by chanting the Devi mantra provided below. Yet another way to perform the ritual is simply by visualizing the pouring of the offering of ghee (sacrificial butter, see recipe on page 329) into the fire, rather than physically doing it. The sages often conducted the ceremony this way.

Every day is the Mother's day, but Tuesdays and Fridays are the best times to make offerings to the Mother, and are the days that the seers devote to her. I celebrate the Mother every day, and so can you, if you choose to, with the Devi fire ritual practice that follows.

### The Practice: Devi Fire Ritual

You will need the following utensils and ingredients, which should be reserved only for performing the ritual. Starred items may be purchased at Indian grocery stores or health-food stores.

- an image of the Mother
- a small earthen pot (6" diameter)
- a small ladle
- pine kindling (tiny pieces called *dhup*\* or fat-wood), or dried sage, or camphor resin\*
- ghee\* (keep a bottle of ghee to be used only for rituals and prayers)
- red or pink flower petals (optional)
- matches

If possible, perform the ritual outside. Otherwise, remember to have a window open so that you do not set off your fire alarm. The ground, a river, or an ocean are the most auspicious places to put your sacred ritual ashes, but you may also add them to the soil of your potted plants.

*Directions:*

Choose a quiet site in your home, preferably facing east, to set up a tray with all the ingredients and utensils. Place an image of the Mother where you can see her clearly. Put a few pieces of kindling, sage, or a cube of camphor into your fire pot and light the fire. With your right hand, use a ladle to pour a tablespoon or so of ghee into the fire, along with the flower petals (if you are offering petals). Allow the kindling to burn out completely. As the offering continues to burn, look directly at the Mother's face and recite the Devi mantra (see below). Focus on whatever you desire from her. You will know when she is pleased with your efforts. Sometimes, she smiles. Sometimes, she winks.

## *Devi Mantra OM SRI DEVI MA*

Invoking Sri Devi Ma will help you to reclaim your maternal memory and intuition—the divine power manifested in all women as the instrument of healing all things within and without. Queen Maladasa's story from the *Puranas* expresses the power of a mother's love and wisdom. Madalasa was an enlightened woman, and each of her children grew up to be enlightened saints. Whenever she was pregnant, she devoted her time to meditating and worshiping the Indwelling Spirit (Atman). After the birth of each of her children, she gently cradled the infant and sang the song of the spirit:

*Shuddhoshi Buddhoshi Niranjanoshi*
*Samsara Maya Parivarjitoshi*

O child, you are not the body; you are the spirit.
You are enlightened; you are pure Atman (Indwelling
Spirit).

You may sing this wonderful Vedic lullaby whenever you
feel yourself losing touch with the Divine Spirit within.

As women, we must strive to re-create our life around our
maternal memory, our innermost ability to heal. Our earthly
mother is the instrument of love and wisdom. We gain joy
when we recognize that our maternal energies are whole and
unbroken within us, and that we can transmit this joy to all
beings.

When you realize your *shakti-prana*, you uncover your
magnificent spiritual female anatomy. Now that you have
begun to tune in to your maternal heritage, it is time to explore your connections to the subtleties of breath, mind, and
consciousness—connections that are shared by all creatures,
whether male or female, of every species.

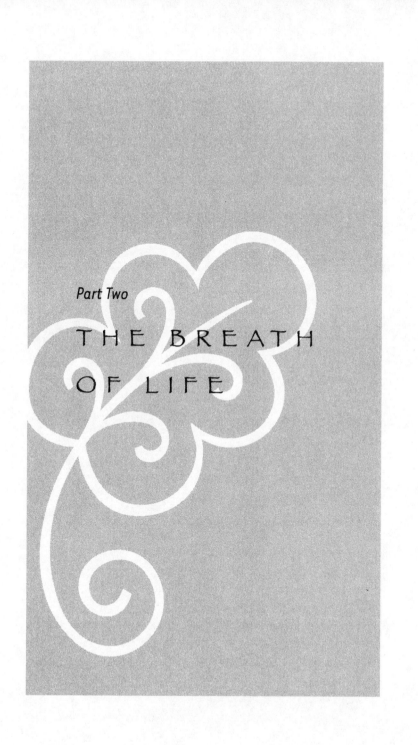

*Part Two*

# THE BREATH
# OF LIFE

# Chapter 5

# THE ANATOMY AND
# PRACTICE OF THE BREATH

*Whatever moves in the universe,*
*Whether it is either seen or heard,*
*Whether it is within or without—*
*It is pervaded by breath.*
*—Maha Narayana Upanishad*

The Vedas tell us that life is defined not by the number of years a person is alive on earth, but by the number of breaths each soul is given for its journey. The *Isha Upanishad* tells us, "Go my breath, to the immortal breath. Then may this body end in ashes." When we expend our ration of breaths, our journey ends. The ancients therefore advise us to slowly synchronize the rhythms of our breath with that of nature. Breath is also an intrinsic aspect of *prana*, our principal life force, which controls the quality of our life as well as longevity. *Prana* is the breath of the soul, a bridge between body and mind, so conscious breathing practices can nourish our spirit and heal even our most grievous spiritual and emotional wounds.

The sages developed a science of breath, called *pranayama*, which literally means "manifestation of ultimate cosmic energy." *Pranayama* encompasses a variety of practices, all of them designed to reestablish the flow of breath in harmony with the rhythms of the universe. "He who has control over his breath also has control over his mind," says the *Chandogya Upanishad*. Swami Rama, a noted contemporary yoga master, describes the mind as "a wall [that stands] between the yogi and the reality. When the student comes in touch with the finer forces, called *prana*, he can learn to control his mind, for it is tightly fastened to the *prana* like a kite to a string. When the string is held skillfully, the kite, which wants to fly here and there, is controlled and flies in the direction desired."

When we aim to control the mind through the various *pranayama* practices, we gradually reduce the constant barrage of intrusive thoughts and ever-changing sensations that keep us from spiritual understanding and consciousness. Thus, *pranayama* promotes the yoga principle of unification of the mind and cosmos; as we begin to transcend the distractions of the mind and body, we move beyond the physical realm to the far greater awareness of our inner oneness and our oneness with the universe. Mircea Eliade, one of the twentieth century's preeminent philosophers of religious history and traditions, describes *pranayama* as "an attention directed upon one's organic life, a knowledge through action, a calm and lucid entrance into the very essence of life."

*Pranayama* is also a wonderful way to extend both the duration and quality of your life. If you have never practiced *pranayama*, your respiratory pattern probably consists of quick, shallow breaths that start and end in the chest. Think back to moments when you felt angry, frightened, or under stress, such as during a fight with your supervisor in which you felt you were treated unjustly, or upon hearing the unmistakable wail of a police siren when you've been speeding. You engage in the sort of shallow chest breathing that is the hallmark of the body's fight-or-flight stress response.

Of course, this physiological reaction is appropriate under extremely stressful circumstances, but the problem in our culture is that we habitually breathe these shallow breaths even under normal, less stressful conditions. Chest breathing does not allow us to take in enough oxygen to feed the lower lungs properly, so that the cardiovascular and other biological systems cannot operate efficiently. Thus, we spend much of our lives unwittingly depriving ourselves of sufficient oxygen—and the *prana* that comes through deep breathing—which leaves us in an energetically and spiritually impoverished state.

We can correct this *pranic* deficiency through the practice of several simple breathing exercises, all of which are rooted in deep abdominal breathing. You may start your practice with diaphragmatic breathing, a method that transforms shallow breathing into a deeper, more expansive rhythm and facilitates the flow of *prana* throughout the entire mind-body system and revitalizes us on every level. The following exercise, known as *shavasana* (literally translated as "corpse posture" or "tranquil posture"), uses diaphragmatic breathing along with a visualization. It is an excellent starting point for other, more advanced breath practices.

Diaphragmatic breathing is easy enough to do, once you become aware of how it differs from chest breathing. After you practice breathing from the diaphragm while lying in tranquil posture, you can begin to incorporate this deeper, more relaxed respiration into your everyday life. You can practice conscious diaphragmatic breathing any time, even sitting at your desk or in your car. I particularly recommend tranquil posture whenever you feel overwhelmed, stressed, exhausted, or simply blah.

### The Practice: The Tranquil Posture

Lie flat on your back on a rug, yoga mat, or any other surface that comfortably supports your body. Put one hand on your chest, the other hand at the bottom of your rib cage just above the belly. Inhale into your belly so that you can actually feel it rising, becoming round and full, while the diaphragm moves downward, allowing your lungs to fill with oxygen. (Never mind what you see in the fashion magazines. If you hold in your stomach in order to look thin, you are cheating yourself of breath, oxygen, and *prana*.) Allow the breath to travel slowly all the way up through the diaphragm, into the chest, and up to the collarbones. Your chest should remain relatively stationary. When you have completed the inhalation, slowly exhale, and feel the belly contracting as your diaphragm moves upward. Continue this practice for several minutes until the process begins to feel natural to you. Now that you have begun taking slow, deep breaths, allow the breath to travel all the way up your spinal column, then feel it circulating throughout your entire body. Position your arms by your sides, with your palms facing up. Stretch out your legs hip-width apart and parallel to each other. Close your eyes and visualize your breath as a stream of cool, tranquil, golden light that flows from your heart and radiates to the farthest reaches of your body. Allow this golden breath to flood your entire being. Feel it in the tips of your fingers and toes, in the crown of your head, in each of your vertebrae, behind your eyelids, and in your throat.

Rest your mind in the serenity of the breath. Let yourself relax as fully as you can in this posture, breathing slowly and peacefully, for fifteen minutes. (It's best to stay awake, but if you fall asleep in this posture, you obviously need the rest, so enjoy your nap!) Now, open your eyes, and gently shake out your hands, arms, and legs. Look around the room, noticing what comes into your mind as you observe your familiar surroundings. Allow yourself a gradual transition to full consciousness by sitting up slowly and taking whatever time you need before you resume your normal activities.

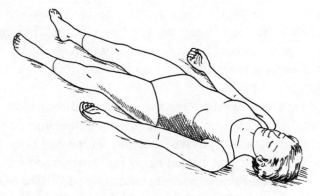

*The tranquil or corpse posture*

These breathing exercises are based on an understanding of how *prana* flows through your body and are designed to enhance your *pranic* energy. Lily, the wife of a mechanical engineer in a Toronto Indian community that I often visit, recently experienced the powerful healing effects of *prana*. Lily was feeling very upbeat as she maneuvered her car along a crowded street not far from her home on a brisk, mid-October night. She had gone shopping for a statue of Saraswati and she was pleased with her purchase, which was now propped up in the front seat of her car. She had bought the statue in honor of Dipavali, the Hindu festival of lights. Soon the streets would be illuminated with strings of bright lights in honor of the holiday. As she braked for a yellow light at a busy intersection, her mind was preoccupied with thoughts of dinner and preparations for the celebration.

The next time she opened her eyes, she was lying in a hospital bed, her right arm set in a cast and pounding with pain. She had no recollection of how or why she had been brought to the hospital, so she was shocked to hear from her husband that a car had hit her from behind with such force that her car had skidded out of control, flipped over, and landed upside down. The car was demolished, and she had had to be rescued from it by the "jaws of life." The emergency personnel on the scene were amazed that she had suffered nothing more than a concussion and a fracture to her arm.

About four weeks after the accident, the cast was removed and Lily just had to wear a sling for her arm. She began working with a physical therapist for the next two and a half weeks but was beginning to feel discouraged because she was hardly able to move her arm. Lily had hoped to take part in the yoga classes I was scheduled to teach at the local Indian community center, but because of the pain and extremely limited range of motion, she couldn't do even the simplest poses.

I explained to Lily that when we sustain a severe trauma to any part of the body, we have to be concerned not only with the pain and muscular damage, but also with the accompanying emotional injury—all of our fears and anxieties that quite naturally arise out of such a situation. Her *prana* had become blocked by the shock of the accident, and the *pranic* flow needed to be reestablished before the physical healing could take place.

With the support of the other women in the class, I asked her to lie on her left side in sleeping-moon posture. This is a simple pose: you lie on your left side in the fetal position, with your forehead almost touching your knees, and breathe normally. Sleeping-moon posture is intended to return you to a psychic state akin to that of an embryo in its mother's womb. It helps restore our *shakti-prana* and is especially useful for women who have had abortions, miscarriages, or other traumas such as Lily's accident.

I covered her with a light blanket and told her to close her eyes, breathe deeply into her belly, and then exhale fully, directing the breath into her arm. As she followed my instructions, I quietly explained that with each of her exhalations, she was sending a message from her womb—the deepest part of her belly—to her arm. I could see her face soften and her limbs relax as she lay peacefully in the posture, taking long, slow breaths that were the only sounds in the otherwise silent room.

After five minutes or so, I had her sit up, cradle her right arm in her left, and rock it as she would a baby. Next I instructed her to inhale deeply, then exhale slowly while simultaneously humming. Humming while exhaling is called "bumblebee breath," because the humming recalls the buzz of a bumblebee; it is a powerful technique. Breath and sound, merged together, alleviate fear, anxiety, and exhaustion. I use a particular combination of humming sounds and *pranayama* practices—my own, unique breathwork practice that I teach to all my yoga students.

After repeating the bumblebee breath for several minutes, Lily stopped abruptly and pointed to her right arm. "It's shaking," she said nervously. "I feel as if some kind of pulse is moving through it." I told her not to worry, that this was exactly the reaction she was working to evoke. The stalled *prana* had been reawakened and was rushing down the length of her arm.

Lily dutifully practiced the two breathing exercises for the next seven days. Each day, the tremor in her arm grew more intense, yet at the same time the pain and stiffness diminished. At the end of the week, she hurried into the yoga class and announced, "Look what I can do."

Lily could now perform the spinal twist, a pose which called for her to extend an arm over her head and behind her back, placing the palm on the floor while twisting her body toward the extended arm. Then this is repeated with the opposite arm. Lily's pain was gone, and the mobility in her arm had almost totally returned. In a few more weeks, she recovered completely.

(In an example of divine synchronicity, the statue of Saraswati also survived the car accident, intact except for its right arm. Lily was planning to discard the statue, but I told her to bind the arm to the body with a cloth bandage and recite healing prayers on its behalf for the next month. I'm still waiting to hear whether the statue's arm has healed!)

How did the breath exercises enable Lily's arm to mend so swiftly? The Vedas tell us that breath is not simply a flow of air that is a by-product of the respiratory process. Breath is also the kinetic life force that drives the dynamic interworkings of all creation. This concept was beautifully articulated by Master Great Nothing of Sung-Shan in the *Taoist Canon on Breathing*, when he stated, "No one has form without breath. Consequently, breath and form must be accomplished together. Isn't this evident?"

*Prana* propels the earth's orbit around the sun and the moon's orbit around the earth. It animates the wind and water, as well as the ebb and flow of the oceans. The wave of *prana* in the body is the basis of consciousness in the universe. Memory rides the waves of breath.

When *prana* is balanced, memories abound. *Prana* and memory together form the second layer of our anatomy—the *pranamaya kosha*, or breath-body. When breath is out of balance, memory suffers, and vice versa. By restoring the flow of *prana*, Lily provided her bodily tissues with the necessary nourishment to overcome her fearful memories of the injury and pain and reestablish the cellular memory of the healthy arm.

# PRANAYAMA: THE FIVE-FOLD SYSTEM

According to Vedic thought, *prana* is composed of five "airs" that have different functions in our body-mind. The sages developed this *pranayama* science of the breath as a way to realign the body-mind so that it can function harmoniously with the universe. The body is constantly revived through the natural rhythm of deep, measured inhalations and exhalations, and each of the five *pranic* energies—*prana, udana, samana, apana,* and *vyana*—directs a different area of the body.

## Prana

The first of the five subenergies, or airs, of *prana* is also referred to as *prana*. Called by the ancients "the soul of the body that sits on the throne of the heart," *prana* is the silent witness to all of our journeys. *Prana* suffuses the region between the larynx and the heart; it sustains the heart, voice, intelligence, and respiration. *Prana* enables each of us to quiet the mind, enter the inner universe, and discover our true nature. When *prana* malfunctions, our very life force is threatened.

## Udana

The second air, called *udana*, or rising air, sustains our voice or individual sound, and the universe's cosmic memory. *Udana* functions through the breath. When the breath is calm, cool, and rhythmic, we are able to increase our life span and better serve our purpose on earth. When the breath is shallow, rushed, and fatigued, we shorten our stay and leave the journey unfinished.

Our voice is meant to be a reminder of our sacred origin, since it expresses, through breath, the sound of the creator. Producing harmonious sounds causes us to resonate with the vast, immutable consciousness. Producing disharmonious sounds disrupts our breathing rhythm and alienates us from the sonorous rhythms of nature. *Udana* also helps to produce and preserve our inner voice or sound, which permits us to cultivate awareness.

## Samana

The third air of *prana* is *samana*, the keeper of balance. *Samana* stimulates our spirit of discernment and flexibility, and rules our metabolism and digestive processes. When *samana* is balanced, we achieve equanimity and satisfaction. The body's sense of reason comes alive, helping us determine what is valid or invalid, valuable or useless, sacred or sacrilegious. *Samana* allows us to be conscious of the Divine and the sanctity of life within us and, as a result, discover a life of balance within nature.

## Apana

The fourth air of prana is *apana*. This air preserves our ability to reproduce and nurture life. *Apana* regulates our spirit of nonattachment to material objects, and also teaches us to nourish ourselves without indulging in excess. The dominant air in a woman's body, *apana* flows downward to help preserve the health of the reproductive organs and tissues, including the mammary glands, and the womb. *Prana* and *apana* work hand in hand. When *shakti-prana*, which works through *apana*, is impaired, *apana* is also weakened. *Apana* acts as a receiver for *prana* in the lower body.

*Apana* rules the colon and promotes the release of whatever is toxic or excessive in our lives, while retaining that which nourishes us. In order to maintain good health in the pelvic region, *prana* and *apana* must flow harmoniously.

## Vyana

The fifth air of *prana* is called *vyana*, which is manifested in the hearts of all living things. *Vyana* helps to distribute the energy extracted from the universe's breath and natural foods within the body. *Vyana* is the power of circulation, and it arouses the desire for personal freedom. It also provides the force of outward movement that teaches us to be charitable and to cultivate goodwill with all of life. Pervasive and gentle, the encouraging nudge of *vyana* makes it possible for us to act harmoniously within the family and community and fulfill the Divine Plan.

The five airs of *prana* not only pervade the region of the heart and chest, but also the face and brain. They help us chew and swallow food and provide immediate nourishment to all the vital tissues of the body. They also support the vitality of our spirit and are the "gatekeepers to the celestial world," in the words of the *Chandogya Upanishad*, enabling us to transcend the notion of dualities so that we merge with the Universal Oneness.

## HARMONIZING OUR BREATH WITH LUNAR AND SOLAR RHYTHMS

Every person is endowed with two main channels of breath—lunar and solar. The lunar breath works in accord with the rhythm of the moon, and the solar breath works with the rhythm of the sun. These two luminous beacons were set out in the sky to safeguard the affairs of creation: As the earth turns on its axis, creating night and day, the cosmic breath moves in accord with the earth. The breath is constantly shifting from left to right channels, and back again. In a healthy body, the lunar breath is more active during the day, and the solar breath is more active at night. Four distinct junctions recur each day—sunrise, noon, sunset, and midnight—marking four definitive exchanges of *prana* as our breath moves from the solar to the lunar cycle. When we are healthy, the two channels of *prana* within the spinal column—the *ida* (left channel) and the *pingala* (right channel)—naturally flow in accord with these changes in the rhythms of the cosmic breath.

The *pingala*, the solar current, is dominant during the day, and the *ida*, the lunar current, is more active during the night. We receive the solar energies of the cosmos through our right breath, and the lunar energies through our left breath. Our solar breath pervades the right side of the body and controls the bodily functions of eating, digestion, and elimination. The lunar breath pervades the left side of the body and controls the functions of ingestion and assimilation of fluids and urination.

Both lunar and solar breaths also serve specific roles in our emotional body. The right breath controls our routine, rational activities—working, thinking, exercising, planning, or what we call left-brain functions. This breath is naturally heightened during strenuous and aggressive activities. The left breath controls our creative functions—meditation, prayer, singing, journaling, or what we call right-brain activities. This breath is generally increased during peaceful and relaxing activities.

When you align your breath with daily lunar and solar rhythms, you cultivate good health and awareness, which provides the basis for your spiritual work and ultimately leads to internal harmony. In balancing both channels of *prana*, our goal is to bring our breathing rhythms into accord with the cosmic breath or universal *prana*. The rising sun, for example, emits powerful solar energies. The left breath must therefore be activated at sunrise, so that the lunar energies in the body increase and complement the strong solar energies. Otherwise, if the right breath remains dominant, aggressive tendencies will be overactive. Although the instructions that follow may seem complicated at first, I promise that these breath practices will increase your energy and give you many more precious moments in your everyday life.

## ACTIVATING OUR LUNAR AND SOLAR BREATHS

The ideal pattern for our breath is an active left breath at sunrise and throughout the day, and an active right breath at sunset and throughout the night. While the solar breath in a healthy organism tends to be more active during the night, in some instances the lunar breath should be activated during the evening. For example: before drinking fluids, because the lunar breath cools the digestive tissues to allow for optimal absorption of the liquid; and before urinating, in order to cool the urinary tract and allow *apana* air to collect the liquid waste and guide it out of the body efficiently.

When the body is not well or engaged in healing, the left breath tends to become more active as the body attempts to use energy to facilitate recovery. However, in the case of a serious disease that requires a lengthy healing process, the regular breathing schedule of an active left breath during the day should be adhered to as much as possible. Once you are able to promote an active left breath during the day, the right breath will automatically fall into correct alignment during the night.

Although the solar breath is best activated at sunset to balance the energies of the moon, certain circumstances require that the solar breath be activated during the day. These include: directly before eating, in order to strengthen the digestive fire; directly before defecating so that the *apana* air can more efficiently collect bodily waste and escort it downward and out of the body; directly before sexual activity, to enhance the downward flow of the *apana* air into the genitals, heightening fertility and the joy of sexual communion. After sexual intercourse, the left breath should be activated to recharge *prana* and bring the body back to a tranquil state.

By regulating and redirecting the dynamic flow of breath from the left and right channels into the central pathway, you intertwine the two breaths and induce an inner state of vitality and harmony. This practice will protect you from anxiety, despair, and illness. It will also give you the necessary foundation for meditation, which you will learn about later in this chapter. The practice of the lunar and solar breaths is also a powerful means for integrating feminine and masculine energies. Once these *pranic* conduits are in a state of balance, they naturally harmonize with the cosmic cycles of *prana* in the universe.


I have found that the most vital key to good health is the revitalizing practice of breathing in rhythm with nature. Consider the case of Joanie, who timidly approached me at a book-signing event I did at a small bookstore in South Carolina. With hunched shoulders and swollen eyes, she seemed miserable. She had come to me out of desperation because she had read my books on Ayurvedic nutrition and healing and hoped that I could help her out of her anxiety and depression. I invited her to have a cup of tea with me and tell me what was troubling her.

"I've been crying nonstop for weeks," she confided. "All I want to do is sleep."

She went on to explain that she had been in a funk for a little over a year. "I'm a teacher, but I had to stop working. I feel like I have a big hole in my stomach, and that the life is draining out of me. I feel physically ill with the pain. I have no energy. All I do is watch TV, day in and day out. My house is a wreck, my husband is angry at me, and my mother says my problem is all in my head."

She slumped in her chair as her eyes filled with tears. "I was also having terrible panic attacks and episodes of claustrophobia, especially in crowds. I couldn't ride in elevators, or go to restaurants or movies, because I'd start to get anxious as the place filled up with people."

Joanie was seeing a psychiatrist because she was having severe mood swings that would often result in furious outbursts during which she would phone friends at all hours of the night and make wild accusations against them. Her doctor had prescribed medication for what he termed "manic-depressive" episodes, but Joanie felt her condition had gotten worse because of the drugs. She also had an antianxiety medication for her claustrophobia. On her bad days, of which she had many, she would swallow the pills as if they were candy.

One day, racked with despair, she downed an entire bottle of tranquilizers. A friend happened to stop by her house, found her unconscious, and immediately called for an ambulance. Joanie had been out of the hospital only a month, and was still feeling very shaky and raw. "I would have died if my friend hadn't dropped by, and lately I've been having lots of moments when I'm sorry she came over that day," she said.

I told Joanie that I knew of a simple breathing practice that I was quite certain would alleviate her painful symptoms. I explained that by balancing her lunar and solar breaths, she would reestablish the proper alignment between the natural rhythms of the universe and her own internal rhythms. I asked her to do the practice every day for a month, no matter how depressed or angry she felt. "It may be hard at first to honor your promise, but soon enough you'll experience some results, and that will reinforce your commitment," I said.

Joanie agreed to practice the lunar and solar breath exercises including the alternate-nostril breathing, three times a day (see below for instructions). "Thank you," she said, as she stood up to go. "I really appreciate your help, and at this point, I have nothing to lose, especially if it doesn't involve another drug."

A month later, I received a letter from Joanie. "I can hardly believe it myself, but I'm feeling so much better," she wrote. "I'm much less depressed, and my energy has really picked up. In fact, my symptoms are so improved that when I went to see my psychiatrist last week, he cut my drug dose in half—and I still feel okay! Even my husband sees a difference. The other day, he and I took a three-mile hike, something we used to do all the time. It was great to be outside, and he was amazed that I could keep up with him."

Joanie has since come to study at the Wise Earth School. Three years later, she continues her daily breath practice and has also incorporated the food and sound *sadhanas* into her life. She is now completely free of medication, has returned to teaching sixth graders, and is fully functional and healthy.

### The Practice: Checking the Lunar and Solar Breaths

In order to align your breath with the lunar and solar rhythms, you must first determine through which nostril you are exhaling the most air.

Press one finger lightly against your left nostril with one finger to block the flow of air, and blow out your right nostril, holding your hand beneath your nose. Feel the force of expelled air. Then do the same on the opposite side, blocking your right nostril and blowing through your left. Your dominant side is the one where the breath is more forcefully expelled. When the air is stronger on the right side, your solar breath is activated. When the breath is stronger on the left side, your lunar breath is activated.

The motive in *sadhana* practice is always to harmonize the body with the environment. We harmonize with the day by activating the lunar breath. We harmonize with the night by activating the solar breath.

### The Practice: Activating the Lunar Breath

Check your breath in the early morning to determine whether solar or lunar is stronger. If the lunar, or left breath, is naturally stronger, you are ready to begin your day in tune with the cosmic rhythms. If the solar, or right breath, is stronger, make a fist with your left hand, and place it securely under your right armpit (see cuffed fist under armpit posture, below). Using your right hand (see hand mudra image, below), alternate your breathing from nostril to nostril for a few minutes, or until you feel the left breath gain more volume than the right (see exercise for alternate-nostril breathing, below). Remove your fist from your armpit and recheck your breath.

Your cooling, lunar breath should now be more active. (Even if it is not, do not do this exercise for more than fifteen minutes. As a general rule, you should not engage in any *prana* practice for longer than fifteen minutes. Doing so can create stress and weaken, rather than strengthen, your lunar and solar channels, and therefore, your breath.)

**The Practice: Activating the Solar Breath**

Check your breath in the early evening to determine whether lunar or solar is stronger. If the solar, or right breath, is naturally stronger, you are ready to begin your evening in tune with the cosmic rhythms. If the lunar or left breath is stronger, make a fist with your right hand, and place your fist securely under your left armpit. Using your left hand, alternate your breathing from nostril to nostril for a few minutes, or until you feel the right breath becoming stronger than the left. Remove your fist from your armpit and check your breath

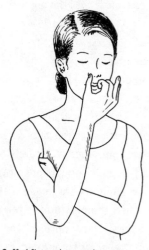

Cuffed fist under armpit posture

Hand mudra for alternating lunar
and solar breaths

again. Your warming, solar breath should be more active. (Do not do this exercise for more than fifteen minutes.)

### The Practice: Alternate-Nostril Breathing

Sit in a comfortable cross-legged position on a meditation cushion or pillow, or in any posture that feels comfortable to you. Block your left nostril with your right ring finger and pinkie, and inhale through your right nostril (see alternate-nostril breathing, below). Then block your right nostril with your right thumb and exhale through your left nostril. Continue alternating right and left nostrils for approximately ten minutes. Be sure to always inhale through the same nostril from which you just exhaled.

The Sanskrit name for alternate-nostril breathing is *anuloma viloma*. The classical formula for length of inhalation versus exhalation is to hold the breath for a period of time that is four times as long as the inhalation, then exhale for twice the length of the inhalation. Once you feel comfortable with the mechanics of the practice, you may want to silently count the seconds of your inhalation, and then try to extend your exhalation for twice that count. As you become more adept, you can work your way up to inhaling for eight counts, exhaling for sixteen. You may then incorporate the more classical techniques, which involve holding your breath between inhalation and exhalation. Begin with a ratio of 4:16:8 (so that the holding is four times the length of the inhalation, and the exhalation is twice the length of the inhalation), and work your way up to a ratio of 8:32:16.

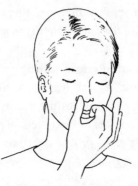

*Alternate-nostril breathing*

### The Practice: Balancing the Solar and Lunar Breaths

As I mentioned earlier, the breath in a healthy person's body naturally tends to be balanced at the four junctions of the day—sunrise, noon, sunset, and midnight. Both the lunar and solar breaths flow in almost equal volume during these brief, transitional periods. For this reason, these daily junctions are also considered the most auspicious times to practice yoga or meditation.

Although attaining and maintaining the inner state of balance is the most healing experience possible, people who are active and involved in the world should not attempt to maintain indefinitely a balanced state of *prana.* Generally speaking, your breath follows the rhythms of your movements. When you are busy, your breath tends to become more active, since the *prana* fuels your activity. If you impose the practices that bring the breath to a place of stasis but ignore the simple notion of living and sitting within yourself that must accompany this balanced breath, you would be misusing the sacred intention of your *prana.* Worldly activity creates a certain chaos in the body, and enforcing a constantly balanced breath would only further that chaos.

We have practiced aligning our breaths with lunar and solar rhythms. Now, we will see how the universe gives us the wonderful opportunity during her junctions to feel her presence and to regain inner balance. At sunrise, noon, and sunset, sit in a comfortable seated posture, facing the sun. At dawn, face east (sun is rising); at dusk, face west (sun is setting); at noon, face north (sun is directly overhead, and north is symbolic of the daytime sun that we do not see); and if you're up until midnight, face south for this practice (south is symbolic of the nighttime "sun" [the moon]). Check the breaths to determine which of the two is stronger.

A significantly dominant breath through one nostril during any of these four junctures is a clear indication that your health is out of balance. If this is the case, make a fist with the hand that is on the same side as the blocked nostril and place that hand under the opposite armpit. Perform alternate-nostril breathing for ten minutes. The blocked or diminished breath should now be more active.

Practice these procedures at sunrise, noon, and sunset, when the two breaths should be closer to a state of balance. Remember to face the proper direction during your breathing practices. Keep in mind that when the body is healthy, the *prana* will be slightly stronger in the left channel during these junctures.

Once your *prana* is in a state of balance, you may sit and enjoy your natural state of serenity, and feel the perfect harmony of your inner rhythms.

A word of caution: If your *prana* is chronically out of sync with the cosmic cycles, spend no more than fifteen minutes exercising the *prana* during the junctions of the day. The practice of meditation, sound, and food *sadhanas* described elsewhere in this book, together with breathwork, will cultivate your innate tranquility of body, mind, and spirit.

The lunar and solar breath exercises can help relieve not only emotional disorders, as in Joanie's case, but also physical symptoms and ailments, as they did for Edward. A recovering alcoholic, Edward is the head of counseling and job opportunities services at the Caribbean community center in a New Jersey town not far from New York City. Edward sought my advice when I gave a workshop at the center, because he had an array of symptoms that included insomnia, depression, and mental fatigue. He also had diabetes, for which he was taking daily shots of insulin. I showed Edward how to check and balance his lunar and solar breaths and told him to do the practice twice a day. I also suggested that he eat healthier foods, specifically whole grains and rice.

When I returned a year later to give another workshop at the center, Edward greeted me with a wide grin. "The depression is gone, and I can sleep nights," he said. "My energy is excellent. Instead of leading two Alcoholics Anonymous meetings a week, now I lead four."

But there was more good news. "My blood sugar is absolutely normal, so I don't need the insulin anymore."

His faithful performances of the practice, at sunrise and sunset, had become the two anchors of his life. Like Edward, each one of us has the capacity to reclaim and perform the *sadhana* of realigning the breath with the day and night. When we are aligned with the natural rhythms of nature, our breath is balanced with the cosmic rhythms so that it automatically safeguards our mental processes, redirecting all thoughts into a state of stillness.

The Divine Mother says in the *Devi Sukta*, "I breathe

out strongly like the wind while clasping unto myself all worlds, all things that are." Once we learn to ride the inner winds of breath and traverse the pathways of the mind, we become the instrument of consciousness. Harmonizing the breath, we become more aware of the harmonious movement of our inner life force. This is the beginning of meditation.

# Chapter 6

## THE VEDIC ART
## OF MEDITATION

*As a weary bird flies hither and thither and
comes to rest on its perch where it is tethered,
so does the mind come to rest at last in its own
Self.*
—*Chandogya Upanishad*

Last year, thirty of my students and I observed the nine-day Navarati celebration of the Divine Mother at the Wise Earth monastery. We chanted to the Mother every morning at sunrise and practiced the various breath, sound, and food *sadhanas* together. On the final day of the program, after conducting a fire ritual in honor of Saraswati—the goddess of wisdom, creativity, and spiritual expression—we had a delightful feast, which we had prepared together over the course of the nine days. The meal was a lovely, joyful occasion, made even more special by the presence of Yogi Ramananda, a seventy-five-year-old adept who was visiting me from Bangalore, India.

By the time we were done, the kitchen counters and the sink were piled high with dirty dishes and sticky pots and pans. We were about to organize a cleanup crew when Yogi Ramananda announced that he wanted to wash the dishes himself. "But you are my honored guest," I protested. Yogi Ramananda smiled and insisted that the job was his. "A few helpers, then," I said. Yogi Ramananda shook his head and shooed me out of the kitchen. He wanted to do it himself.

Finally, I gave in and went off to do some chores. I returned an hour later. All the washing was done. Yogi Ramananda was just putting the last of the pots into the cupboard.

"How on earth did you finish up so quickly?" I asked.

"From beginning to end, only one thought crossed my mind," the yogi replied. "Wash the dishes."

Yogi Ramananda understood that thought and action must flow together. After years of practicing meditation as *sadhana*, he had attained a state of equanimity that was apparent in the way he performed even the most ordinary tasks. His mind was tethered to his breath, regulating and energizing his every undertaking, whether he was taking a walk in the woods, practicing yoga postures, chanting the Vedic mantras, or sweeping the kitchen floor.

The *rishis*—the ancient seers whose inspired visions became the wellspring of Vedic tradition—called meditation the fundamental practice for everyday life. They extolled it as the primary *sadhana* for exploring, developing, and expanding the mind and its inner pathways of consciousness. Meditation is pure concentration, directing the mind to stillness and keeping the internal focus absorbed in consciousness. The Upanishads say, "meditation reveals the mind." British psychologist John H. Clark, in his book *A Map of Mental States*, put it this way: "Meditation is a method by which a person concentrates more and more upon less and less. The aim is to empty the mind while, paradoxically, remaining alert."

Over the centuries, many schools of meditation have arisen, including Zen, Buddhist, Vipassana, and Transcendental Meditation. Many schools advocate meditation as an exercise, as the means to achieve something—clarity and peace of mind; transcendental experiences; spiritual enlightenment. You can greatly benefit from making a concerted effort to cultivate this state of quiet and awareness at regular times during the day or night. But as you become more adept in the practice of *sadhana*, you will want to carry your meditation beyond these set times. Meditation as a practice is not meant to be viewed as separate from your normal daily activities.

The Vedic explanation of "to meditate" is "to discern, measure, ponder, contemplate, and ultimately to be free from all limitations and standards by which we measure ourselves." Meditation leads us to the universal consciousness that resides within us, to the selfless awareness of that which is greater than our body-mind, and to a reality and plane beyond material wealth and success. Through meditation, we are able to intuit our individual purpose. We learn to step away from the engaging mirages and delusions that encumber daily life.

The Vedic seers tell us that we must protect, nurture, and preserve both the internal truth of the self and the cosmic truth of nature. Part of our spiritual purpose entails finding the courage to present to the world our genuine faces. I learned this lesson under the most extreme circumstances, and I fully understand how very painful and difficult it is to embrace authenticity. You can probably recall instances when you stopped yourself from speaking up because you were afraid of losing a job or hurting someone's feelings or losing someone's approval. To keep the peace, you compromised your inner truth. We learn to do this over the years almost naturally because most of us are accustomed to performing certain roles and hiding behind an assortment of guises.

Meditation can help us rediscover our authentic selves. It can help us put aside the masks that keep us from our essential nature and our innermost desires. In helping us uncover our core truth, meditation allows us to integrate our energies of mind, body, and spirit, to reunite them into wholeness and health. Meditation is also the greater task of inquiring into, and serving, the Universal Self. The true practice of meditation entails nothing less than the day-by-day, moment-by-moment observance of *sadhana*.

During meditation, we travel inward to explore the mind's true nature, not the obsessive or mundane distractions that can plague us. My teacher, His Holiness Swami Dayananda, tells us that the seers who cultivated the principle of meditation "sat in themselves," and this sitting pervaded their every action and word. The highest goal of meditation is to surpass perceptions, thoughts, imaginings, and even visions and revelations. Meditation takes you past the mind's input of the five senses. To get to the inner universe, you must ultimately move beyond your common perceptions of sights and sounds, beyond the elements, beyond even the grasp of intelligence, into the realm of pure consciousness which the *rishis* call *anandam*, "the abiding joy and complete fullness."

In the more than twenty years that I have been practicing meditation, I have experienced numerous distinct leaps of consciousness. Often in my inner universe, the deities come alive, and sometimes they speak to me. I've seen wondrous, magical light-shows, accompanied by the high-pitched tones of wind instruments. The more seasoned I have become in my practice, the more silence and abiding serenity have grown within me. As you move deeper into your meditation practice, you, too, will discover that your consciousness takes on a life of its own. You will begin to eagerly anticipate the time you have set aside for meditation. You will experience long periods of lucidity and clarity. You will gain in your intuitive powers, and know who is calling you before you pick up the phone. When the unexpected happens you will not be surprised or worried or thrown.

Today, an ever-increasing number of mainstream physicians and health practitioners are recognizing the value of meditation. In May of 1998, the Beth Israel Medical Center in New York City invited His Holiness the Dalai Lama, the spiritual leader of Tibet, to speak with a group of leading neuroscientists, physicians, and mind/body clinicians about the value and possibilities of using meditative practices in hospitals and other health-care settings.

Western doctors and thinkers are starting to recognize what the *rishis* saw many centuries ago: Nature is a unified whole and the human mind and body are inseparably linked to her, as well as to each other. The age-old practices of yoga and meditation are now being used by neuroscientists to track the biochemical pathways of the brain, and they are discovering what the Vedic seers have always understood: Meditation stimulates knowing, intuiting, and healing.

Meditation works for everyone who is willing to devote some time to the practice. Patanjali, the third-century scholar, teacher, and author of *Yoga Sutras*, the earliest and classic text on yoga and meditation, wrote, "Through absorption and concentration, the processes of meditation, we may go beyond sensory perceptions." You, too, can journey past the five-sensory mind. At the very least, you can reach a point where you can observe the way it works.

For a beginner, a successful meditation is simply one that leaves you feeling tranquil and rested. As your mind empties itself of distractions, your inner energies start to flow in harmony with each other. You take away from your period of sitting in meditation an enhanced ability to focus completely on the activity in which you are presently engaged.

The *Svetasvatara Upanishad* says, "With conscious effort hold the senses in check. Controlling the breath, regulate the vital activities." As the flow of breath becomes more measured, the heart begins to beat more slowly and the emotions grow calmer. Riding the waves of breath, our thoughts become less frantic and scattered, and the mind moves toward a state of stillness.

The exercise that follows is an excellent preparation for

meditation because it helps you become more aware of the movement of your breath. The practice is also very useful whenever you feel anxiety, anger, or any other kind of emotional distress. The beauty of this practice is its simplicity. You can do it anywhere, at any time, to promote relaxation and ready your mind and body for meditation. Remember: Whatever your condition, wherever you are, you can always breathe and bring your attention to your breath.

### The Practice: Take a Simple Breath

For your first practice, find a comfortable place to sit, whether on the floor in a simple, cross-legged position, or in a chair with your feet flat on the floor. Close your eyes and place your hands on your knees or in your lap. Take a long, slow inhalation through your nose. Exhale through your nose, making short hissing sounds as you release the stale breath. Repeat this breath two more times. Become aware of how you feel as you inhale and exhale. Does your heartbeat become slower? Are you more conscious of the tension in your shoulders, or any other part of your body where you hold your stress and other negative emotions? Take full, diaphragmatic breaths and feel the difference in your chest and belly.

Inhale again, this time allowing the breath to flow from the base of your spine and circulate through your entire being, from the tip of your toes to the crown of your head. Exhale slowly and silently through the nose, from the deepest place within you. Continue breathing through your nose, allowing the air to flow easily and naturally. Try to experience the breath without controlling it. As the inhalations and exhalations become quieter and less frequent, you will start to feel calmer and more relaxed.

The next step in preparing for meditation is to learn the classic yoga sitting posture, *sukhasana,* or "posture of ease."

Seated in *sukhasana*, your back remains erect, which simultaneously facilitates the flow of breath through the main pathways along the spine and cultivates the *prana*. As your practice evolves over time, you will discover the true meaning of *sukhasana*—lightness and happiness in the sitting posture.

If you are uncomfortable sitting on the ground, you should feel free to do the meditation and breath practices sitting upright in a chair, with the soles of your feet on the floor. Twenty-one years ago, when I first started *sukhasana* practice, I was so stiff that I couldn't get my knees anywhere near the floor. My yoga teacher, Dr. Narasimha Rao, would say, "*Abhyasa, abhyasa, abhyasa!* Practice, practice, practice!" As with so many other things in life, yoga does, indeed, require *abhyasa*. Even a few minutes of daily practice goes a long way. Once you begin to move the *prana*, you will become more limber, and the stiffness will gradually disappear.

### The Practice: Posture of Ease

Sit on the edge of a medium-sized cushion or folded blanket that you've placed on top of a mat or carpeted floor. This will help you keep your bottom from rolling under you and curving your lower spine. Keeping your back erect, sit in a cross-legged position. Lower the chin slightly to release the back of the neck, and bring it into alignment with the rest of the spine.

Silently count to six as you slowly inhale; then exhale, extending the exhalation twice as long as the intake. Center your awareness on the flow of *prana* along the spine. With each breath you will find your body relaxing into the *sukhasana* posture.

*Sukhasana* posture, one of the primary postures for meditation and breathing practices, strengthens the body's life force. I recommend it for relief of mental and emotional distress, as well as disorders of the reproductive organs and tissues. A regular practice of sitting in *sukhasana* posture may also greatly improve conditions such as insomnia, lethargy, heart disease, memory loss, eating disorders, and attention deficit disorders.

Kathryn, the younger sister of one of my students, is a wonderful example of someone whose symptoms were relieved by the simple act of sitting in *sukhsana* posture. I caught my first glimpse of her on a beautiful spring day as she trudged up the hill to my cabin, her shoulders hunched to her ears as if she were toting a sack of bricks on her back. As I opened the door to let her in, I could see that her face was etched with worry lines and her eyes were red with exhaustion. I didn't have to ask the reason for her visit. The words came spilling out of her before I even had a chance to say hello.

"I'm a grad student in chemistry," she said, perched at the edge of her chair and tugging nervously at her long hair. "I've done all my course work for my Ph.D., but I have a long way to go in writing my thesis. I can't concentrate, I can't sleep, and I've just been diagnosed with A.D.D.—attention deficit disorder." She threw her hands up in the air. "Look at me, I'm a nervous wreck! I'm so desperate that I drove forty-five miles into this wilderness because I thought you could give me herbs or something to make me calm down."

My impulse was to tell her, "Kathryn, you have to slow down," but the obvious is usually the last thing we want to hear. "Let's start with a cup of tea," I suggested. As I filled a kettle with water, I saw that Kathryn was breathing rapidly, almost as if she were racing to keep up. The metaphor seemed apt. She had told me a little bit about herself on the phone when she'd first asked to visit me, and I sensed that she was "running scared" from all the pressure on her.

Through the window, I saw that the sun was shining and

the trees were blossoming with extravagant white flowers. In her present state, Kathryn could see none of nature's bountiful beauty. I wondered whether she was even aware of the scent that lingered in the room of sandalwood incense from my morning prayers. While I prepared the raspberry tea, she chattered nervously, answering my questions in quick bursts as her eyes darted around the room. I put on a tape of Vedic chants to play in the background, handed her a mug, then stepped outside to pick some flowers and give her a few moments alone.

She had leaned back in her chair and even managed a smile when I came back inside. "Your place is *so* peaceful," she murmured, sipping the tea. "I wish there was a way to create some calm in my life."

"Tell me more about your work," I said, arranging the wildflowers in a vase.

Kathryn tugged again at her hair, and I could hear the anxiety creep back into her voice as she dutifully responded to my question. She spoke in quick starts and stops, then finally said, "I just have to get through these next few months, and then I'll be okay. But I can't believe that I have A.D.D. I never had trouble studying in high school or college, so how did this suddenly happen to me?"

I suspected that she had been misdiagnosed. Kathryn was not breathing properly or giving herself time to relax and simply be, and was in a constant swirl of worry, fear, and self-doubt. Rather than explain any of this, I asked, "Are you willing to try a simple meditative posture and some breathing techniques to provide more oxygen to your mind?"

Kathryn seemed disappointed. She probably knew from her sister that I used various herbs and other preparations for healing, and I suspected that she had come in search of a quick remedy—some kind of pill or oil or herbal concoction that would be the panacea for all her complaints.

"Sure, I'll try breathing, but I'll need a lot more than meditation to cure my problems," she said.

*A lot more than meditation?* I could not imagine what that might be. But Kathryn would have to discover for herself that a regular meditation practice is a far more potent healing tool than a whole cabinet full of tranquilizers, antidepressants, antianxiety medications, and any other drugs for that matter.

"If the meditation and breathing don't help, we can discuss other remedies," I said. "Just give this a chance, and let's see what happens."

First I taught Kathryn the simple, diaphragmatic breathing practice, as described in chapter 5. Then I put my yoga mat on the floor, handed Kathryn a meditation pillow, and showed her how to position her legs in *sukhasana* posture. "I can't make my legs lie flat like yours do," she said, struggling to get comfortable.

"Just do your best," I said. "The flexibility comes over time, with practice."

We had been sitting with closed eyes, breathing in *sukhasana* posture for about fifteen minutes, when I was startled out of my meditation by a gentle snoring sound. I looked over at Kathryn and saw that she was fast asleep. Tiptoeing out of the cabin, I went to weed my garden, came back inside, and answered some mail. An hour passed before Kathryn reawakened.

She raised her head suddenly and looked around the room. "I'm so embarrassed," she said. "Sorry, I fell asleep."

"How do you feel?" I asked.

"Terrific," she said, stretching her arms. "Best sleep I've had in days. Will I fall asleep every time I practice the meditation?"

"Only if you are exhausted," I said.

"Will it help the A.D.D.?"

"I'm sure your ability to concentrate will improve," I said.

"Call me in two weeks to let me know how you're feeling. And don't forget to breathe!"

Kathryn phoned me exactly two weeks later to report that she was feeling much more energetic, and that she was having far fewer problems with focus and clarity. In fact, the symptoms related to A.D.D. were so infrequent that she had decided not to take any medication, at least for the time being.

I was delighted to hear she was making such good progress. "But please, pace yourself," I cautioned, "so you don't get weighed down again by the pressure."

Six months passed before I heard from Kathryn again. This time, she was calling to say she had just finished writing her thesis and had been offered a part-time teaching position at the university. She felt wonderful and no longer suffered from insomnia. Her doctor now thought that the A.D.D. diagnosis had been a mistake. Kathryn was also eager to learn more advanced meditation techniques, so I suggested that she come study with me at the Wise Earth School, if her schedule permitted.

Soon afterward, Kathryn found the time to attend one of my weeklong courses, where she learned other meditation and *sadhana* practices. She has since become an enthusiastic yoga student, as well. I still hear from her about twice a year or so, and although her life is very full and active, she no longer complains about fatigue or lack of focus.

## HOW TO MEDITATE

Find a place in your home where you will not be disturbed by anyone or anything, including the telephone, fax machine, or television. Keep a notepad and pen by your side so that when you first sit down, you can jot down any pieces of unfinished business that are in your head: the list of groceries you have to pick up at the supermarket, the menu for the dinner party you're giving next week, the errands you're planning to do as soon as you're finished meditating.

Sit in *sukhasana*, with your hands in *shanti* mudra, resting on your knees, your palms facing toward the ceiling to receive energy, your index finger and thumbs touching lightly to form a circle.

Begin by closing your eyes and being mindful of your intentions. Silently remind yourself, "I am sitting in meditation. I am meditating. I am where I am." This intentionality and witnessing of yourself will keep your mind from veering off into "I am sitting in meditation, but my thoughts are in Hawaii. . . . I wonder what my friend Karen is doing on her vacation. . . . Oops, almost forgot I have a dentist's appointment today. . . . Did I turn off the stove?"

Of course, thoughts will continue to come up, but don't try to force them to disappear. One of the most important points to remember about meditation is that you should not engage with or dwell on whatever specific thought arises. Let it be, and it will move on. Another one will come up. Witness it, then let it go. Concentrate on the breath, rather than on the thought, and the thought will dissolve.

No matter how quiet your environment, you are surrounded by noise of one sort or another, including the noises that issue from our own inner agitation. Don't try to shut out the sounds. Focus, instead, on your exhalation. In time, you will discover that even the most dissonant noises become harmonious with the sound of your breath.

Begin your practice by sitting for ten to fifteen minutes at a time. When you feel ready, lengthen the time to twenty minutes, then to half an hour. Keep a clock or watch nearby. You will probably find that after several sessions of sitting in meditation, you will know exactly how much time has passed and when you are ready to end the meditation.

You can meditate at any hour of the day or night, but the optimal time is during the junctions of the day when the lunar and solar breaths are in a state of balance. For most of us, the best junctions are sunrise, noon, and sunset. According to the Vedas, the most auspicious time for spiritual practice is *Brahmamuhurta*, around four A.M., when the mind is in its most lucid and tranquil state. Unless you are an early riser, however, a predawn meditation practice is probably an unrealistic ideal. Set yourself the more practical goal of trying to meditate at the same time every day, whether it's in the morning, late afternoon, or evening. As noted earlier, after years of following this practice, if I postpone my meditation for more than a few minutes, I get a pulsing energy in my right temple that becomes more persistent the longer I try to ignore the sensation. I feel I am being called to meditate, and I have to stop whatever I am doing in order to sit and give full attention to this call and to the flow of *prana*.

As I mentioned earlier, some people find it difficult to sit cross-legged on the floor. It is perfectly fine to meditate while seated in a chair. The key is to keep your back erect. Meditation is not intended to be punishment. When we meditate, we aim for fullness of self, not a void. You want to become aware of the self, without engaging in blame or recriminations. If you develop a pain in some part of the body, do whatever you need to do to relieve the pain. If your foot falls asleep, move it. Do this with awareness. Send your breath into the leg or whatever part of your body is in pain. Move quietly, then resettle yourself. If your discomfort becomes intolerable, quietly get up, leave the room, and walk around carefully, keeping your awareness on your breath, until you restore the circulation.

A regular, ongoing meditation practice can benefit you in many ways. On a physiological level, your breath will gradually and naturally become deeper and more balanced for longer periods throughout the day and night. If your blood pressure is high, it may decrease; your heart rate and oxygen consumption will be lessened; and muscular tensions will be released. On the mental level, you will develop a sense of clarity about everyday issues and events. Rather than throwing yourself into family, work, or social situations that are stressful or otherwise emotionally charged, you can more readily become a nonjudgmental witness, standing apart from the chaos and confusion. You may be released from the grip of addictive and compulsive behaviors. You can attain an enduring sense of peace without the need for substances, material goods, or unhealthy relationships.

With regular practice, you begin to feel joy in small, everyday, seemingly trivial events. What was formerly hidden now becomes obvious and apparent. Your awareness is both sharpened and nourished as you fully attend to the joyful nuances of everyday life—the shapes, colors, sounds, smells, and feel of the world around you. Each moment, each minor event, becomes a source of wonderment, an occasion for a deepening appreciation of your self and your oneness with the universe.

### A Meditation Tool: Keeping a Journal

As you can see, meditation practice brings forth a rich trove of material from the mind. In my experience, one of the most helpful tools to mine that material, and at the same time maintain inner balance, is to keep a meditation journal. During my first year of meditation practice, I kept a written record that enabled me to bear witness to my shifts in consciousness. I named this journal my *Celestial Companion*, and it became a daily account of my spiritual and physical progress. In it, I noted changes or improvements in my breathing, energy, and health. My eating patterns were gradually changing, as I began to notice the types of food and quality of the food I was putting into my body as documented in my journal.

I was especially keen to observe the flow of my thoughts, paying special attention to ongoing transformations in my mental processes as my practice deepened. For example, within the first month of my practice, I found myself becoming less judgmental and less likely to engage in idle chatter, both in my own mind and with others.

During my first year of meditation, my journal became my confidant and trusted ally. As my well-entrenched habits and lifestyles began to give way to new patterns, I often felt flustered and unhinged. During these times, I turned to my journal. When I was too tired to sit and meditate, I would lie in bed and review or write in my *Celestial Companion*. Whenever I confided my tears and fears to these pages, I was better situated to surmount the challenges and obstacles in the way of my spiritual progress.

As my spiritual experiences became more profound, I felt as if I were climbing a ladder of inner consciousness, until one day I found myself soaring to new heights of awareness and serenity. Now, many years later, as I reread my old diary, I see the remarkable progress I made during that first year. Revisiting my writing, I realize that my meditation practice— and my willingness to unburden my heart on the blank pages of my journal—enabled me to push aside the boulders that were blocking my life's path.

I invite you to keep a diary in which you record your meditation journeys. On the first page, you may wish to write the Vedic mantra for Goddess Saraswati that follows, or you may choose to write a prayer or invocation of your own creation or selection.

### Saraswati Mantra AIM SARASWATYAI NAMAHA
(ah-eem sah-rahs-wat-yi nah-mah-ha)

Saraswati is the goddess of wisdom, creativity, and light. Her mantra helps the mind to merge with its innate intuition, or *buddhi*. Invoking Saraswati will enable you to feel refreshed, open, and ready to express your thoughts on paper.

Before you begin your journal, ask yourself these key questions: What does meditation mean to me? How do I feel about embarking on a spiritual journey? What are some of the changes I would like to bring about in my everyday life? What desires and goals would I like to fulfill? What image of myself would I like to see realized a year from now?

Begin your initial entry by noting the time and place of your first meditation practice. Do not censor yourself by worrying about grammar, punctuation, literary style, or whether or not you are "doing it right." Do not prejudge the content; whatever comes to mind is worth recording and investigating. After you have completed your meditation, pick up your pen or pencil and just keep it moving on the page. Allow your feelings and motives, thoughts and reactions, to float lightly on the surface of your consciousness as you record your meditation experience. Did you find your first meditation easy or difficult? Did you settle into awareness of your breath quickly or did it take a few minutes? Were you distracted by noises outside the room or were you able to tune them out? Did your body feel comfortable in the position or did your back hurt, your foot fall asleep, your shoulders ache? Were you impatient or calm? Try as best as you can not to get caught in one endless loop of thoughts or feelings. Give yourself ten to twenty minutes of meditation as a reasonable period at first.

Your journal is a powerful way to witness your meditation progress. As the rhythms of your breath and consciousness become more synchronous with nature's rhythms, you become more aware of your individual nature and purpose, your authentic self. Yet simultaneously, you become more receptive to the sacred transmissions of the universe.

# Chapter 7

## AWAKENING YOUR COSMIC
## MEMORY AND INTUITION

*He who has crossed the boundary and has
realized the Self, ceases to be wounded or
afflicted. When the boundary is crossed, night
becomes day; for the universe of Brahman is
light itself.*
—*Chandogya Upanishad* (8.4.2)

The elephant has been worshiped by Hindus for thousands
of years as a sacred being. It is the earth's oldest animal ancestor, according to Vedic tradition. Two icons—Gajendra,
Lord of the Elephants; and Ganesha, the elephant-headed son
of Shiva, bestower of success in new endeavors and remover
of obstacles—are honored by millions of devotees every day
in the temples of South India. Until very recently, you could
hear the thundering sounds of elephants foraging for food in
the dense forests, deep in the Nilgiri Hills of South India. But
on my most recent visit to this once-peaceful region on the
Kerala border, the atmosphere was tainted by the fear and
grief of the elephants. Since the late 1990s, poachers have
killed more than 20,000 elephants for their precious tusks.
People in the surrounding villages tell horrifying stories of
the animals' suffering and their terrified exodus from the forest that was once a safe haven to them.

Two weeks before my most recent trip to my teacher's
ashram in Coimbatore, a wounded elephant calf left its
home in the hills and traveled some three miles to the near-
est temple that had been erected in honor of its ancestors in
the small village of Anaikatti. The calf had apparently been
injured when it had tried to break through the barbed-wire

fences set up by the forestry service to ward off poachers and contain the elephants within the forest. Its wound had become infected. Local residents reported that the calf limped into the sacred grounds of the temple and lay prostrate before the image of its god ancestor, Gajendra.

Thousands of devotees and holy men flocked to the temple to try to nurse the elephant calf back to health. Although prayers were offered to Shiva, Ganesha, and Gajendra for three days and nights, the calf could not be saved. No one in South India questioned why a wounded calf would walk three miles to die in the presence of its sacred ancestor. They understood that each being and creature carries within its brain the instinct of its own species, formed by the cosmic memory of all the matter and energy in the entire universe from the beginning of time. Because of its cosmic memory, the wounded elephant calf felt called to make its way to the temple of its ancestors, to die on sacred ground.

Cosmic memory is my own theory, informed by the Vedas, and one of the foundations of the Wise Earth *sadhanas*. It is roughly analogous to Carl Jung's concept of the collective unconscious, only greater in scope, encompassing not just the memories and cultural and spiritual associations of all people, but of all living beings as well as all inanimate energies. Another version of cosmic memory is reflected in British biochemist Rupert Sheldrake's theory of morphic resonance. His theory holds that learned behaviors are passed on to different groups of a species in disparate locations through an energy field, without the need for direct physical communication or influence. Sheldrake proposes as his basic hypothesis that "memory is inherent in nature," and that "natural systems such as termite colonies, or pigeons, or orchid plants, or insulin molecules, inherit a collective memory from all previous things of their kind, however far away they were and however long ago they existed." Thus, the palm tree does not need to remember how to produce coconuts, nor does the horse doubt that its young will be born in its image and not that of a geranium.

The Vedas tell us that our tissues remember their preordained functions, just as the food we eat remembers its structure and purpose and conveys that information to our bodies. Cosmic memory is held and refined by the genetic code, the DNA, or molecular structure of all life-forms. We call our own genetic memories into consciousness and honor them by the foods we choose and how we prepare them, how we treat the land, how we breathe, and how we listen to ourselves and the living universe around us. The key to healing our physical, psychological, and spiritual maladies is through the evocation of these genetic or ancestral memories that are imprinted into our individual body-mind and spirit.

In addition to ancestral memories, each species carries its own block of cosmic memory. More than the inherited knowledge necessary for that species to survive, this cosmic-memory block is the gift that each species brings to the planet. For example, spiders spin webs because of instinct within the brain, an instinct informed by the ancestral memory of this species. Some furry creatures build dams. Some feathered creatures fly south in autumn. Bats home in on flying insects using their sonar skills. Mountain goats are able to defy gravity and stand upside down on Himalayan peaks. All these ancestral skills are also carried in the greater cosmic memory.

The instinctual skill of human beings is intuition, which, in Vedic tradition, is a richer mental and spiritual function than is acknowledged in Western cultures. The Sanskrit term for intuition is *buddhi*, which means individual knowledge, consciousness, and memory. The *rishis* revealed that human consciousness emerged from the memory of the cosmos itself, the greater consciousness that is everywhere. Every cell of our being is formed from the essential memories existing within all of creation. Every species is further formed from its own set of memories. Memory contains the truth of the universe. It is both the inner guide for each life and the means of exchange with all other beings.

The first human tribes knew the memory of the universe because they observed the wild animals with whom they shared the earth. By hunting and eating wild animals, the early humans inherited animal powers, their instinctual memory. The *rishis* themselves emulated the movements and postures of the animals and created hatha yoga—a practice through which we can enhance the movement of *prana* in accord with the cosmic memories. Animals and plants are wonderful guides. When we learn to observe our surroundings consciously, every grain of sand can help us get in touch with our own memories.

Both cosmic and individual memories express themselves through our bodies. Our tissues carry the memories, both collective and individual, that shape our unique body-mind. Through these memories, each life-form is able to adapt to the demands of its present environment and to function through all rebirths. Specific cosmic rhythms have also been encoded in our memory banks: the cycle of the seasons, the energies of the seven chakras, the stages of aging, the daily rhythms of breath, and our vital tissues. The memory of each individual life along with the collective memory of the universe are forever braided into the fabric of our being.


## AWAKENING INTUITION

The *rishis'* hearts were open to nature and so they were able to master perfect communion with her through their interior language of intuition. As Steven Pinker says in his book *The*

*Language Instinct*, "We are a primate species with our own act, a knack for communicating information about who did what to whom." We can do this because of the cosmic and ancestral memories that we as a species carry within us, from life to life, in our intuition, or *buddhi*. Physically, this intuitive mind or block of cosmic memory is located in the frontal part of the brain, and is sometimes called the greater mind. The sages say that through meditation we develop our individual wisdom, intelligence, and memory—the *buddhi*—which is our vehicle for connecting the ultimate vision of being One with the Whole, or as the *rishis* put it, the whole in the one and the many.

The *buddhi* is a conscious intuition and an intuitive consciousness, filtered down to us humans from the cosmos. It can become our inner guide. It enables us to express our consciousness in authentic ways. Our individual mind governs how we express the memories held within our consciousness or *buddhi*. When the mind is aligned with the *buddhi*, we express ourselves consciously, as when we cultivate compassion or spiritual practices. As we awaken to the power of our *buddhi*, we become more sensitive, introspective, and sentient, flowing in harmony with nature's cosmic rhythms. When we move in harmony with cosmic rhythms, our thoughts reflect the pure, unwavering consciousness of the *buddhi* and we are guided by it.

By the same token, when we are out of balance with these rhythms, the mind becomes distracted, and abundant thoughts arise, blocking our power of intuition. Meditation and breathwork—*sadhana*—are the most effective means of connecting to our innate intuitive abilities and of developing them. Meditation allows us to wake up internally so that we can act consciously in the external world. The *buddhi* allows us to be spirit or consciousness in action.

We are often unconsciously guided by our intuition in ordinary life. When someone close to us is injured or ill, we sometimes know it, however geographically distant we may be from that person. My neighbor Jane was preparing lunch when she slipped and fell on the kitchen floor. A few minutes later the phone rang. Her daughter's teacher was calling from school to say that Sarah had taken a bad fall down the stairs. Jane remembered that just before she slipped and fell she had felt deeply concerned for Sarah.

With the practice of sadhana, the power of buddhi has grown in me over the years. What once would have taken me a few months to accomplish, I can now do in only a few days. I experience the miracle of buddhi every day in my own life. Recently, I happened to be in a grocery store when an elderly woman had a convulsive fit. The store manager and several shoppers rushed to her aid, but as they stood around her, the convulsions worsened. I realized that I could best help her by entering a meditative state and sending her light. I stood back and closed my eyes. I visualized her in a white light, which I began to project to her. After a minute or two, the convulsions stopped. The woman stood up, walked over to me, and took my hands. She did not need words to thank me for the healing energy I had sent her.

Angelica, who has been studying with me for the last five years, teaches the Wise Earth sadhanas in San Francisco and at conferences all over the country. About a year ago, after months of simultaneously chanting and practicing the breathwork meditations for several hours a day, Angelica felt a new awareness of the world around her, as if her consciousness had greatly expanded. Soon thereafter, she was taking a walk on an unfamiliar street when she noticed a beautiful, old Victorian-style house. As she stopped to admire the architecture, she saw an image of Hanuman, the Vedic monkey god, poised above the house. She was so struck by the image that she called me to ask what I thought of it.

I knew that Angelica had been planning for some time to find a new location for her *sadhana* studio, and I took the appearance of Hanuman as a sign that her intuition had drawn her to that particular house. "I could never afford such an expensive place," Angelica said wistfully when I told her my interpretation. The next week, a letter arrived from a mortgage company, stating that a loan application she had submitted weeks earlier had been approved. Angelica was stunned, because she'd been sure that her minimal annual income would prevent her from qualifying for a loan.

She bought the house where she visualized Hanuman, and has since had many other visions, including frequent visits from my teacher, Swami Dayananda, whom she has never met, as well as from me, whenever she has questions she wants to ask one of us.

## THE WAY OF *BUDDHI* YOGA

In the *Bhagavad Gita*, Lord Krishna teaches about the inner attitude of tranquility and compassion behind all actions, which he refers to as *buddhi* yoga. "Attributing in thought all actions to Me, intent on Me, resorting to *buddhi* yoga, be constantly focused upon Me." Thus, when we operate through the *buddhi*, instead of the rational mind and ego, we continually recognize the Self to be an instrument of the Divine will and all our actions to be the consequence of Divine Grace. Whenever my teacher receives a compliment, he always responds in the same way: *"Isvara's Daivam,"* "Everything comes from the Divine." The attitude of ceding all human accomplishment to the Divine comes from the *buddhi*. As possessors of this block of cosmic memory, we are intended to preserve and sustain it, and thus to help all species refine their particular blocks of cosmic memory.

The ancients advocated *buddhi* yoga (the selfless meditation that you learned in the preceding chapter) as a primary means to rejuvenate the mind, recall memories, and enhance our intuitive power. When we perform any activity to excess, whether it is thinking, working, sleeping, or playing, we create mental toxicity and block intuition. The purpose of *sadhana*—and of spiritual practice in general—is to awaken the *buddhi*, become conscious of its function, and place ourselves at its service. That is why so many spiritual exercises, such as meditation, yoga, mindfulness, chanting, or the use of Zen koans, are designed to get us beyond the busy, distracted, five-sensory mind and allow the *buddhi* to prevail.

*Buddhi* yoga calls upon your individual intuitive powers to transcend rational thinking, so that you allow the collective consciousness of the universe into every atom, cell, tissue, and memory of your being. As your meditation practice becomes deeper and you develop greater insights and intuition, you start to move outward as well, bringing unity and wholeness to your family and the larger communities in which you live.

Alice came to the Wise Earth School to study meditation. A social worker in the New York City welfare system, she had become so utterly consumed by her clients' problems that her marriage was beginning to suffer. Alice would sit at dinner with her husband night after night and repeat to him the heart-wrenching stories she had heard that day at work. Often, the phone would ring, and one of her clients would be calling to ask her advice or report some new crisis. Her husband repeatedly asked her to let the answering machine pick up the messages, so that they could have some time together to relax. But Alice could not ignore the cries for help, and her around-the-clock dedication to her job was becoming a source of friction between her and her husband.

A friend suggested meditation as a way to clear her mind and find some tranquility amidst the life-threatening issues facing her clients on a daily basis. Alice had heard me speak at the Open Center in New York City. With her husband's encouragement, she decided to take a week off to study meditation with me. She particularly responded to the *Bhramari* breath meditation, which I describe below, and continued the practice after she returned home.

Alice wrote me a long letter about six months later, letting me know that she had implemented some very positive changes in her life: she was now able to curtail the long, work-related conversations with her husband and she no longer took calls at home, except in extreme emergencies. The meditation, she said, "has become a valued part of my morning routine. I wouldn't think of starting the day without it. This practice has given me a new level of energy. At the end of a fourteen-hour workday, I feel little or no exhaustion."

Her coworkers were so impressed by her newfound energy that they asked her to share the meditation with them. "Once a week, we practice it as a group, and we're working more effectively as a team."

Alice was able to detach herself from her work in a healthy way. During her meditations, she sometimes had images of her clients flash into her mind. Instead of pushing them away, she was able to acknowledge the images, understand how she might better handle a given situation, and then let go of the thought. This enabled her to become more solution-oriented about her work, rather than dwelling obsessively on the clients' problems, as she had in the past. Instead of being anxiously preoccupied with these issues, Alice became more compassionate and more effective on the job. Mindful of how profoundly she'd been helped by her meditation practice, she persuaded her supervisors to let her teach meditation to a group of women and children at a home for battered women, all of whom had experienced severe stress, trauma, and chaotic living conditions.

As Alice's story demonstrates, meditation is not an escape hatch from our problems, but rather a pathway to far greater clarity, which leads us to behaviors in the world that help to resolve conflict and difficulty. It also shows how meditation practice not only fosters such intuition and lucidity, but also broadens our awareness, connecting us with those in our social environment and, even more expansively, with other living creatures on the planet. Thus *buddhi* yoga is a first step toward helping you cultivate your cosmic memory and intuition. The more we practice meditation, and *bhramari* specifically, the greater our field of awareness, and the deeper our connection to the subtle body.

## BHRAMARI BREATH MEDITATION: LAYING THE GROUND FOR COSMIC MEMORY

*Bhramari* breath meditation is a meditation or a *buddhi* yoga practice that links us directly to the Divine Mother. Apart from helping us toward the ultimate goals of self-awareness and a heightened consciousness of our selfless relationship to the Divine, *Bhramari* breath meditation, which connects sound, breath, and posture, has numerous other benefits. It balances the immunological and nervous systems; strengthens *prana* breath that flows to the heart and brain; and resonates in the energy center located in the midbrow, the point where mind merges into *buddhi* (*ajna,* the sixth chakra).

The Sanskrit verbal root *bhram* literally means "bees" and refers to the resonant hum of inner consciousness, reminiscent of the sound of buzzing bees. As *Bhramari-Devi,* the Mother took the form of the queen bee. Surrounded by bees, *Bhramari-Devi* is symbolic of the mind's rise to the summit of its awareness.

According to the seers, sound can be used in conjunction with only a few specific postures. This age-old meditation practice is among the foremost of these and is an essential part of the Wise Earth meditation *sadhana.* In *Bhramari* breath meditation, we vibrate the vocal cords through buzzing sounds, thereby activating the nervous system and brain and bringing the mind into a state of balance. The buzzing process also purifies the lunar and solar pathways of breath, which has a dramatic clarifying influence on the mind.

### The Practice: *Bhramari* Breath Meditation—Developing the Subtle Breath

Sit in a comfortable meditative posture where you will not be distracted. Release the stale breath from the body with a forceful exhalation through the nostrils and proceed with the meditation practice.

Use the fingers of both hands to close your eyes, nostrils, ears, and mouth, as shown in the diagram below.

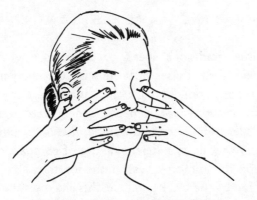

*Hand posture for* Bhramari *breath meditation*

Once the apertures to the sensory organs are sealed, lock your anal muscle by contracting it. Slightly relax the fingers on the nostrils and inhale deeply into the belly. Close the nostrils and maintain your hand position, or mudra. Keeping the anal muscles locked, release the breath slowly while humming on the exhalation. You may not actually hear the sound you make, but you will feel its deep vibration resonating within your *ajna* chakra.

Release the anal lock and mudra. You will experience a surge of energy rushing through your body, followed by a sense of calm, and awareness of everything around you. This awareness is produced by the potent combination of oxygenated breath and inner sound vibrations, vital conduits of energy to and from your subtle body. This breath meditation actually connects you to your subtle body. The rhythms of breathwork and vibration help you move beyond the temporal five-sensory mind to a deeper peace within yourself. This heightened awareness beyond your rational mind is the beginning point of intuition. Each one of us holds this capacity to awaken into intuition, or the *buddhi*, and enter its realm of silence and knowing.

## CULTIVATING INNER SILENCE

All spiritual traditions speak of the silence within. The *Shukla Yajur Veda* advises, "Let the wise, the knower of Brahman, realizing Him, practice their wisdom. Let them not ponder many words, for in speech is mere weariness."

Inner silence transcends the mind, making it possible for the heart to recall its inherent nature of compassion. Vedic lore locates the immortal heart in the fourth chakra, *anahata*. Symbolized by the black antelope, this chakra is the abode of cosmic love in the body. When we enter silence, we enter the heart and the primordial sound that reverberates there. *Anahata* actually means "unstruck" and refers to the pure sound of all creation.

Silence is an integral component of meditation, or *buddhi* yoga. At the beginning of your practice, silence is a way of letting the mind fast, much as you might observe the occasional food fast to rest, cleanse, and rejuvenate the digestive system. Cultivating inner silence is a powerful means of awakening intuition, and hence, cosmic memory.

My own spiritual journey taught me the value of silence, how it can awaken intuition and cosmic memory. My first long period of silence was during that secluded winter interlude when I was diagnosed with cancer. But I first undertook silence as a spiritual practice when I went to study at my teacher's monastery in India.

I experienced some difficulties adjusting to Indian culture when I first arrived there because of the language barrier. The fact that I was of Indian origin but could not speak the language only exacerbated the problem. I finally decided that while I was at the monastery, in order to escape the constant barrage of questions from my teacher's well-meaning devotees, I would observe complete silence.

The longer I practiced, the deeper the silence became. I watched my thoughts transform themselves, so that in time, I was exploring the consecrated territory of heart and *buddhi*. After some months of silent contemplations, I began to experience a dramatic shift of mind that gave birth to a host of visions. On the third anniversary of his death, my father came to me during my meditation. He had ascended to the celestial abode, where he was serving water to children at the gate of a beautiful alabaster-white temple. Austerely dressed in white, he, too, was silent. Later, he moved to second level of the abode, where I saw him sitting in profound silence. Then he ascended to another place, where I was no longer able to connect with him. I knew, however, that he was well and that his spirit was continuing to safeguard each member of his family and of his flock.

My father reappeared in a subsequent meditation. This time, he revealed to me a tumultuous river, red as vermilion. He sent me this wordless transmission: "This is the river of your heart. Care for your heart, for it is the keeper of the Sound. If you do not, you will have to cross this raging, red river after life. I know, because I have just emerged from the crossing."

One week after this meditation, my teacher's guru had a massive heart attack. The synchronicity of this vision of my father, who had died of a heart attack, felt like a revelation from my *buddhi*. I understood it as a warning that the spiritual facilitators and teachers who give so much of themselves must be especially mindful of the health of their own hearts and bodies. Since then, as I myself have become a teacher and healer, I have often recalled the message of these visions. They are profound instances of cosmic wisdom, intuition, and memory transmitted through the *buddhi*.

Cultivating periods of silence in my life has also brought me closer to knowing my heart's desires, which has led me further along the pathway to intuition and inner freedom. It is said in the *Chandogya Upanishad*, "A person is what his desire is. It is our deepest desire in this life that shapes the life to come. So let us direct our deepest desires to know the Self"—a Self that is born of silence and song. We need only recognize this wondrous divinity within to receive the celestial bounty that lies in the heart.

### The Practice: *Pranava* Meditation

Swami Jyotirmayananda writes in his book *Mantra Kirtan*, "Om is the mother of all mantras. It is the source of all words and sounds. Therefore, Om describes the most perfect symbol.

It is the mystic name of God." Reflecting on the sacred syllable om is the most direct pathway to quieting the mind, which is the focus of *buddhi* yoga. When we pronounce om, we use the entire spectrum of vocal range from throat to lips. Om recalls the most ancient phenomenon—the cosmic sound of consciousness. *Pranava upasana,* a *buddhi* yoga practice based on the contemplation of om, calms the mind and opens the gateway to the vast inner realm of silence and cosmic memory. The *buddhi* assumes dominance as we enter silence.

Try to take a day (or several hours) once a month to practice silence. Start the day with twenty minutes of *pranava* meditation. Spend approximately five minutes at each of the four stages of this meditation. As your ability to quiet the mind improves, you may wish to extend the meditation to an hour.

Sit in *sukhasana* (cross-legged) posture on the floor or in an upright chair with your feet firmly planted on the ground. Concentrate on the first syllable of om, which is *ah*. (In Sanskrit the word "om" is composed of three syllables, *ah-ou-m*. The *ah-ou-m* sounds represent the three states of consciousness in the cosmos. The *ah* aspect of om refers to the physical body and universe and the waking state.) Say *ah* for the count of one, then pause for the count of one. Concentrate on the silent pause between the repetitions of *ah*. Do this for five minutes.

Now, focus on the second syllable of om, which is *ou*. (The *ou* aspect of om refers to the subtle or astral body and the cosmic mind. It also refers to the dream state.) Say *ou* for the count of one (pronounced by puckering your lips into a circle), then pause for the count of one. Concentrate on the silent pause between the repetitions of *ou*. Do this for five minutes.

Next, concentrate on the last syllable of om, which is *m* (pronounced with the lips closed). *M* represents the causal body and the state of sleep. It also refers to the state of cosmic stillness—the unmanifest. Say *m* for the count of one, then pause for the count of one. Concentrate on the silence between the repetitions of *m*. Do this for five minutes.

Lastly, focus on the whole syllable om. Say om for the count of one, then pause for the count of one. Concentrate on the silence between the repetitions of om. Do this for five minutes.

Observe silence as you continue with the rest of your day.

During a recent silent retreat, I was able to reaffirm the importance of resting and fasting the mind periodically and keeping in touch with the *buddhi*. I soon left behind the incessant chatter of the mind, and came to rest serenely beneath the surface of everyday awareness. No longer engaged by superficial thoughts and stimuli, my senses retreated into their source within the *buddhi*, where they were reconnected—through cosmic memory—to their original, vital receptivity. Objects became luminous and vivid. I saw that each blade of grass wore a neon aura. I heard a hawk flying miles away and worms crawling underground. I became aware of a seamless union between Creator and creation, and I knew that the light of the *buddhi* would always help me see my purpose.

## KARMA, REBIRTH, AND THE ROAD TO ANCESTRAL MEMORY

As a Hindu, I believe in the laws of karma and reincarnation: Every act performed in this life shapes our future and our future lives, just as our present life is the cumulative result of past actions and past lives. The Vedic seers inform us that each soul has to move through many lives and manifold occurrences in order to achieve consciousness. The knowledge we gain from life experiences enables us to know our karma, or personal rhythms, so that we can redirect our journey. A spiritual heritage, fame and good fortune, disease and despair, have all been part of my karmic legacy in this life. Joyous or painful as they have been, these events have all led to my rebirth and awakening. Recognizing the events of my personal history as the stones that pave the path to wisdom, I have come to cherish my karma.

Your experience is your gold. When you recognize the value of your karma, you can mine it. Our experiences in this life, from the womb up to the present, become consciously and unconsciously encoded in our cell tissues, giving rise to attitudes and beliefs that affect our lives positively and negatively. Healers are aware of these stored impressions which dwell in the muscles and deep connective tissues. Many ancient impressions live on in the genes we inherited from our parents and ancestors, going back countless generations. These, too, need to be made conscious, lest they manifest as disease or as seemingly inexplicable urges to behave in certain ways or to pursue certain ideas.

The *Rig Veda* says: "When a person comes to weakness, be it through old age or disease, he frees himself from these limbs just as a mango or fig or berry releases itself from its limb, and he hastens again, according to the entrance and place of origin, back to life." Even if you do not believe in the literal truth of past lives, you may find it a helpful metaphor for the phenomenon of being reborn periodically to different roles and missions in your present life. You may have already undergone career changes, or an attraction to different belief systems, or a shift in perspective of yourself and the world.

Past-life regression has become a widely practiced form of therapeutic treatment. Two experts in this field are Roger Woolger, Ph.D., and Brian Weiss, M.D. Although I do not agree with everything they say, some of their ideas may help you work with the teachings I present. According to Woolger, conscious memories of past lives can be seen as representing significant states of the unconscious that have a bearing on your current life situation. "The unconscious mind will almost always produce a past life story when invited in the right way," Woolger writes in *Other Minds, Other Selves.* "Even if the conscious mind is highly skeptical about the reality of past lives as historical memories, the unconscious is a true believer and is simply waiting to be asked."

The wheel of karma turns and brings us to a new beginning of the ongoing cycle. We are licensed by the Creator to enter the physical body and to continue our training in the lessons of the soul. Even if we are wholly unconscious of our connection to all that is, even in our most profound ignorance, the *buddhi*'s light is able to seep through and help us. When we actively seek a connection to the realm of intuition and consciousness, we discover the One spirit that pervades all experiences. As we reach the end of life or the end of a learning cycle, another appears to move us into further self-realization. These cycles continue until all individual karma is fulfilled and unconditional self-knowledge is gained. At this final junction of the soul's life, the individual dissolves into illumination. Absolute consciousness, *moksha,* is attained.

According to the Vedas, the human embryo remembers all of its past lives in a flash at the exact moment it leaves its watery domain and emerges into the open world. After this passage, we gradually lose awareness of our magnificent inheritance and begin to function experientially, under the illusion that we are isolated, separate egos.

To fully reclaim our extensive power of cosmic memory (intuition or *buddhi*) and consciousness, we must first recover, honor, and heal ancestral memories. They are the primary building blocks of our lives. Without addressing the ineffable bond we share with both our male and female forebears, we continue to come up short in our prayer and purpose, sanctity and success, desire and destiny. As you read further in *The Path of Practice*, you will learn how you can recover your ancestral memories—and thus facilitate healing—through *sadhana* and the practice of rituals expressly designed to honor the legacy of your ancestors.

# Chapter 8

## RECOVERING YOUR ANCESTRAL MEMORIES

*Let there be no neglect of the duties to the
Gods and the forebears. Be one to whom the
mother is God. Be one to whom the father
is God.*
—Krishna Yajur Veda
Taittiriya Upanishad (1.11.2)

According to Vedic thought, birth and its resulting shock cause us to lose our memory of our extensive past lives and lessons. These ancestral memories are blocked and we forget who we are. Part of our psyche is also blocked, and therefore we lose our ability to tap into the innate intuitive guidance that keeps us on our life's path. We forget our sacred purpose and authentic nature.

Honoring your ancestors is the first step in reclaiming your spiritual heritage. As you begin to recover your ancestral memories, you will also uncover unconscious, troubled memories that prevent you from knowing the truth of who you are. According to the Vedic sages, we humans are the only species which has the power of intuition. Yet too easily, we forfeit our sacred birthright and with it the ability to change and grow, create, and strive for inner freedom. We have largely forgotten the joy, love, and wellness that are intrinsic to human nature.

Our contemporary culture is so preoccupied with the pursuit of health that we seem to function from the debilitating premise that something is wrong with us. We must shift this false image of ourselves as inheritors of disease and pursuers of wellness. We *are* wellness. We *are* consciousness. These are our natural states. Disease is an imposter, a force that thrives on loss of memory. A crisis provides us with both the urgency and spiritual imperative to explore our past, but we do not have to wait for illness to occur before we undertake to recover ancestral memories.

In ancient India, the royal sage Bhagiratha stood on one foot for a thousand years as penance for having liberated his ancestors from the netherworld. He held both arms high toward the heavens for another thousand years. He performed these sacrifices, called *tapasya*, as a prayer to the gods and goddesses to release the waters and revive the drought-ridden earth. Goddess Ganga agreed, but warned that Her force would destroy the Earth, so God Shiva interceded. Shiva had to break the torrential flow of the great river goddess by catching her waters in his hair. This outpouring formed the Himalayan River and its estuary, the Ganges.

Indian ascetics commonly performed rituals similar to Bhagiratha's sacrifice as a way to show respect for their ancestors and to serve the earthly community. These ancient *munis*, ascetics from India's shamanic culture, had one purpose in life—to develop and refine their inner consciousness through disciplined spiritual practice. In so doing, they influenced the community around them, and all of humanity, with their beneficent energy and vibration. It was in this tradition of self-sacrifice that my great-grandfather fasted to bring the rains one hundred years ago in Guyana. The *Shatapatha Brahmana* tells us: "Sacrifice has only one sure foundation, only one destination, the heavenly realm!"

The Vedic people understand that none of us exists as an independent being; we are all linked to the universe through our ancestry. They believe that the act of sacrifice keeps us in harmony with our society and lineage. The *Rig Veda*'s "Hymn of the Longhair" speaks about the *munis* who rode the winds (the internal life force) to benefit their fellow beings. Although you may be beginning to learn to ride the inner breath, you can honor your ancestral spirits by giving of yourself. As my brother, a Brahmin priest and pundit, has said, "Appease the ancestors so that we may live happily."

You can begin your personal practice of honoring and appeasing your ancestors by making small personal sacrifices on a daily basis. Offer your seat to an elderly or disadvantaged person on the bus or train. Devote an hour a week or month to community service. Say a prayer to alleviate the suffering of others. Offer a pound of rice to a homeless shelter. Visit a nursing home. Fast one day a year for world peace. Make a conscious effort not to injure, pollute, or otherwise compromise the earth, rivers, animals, plants, and environment. The highest personal sacrifice we can make is to embrace a spirit of reverence for nature and work toward healing the indescribable damage we humans have wreaked upon our planet. In the words of the great American naturalist John Muir, who envisioned our national parks system, "When a man plants a tree, he plants himself." Likewise, when he uproots it, he uproots himself.

Disparate cultures such as the Vedic people, Native Americans, African tribes, and the Guyanese Amerindians share similar beliefs about the tremendous problems we face today: pandemic illnesses, pollution, genocide, violence, poverty, and crime are all due to the unhappiness of our ancestors' spirits, and the loss of their protection. If we allow such conditions to continue unchecked, they will bring about a devastating loss of human memory and, ultimately, the destruction of the earth.

With a personal sacrifice, we give back something of

ourselves—our attention, time, or money. The Vedic seers teach that "Sacrifices are the actions through which we receive sustenance from the earth and by which we return equal nourishment back to her." They tell us that giving back to nature not only pleases our ancestors' spirits but helps us develop inner consciousness. As we awaken to our ancestral memories, we remember the meaning and purpose of our lives.

The *Yajur Veda* instructs us in this regard: "To you, most luminous God, we pray now for the happiness of our ancestors and friends. Listen attentively to our call and protect us from those who go against the cosmic order." The collective grief of the modern world is due to the loss of our ancestral memory. This loss is the most basic cause for the breakdown of dharma (which means cosmic laws and life values besides life purpose) in relation to our family, global community, and nature.

Sir James George Frazer, the noted British anthropologist, wrote in *The Golden Bough* that human evolution has gone through three stages: the age of magic, the age of religion, and the age of service. According to Vedic thought, we have arrived at a fourth and final stage, the age of understanding, called *kali yuga* (darkness time). During this time, we will see a breakdown of everything that runs counter to the cosmic order. This breakdown will allow a spiritual breakthrough—an opportunity to ignite the light of unity and understanding among all creations. We can begin to unite by embracing our ancestors and honoring the earth.

We start this process by remembering our indelible link to our past. When we fail to recall these sacred ties, we lose touch with the onrushing stream of consciousness that flows from generation to generation. Without this memory, we cannot hope to sustain our present or know our purpose as human beings. Meditation teaches us to live in the present moment, and as my father taught me, "the past and the future are in our present."

## HONORING THE ANCESTORS

Through ancestral memories we can recall the world's oldest rituals and ceremonies. These rites kept our people connected to one another and to the greater energies of the universe. In everyday Hindu rituals, the ancestors play a significant role. The Vedas inform us that one of the highest universal laws is *Pitri Rina*, repaying our debt to the ancestors: our parents, grandparents, and spiritual teachers. Our ancestral lineage is not limited to those with whom we share a genetic heritage. Teachers, mentors, and older friends who inspired and shaped our lives may be included in the ritual honoring of the ancestors. This, and other practices I describe, strengthen the link to those who sustain us with their spirit and energy.

Our cosmic obligation must be tended so that the influence of the ancestral spirits will grace our lives and purpose. The Vedic ritual practice for ancestors, called *Pitri Paksha*, is observed during a particular time period each year to help revive within us the memory of our people, and to keep their spirits happy. The practice involves two weeks of reciting special prayers prior to the actual day of observance, as well as offerings of grain, water, and milk to appease the ancestors. These offerings are said to give nourishment and strength to the subtle or etheric body of the ancestors and to ensure their safe travel to the blissful abode among the *Petris*, or Divine Fathers. A portion of the food offering is also given to the cows and crows, animal friends we connect with the ancestral spirit.

On the day of *Pitri Paksha* in 1995, I was in Katmandu,

Nepal, observing my last hours of a five-month silent retreat. Early that morning, I heard gleeful shouts coming from the Agni Temple across the street. One of my neighbors came to my door to tell me that the temple's statue of the elephant-headed god, Ganesha, was "drinking" milk. Eager to witness this miracle with my own eyes, I joined the excited throng that had gathered in the temple and slowly made my way through the crowd toward the statue. Indeed, Ganesha did appear to be absorbing the cups of milk held up to his trunk by his eager devotees.

Later that day, I took a three-mile trek to the vast compound of the temple of Pashupati (the god Shiva represented as the protector of animals). After waiting for three hours along with thousands of other Hindu pilgrims, I entered the sanctum where several statues of Ganesha were also drinking milk. Some days later, *Hinduism Today* estimated that some million gallons of milk had been absorbed by a billion Ganesha statues all over the world. My mother told me that the miracle of the milk had also occurred at the small temple in my grandparents' village of Port Mourant, Guyana. And at our family temple in Ontario, Canada, Ganesha's "parents," Shiva and Parvati, were also seen to have taken in milk.

A Brahmin priest in Katmandu quoted me a passage from the *Dharma Sastra*, which states that from time to time, the gods and goddesses make their presence on earth known through the medium of statues, which are imbued by the daily rituals of the priests with *prana*, or life force. However, the *Dharma Sastra* says that this manifestation of a statue's *pranic* power is an inauspicious sign, a stern warning from the celestials that the earth's dharma is being violated. My own interpretation of the milk miracle came to me in a meditation when my ancestors appeared and told me that Shiva was very unhappy because we humans had forgotten our sacred duty to our ancestors and the animals.

*Pitri Paksha* is observed each year during the dark moon phase of the lunar month *Ashvina*. In the Western calendar, this coincides with the dark cycle of the moon that comes at the end of September or early October. The last and most significant day of *Pitri Paksha* falls on the new moon, when prayers and offerings are deemed most necessary. Perhaps there is an ancient link between *Pitri Paksha* and the Day of the Dead or All Souls' Day.

During my most recent observance of *Pitri Paksha*, I was in California, preparing to give a *satsanga* for cancer patients at the Healing Journeys conference. Early that evening, as the sun dissolved beyond the horizon, I performed a brief Vedic ritual on the lawn of the guest house where I was staying. I recited my daily prayers for my ancestors while making an offering of water and black sesame seeds.

That night, I dreamed of my maternal grandmother. She was dressed in her familiar long white smock with its embroidered lace collar, and her hair was pulled back in a bun, just as she had always worn it. She walked over to me and placed her right hand on my forehead as she pressed the left side of my throat with her left thumb. I had returned from India two months earlier with a persistent dry cough. The next morning, after my dream/visitation, the cough was gone and my throat was completely free of any irritation. So real was the dream that immediately after I woke up, I could still smell the beautiful jasmine scent that I had always associated with my grandmother. I believe that my prayer in honor of my ancestors was recognized and responded to by one of their representatives, my grandmother.

Many religions and cultures have their own specific rituals in memory of loved ones and ancestors. You may want to learn more about the practices from your own ethnic or religious background. You may also wish to honor your ancestors on this day of *Pitri Paksha* in particular, when millions of people around the world are doing so, as they have for thousands of years.

Uncovering and gathering information about our ancestral past is not always an easy task. Many of us have lost the connection with our ancestral lineage through adoption or migration. The *Pitri Paksha* is a good way to reconnect emotionally and spiritually to the memory and vibration of our forebears, even if we do not have specific historical details. We may begin to resonate with them through our dream state, or feel drawn toward the ways of life of a certain culture or tradition.

The following is a simple ritual that you can perform at home.

### The Practice: Offering to the Ancestors

1. On your lunar calendar, find the date of the last new moon in September. (This moon sometimes occurs at the beginning of October.) You may, of course, celebrate this ritual and recite the mantra below on any day of the year; the September date is when the offering is required.

2. Make a list of the names of as many of your ancestors as you know.

3. Place a small handful of black sesame seeds or uncooked rice in a brass or bronze bowl. (Black rice, which may be purchased at gourmet or health food stores, or wild rice may also be used.) Fill a brass urn or pitcher with water or organic milk, and place it in a large bowl. (An Indian bronze or brass goblet, or *lota*, and a brass or bronze tray, or *tali*, is used traditionally.)

4. Sit at your altar, or in a clean space inside or outdoors, facing south. Mix the rice or seeds with the water in the urn. Use your right hand to pour the mixture slowly into the large bowl, reciting aloud the names of your ancestors as you pour.

5. The next step involves the use of a mantra. The Upanishads

say, "*Mananat Trayate Iti Mantrah*"; a mantra is that which heals a person through repetition and reflection. Mantras, which are sacred Sanskrit chants and one-syllable sounds, play a profound role in healing, and I will discuss their uses more fully in chapter 10.

Repeat the following mantra nine times, staying mindful of your ancestors, known and unknown. Pray for their well-being and their safe travel in the celestial sphere.

*Om namo vah pitrah saumyah*
(ohm nah-mo vaph pi-tra saum-ya-ha [saum pronounced as in "sour"])
Obeisance to you, O gentle ancestors.

6. Take the offering to a place where birds and animals can partake of it. Do not discard it in the garbage.

## RECONNECTING WITH YOUR MOTHER AND FATHER

Before we examine our own unconscious memories, we must first inquire into the lives of our relatives in order to find out what memories—happy and unhappy—we have inherited. Begin by talking to your parents. Together, you may recall shared experiences, and at the same time receive the support you need to delve into your long-forgotten past and ancestral memories. (If they are willing, you may wish to record your discussions, creating an account for future generations.)

Ask your parents to talk about their greatest challenges and victories. Begin with the easy questions, and, as respectfully as you can, pursue areas that they may try to avoid discussing with you. What made them joyful? What made them sad? Who did they admire? Who did they resent?

Talk to them about their dreams and desires. Are they happy with what they have accomplished? What regrets, if any, do they have? What sacrifices did they make for you? What are their memories of their parents? What difficulties and obstacles did their parents have at different periods in their lives?

If you cannot interview your relatives, undertake to research the experiences of your ethnic group. Use the resources available at your public library to investigate the historical, cultural, and social settings of your ancestors' lives. If some of your family members were immigrants (which includes all of us in the United States except for Native Americans), you will find that their experiences were very different from your experience of growing up here.

To know your ancestors, be they saints, sinners, or average folks, you need to keep an open mind that neither judges nor condemns. Be prepared to accept their strengths and weaknesses. Remember that because of their sacrifices, you have been given life and the sacred opportunity to regain the knowledge of your spirit. Your parents' and grandparents' strengths give you the power to repair your inherited weaknesses. Their weaknesses enable you to see your own and strengthen your resolve as you journey into consciousness.

As part of the law of karma, we all carry memories of pain and conflict passed down from our immediate family. As long as we do not face these memories, we cannot embark upon our own true path. The open and honest acknowledgment of our people's spiritual, emotional, and physical trials allows for healing and resolution. As the philosopher George

Santayana wrote, "Those who cannot remember the past are condemned to repeat it."

Bob, a friend of one of my students, was suffering from exhaustion and a bad case of frayed nerves. He told me that he was desperate for help. He had been adopted when he was just a few weeks old and had no information about his biological parents. "This has haunted me all my life," he told me, his eyes downcast. "I desperately want to find out who my birth parents are, but my adoptive parents don't know anything about them."

Bob was a talented classical violinist who had begun playing at age nine. The demands of his training were rigorous, and now, at age twenty-six, he was in a chronic state of emotional upheaval. Like many artists, he had a deeply sensitive personality. For many months, he had had trouble sleeping and he had lost his ability to concentrate—both on- and off-stage. After seventeen years of pushing himself to the limit creatively, he had lost his desire to express himself through his music. He could no longer perform in public, and even practicing privately felt like a tremendous chore.

The crux of Bob's problem was his longing to know his ancestral roots. To give him some immediate relief from his chronic state of tension, I led him through the focused-breath meditation (see page 198), and urged him to practice it on a daily basis. I felt that the simple act of paying attention to his breath and its effect on his body could produce profound changes in his physical and emotional health. I also gave him an Ayurvedic herbal tonic for relieving nervous tension that consisted of ¼ teaspoon *ashwagandha*, ¼ teaspoon *bala*, ¼ teaspoon *jatamansi*, and a pinch of nutmeg. Finally, I provided him with the number of a search agency that might help him find his biological parents. As he said good-bye, his smile seemed less forced, and his hunched shoulders had relaxed somewhat, as if perhaps a small part of the burden of grief he carried had been lifted.

Five months later, he called to tell me his good news. "I found my mother," he said. "Now I know who I am." He had just returned from meeting his birth mother in Germany, where he discovered that he came from a long line of classical musicians: his grandfather had been a pianist and his mother was a violinist.

Bob's mother had willingly told him the circumstances around his birth. She had been sixteen, a student at a boarding school in New York, when she had become pregnant by her high-school sweetheart. After she had given birth to Bob, her parents had insisted that she give him up for adoption immediately. As soon as she was well enough to travel, she had gone back to Germany and immersed herself in her music studies. She had never married and told Bob that she had wanted no further romantic involvements; giving up her infant son had been such a traumatic experience that she had thought she could never recover from it. But seeing him now, a handsome young man who looked like her father and had inherited her musical genes, had helped to begin to heal her own terrible wound. Now, they could both move forward.

Bob had discovered the ancestral wellspring from which his love of music flowed. In a sense, he had found his purpose. When he came to see me again several months later, he looked very different from the wan, troubled individual whose eyes hadn't been able to meet mine. He was in vibrant health, happily practicing the violin for many hours every day, eagerly anticipating his next stage appearance. He had incorporated the focused-breath meditation into his daily routine, as well as several of the Wise Earth *sadhana* practices which I describe in this and subsequent chapters. Recently, I received a short note from him. I could almost feel his joyful energy as I opened the envelope. He was writing to thank me for helping him to connect with his past and fulfill the promise of his present. Also enclosed was an invitation to his solo violin debut at Lincoln Center in New York City.

When we connect with our close relatives, as Bob did, and learn more about their gifts and their burdens, we invariably find an underlying common force of desire and purpose. Once discovered, that purpose is the key that opens the floodgates of creativity, passion, and intuitive understanding. Unlike Bob, most of us were brought up by our biological parents. Still, we may not truly know them, and we often take them for granted. I cannot imagine how I would have found my life purpose if I had not reconciled with my father before he died, or if I could not regularly experience the love and support of my two mothers. Yet I know many people who did not have these blessings in their lives and are still able to find their dharma and their path of healing.

Even if you do not know your biological roots and have no way of finding out about them, you can follow the instructions in these pages. Keep in mind that the intention of this *sadhana* is healing for both yourself and your ancestors. As you discover ancestral memory, your power of intuition will grow and you will be given insights about your forebears. You may even discover their strengths and vulnerabilities as you begin to examine your own.

## INQUIRING INTO YOUR ANCESTRAL PAST

Once we see the patterns that connect you to your immediate family, you can proceed to evoke the larger scope of ancestral memories. This will help you reclaim your legacy and reconcile the ways in which you are affected by your heritage. When I first set foot in India—the homeland of my people—I knelt down and smelled the earth. I held the soil in my hands and gathered some of it to keep with me. I tasted the water of their wells and poured some of it into a small vial. I heard the sounds of the motherland resonate in my heart. I carry these vibrations with me wherever I go.

Here are some of the steps I took that led me back one hundred years into my ancestral past:

1. Keep a journal. (Read below for more discussion about journaling.)

2. If possible, collect photographs of your ancestors, going back as far as your great-grandparents. Familiarize yourself with their faces. Notice any similarities between them and yourself.

3. Take a trip to your ancestors' place of birth. This may seem arduous and possibly expensive, but it could be an opportunity to discover a deeper resonance in the experiences of your family. You can plan your trip while carrying out the steps that are within your immediate grasp. (I have heard wonderful, healing stories about people who have traveled with one or both parents to their family's country of origin. These journeys into a shared past inevitably transform the way in which both the parents and their children understand themselves and one another.)

4. Prepare your ancestral foods, using what is wholesome from your tradition. Give some thought to what are the true roots of your cultural cuisine. (Regardless of your ancestral habits, however, it is best to refrain from eating flesh foods.)

## ANCESTRAL JOURNAL-KEEPING

My own ancestral pilgrimage has taught me the value of keeping a written record of my thoughts and emotions. My journal had been my constant companion as I retraced my ancestral origins throughout my journey in India. You, too, may consider keeping a diary to chronicle your discoveries, or perhaps you began doing so as I suggested in chapter 1. Write down the stories and events of your family history as you uncover them. Also record your thoughts, feelings, and dreams as your journey evokes them. Express all the emotions that surface.

Recovering ancestral memories can be upsetting, especially if these memories connect you to painful experiences in your life. Ancestral memories often begin to flow in the form of tears. All tears are memories returning; all laughter is memory becoming delighted and awakened within us. Cry as much and as often as you like. Pain is a natural part of your human journey. The Buddha is depicted as a laughing buddha, but also as a gaunt and suffering being. All emotions are important parts of the path of practice. It was pain that led me back to the ancient roots of my ancestry, and pain that gave me insights into my people's greatness and sorrow. This understanding helped me to heal my own pain. My journal kept the memory of my discoveries fresh and became a trusted friend. You may find, however, that joyous memories help you along your path.

This work will dig deeply into your core, and you may dislike churning up old memories. Express all these feelings in your journal. You may be resentful or angry at having to shift your habitual perspective to accommodate the reality of who you are. Whenever you feel this way, you may find it particularly useful to follow the focused-breath meditation.

At any point when feelings of anger, hurt, or humiliation arise, keep in mind that negative emotions consume our healthy life force. Visit with your anger, bear witness to it, explore it, and give voice to whatever provokes you about a particular situation or person. Set a time limit after which you can leave that emotional place. You do not want to dwell in these emotions, but find them and free them from your body-mind so that you can be at peace.

If anger or any other emotion prevents you from being able to write, put down your journal and practice a food, breath, or sound *sadhana*. When you engage in this practice, you move energy and breath through your body, which allows the rhythms of your thought processes to become more fluid. A fresh, new set of ideas is likely to arise in your mind. You may find positive solutions to problems or emotional issues that seem insurmountable and have made you feel struck.

### The Practice: Keeping Your Ancestral Journal

The following schedule will help you with the potentially challenging task of keeping an ancestral journal. For six weeks, once a day, preferably just after dawn or before dusk, spend fifteen minutes writing in your journal. Disregard all rules of grammar or proper usage while recounting your memories of people, places, and emotions, and follow the schedule below. Do not edit or censor yourself. Keep your pen moving across the page until the full fifteen minutes have passed. (This may, at first, seem like a very long time.)

You can combine this writing time with writing in your meditation journal since, after you have been practicing meditation regularly and have also formed the intention to uncover ancestral memories, your meditations may reveal ancestral memories to you.

Begin with a prayer. You may use the following invocation or create one of your own: "May the Divine grant me the courage to be honest. May I learn more about my people and my connection to them. May I learn from their experience. May my heart become gentle as a result of this *sadhana*."

**Week One:** Recall a few childhood memories of your mother. What did she look like? How did you feel in her presence? What are some of the things you did together? In what ways are you like your mother?

**Week Two:** Recall a few childhood memories of your father, as above.

**Week Three:** Describe your earliest memories of happiness and joy.

**Week Four:** Describe your earliest memories of people, places, or situations that you feared the most.

**Week Five:** Describe your earliest memories of pain.

**Week Six:** Describe your health. If you have a serious or chronic health problem, inquire into your family history and see who else has or had this problem. Connect the links of your ancestral health chain.

At the end of six weeks, put away your journal. Allow yourself a couple of weeks to assimilate its disclosures before you reopen it. In just a few weeks, you should begin to remember your ancestral past. Memories may appear in your dreams. As you meditate, you may see your ancestors' faces during your meditation. When I am about to embark on a challenging task, my paternal grandfather often appears in my meditation. At other times, if any dark energy is coming my way, my father and my maternal grandmother appear in my dreams. If I fail to heed their warnings, I receive a visit from the god Ganesha.

Once you start to recollect your forebears, you will gain a better perspective on your life. Any unconscious, troubled memories will surface, and the lessons behind them will become clearer. This clarity readily dissolves pain into that splendid substance that is your strength, tenderness, and joy. When you reconnect with your ancestry, you will notice that obstacles and problems are resolved. You will stop looking at a given situation as problematic and discover instead a lesson to be learned or a challenge to be met.

## INDICATIONS THAT YOU ARE CARRYING ANCESTRAL BAGGAGE

All negative emotions, feelings of alienation from the Divine, restlessness, mental hyperactivity, and unhealthy activities and food habits are indications that your ancestral memories are blocked.

Are you obsessed with trying not to be or think like your parents? Are you uncomfortable with your heritage? Your ancestral memories may also show up in your relationship to food. Do you constantly crave junk food? Do you find yourself on a treadmill of eating disorders? Do you dislike to cook? These are all indications that you need to examine your ancestral memories.

I have observed that unresolved ancestral memories lodged within us become more and more tenacious over time. They express themselves in our lives by presenting us with the same problems, cloaked in different circumstances, over and over again. These challenges or issues will also recur with each successive generation.

I met Rose some years ago when she was already exhausted and depleted from five years of being treated for Hodgkin's disease. Her system had become so weak that she could no longer absorb any nutrients, and her once robust body had been reduced to a fragile ninety-eight pounds. As we sat together drinking tea, we chatted quietly, and I asked her about her family.

In a low, quavering voice, she explained that her parents, who had come to the United States from Eastern Europe after World War II, were both survivors of the Holocaust. As a child, she had heard terrifying stories about their experiences in German concentration camps—stories so devastating that night after night she had silently wept herself to sleep. Determined to shield her own three children from the agony of her parents' heritage, she had hidden the scars of the ancestral memories she had inherited at birth from them and her husband.

She had paid a huge price, however, for keeping so many bitter secrets. Her denial of the past had created an emotional barrier between herself and her family that had seemed as insurmountable as the barbed-wire fence that had surrounded the concentration camp in which her parents had been imprisoned. The children, now adults, rarely called or visited; her older son had not invited her to his wedding. Her marriage, too, had been destroyed by her misguided decision to bury her grief: Her husband had cheated on her for many years and had left her shortly before she was diagnosed with cancer.

Now, too weak and tired even to shed tears, Rose listened with dry eyes as I shared my own cancer story and spoke of how our ancestral memories function. I recommended that she keep a journal in which she could record her thoughts and feelings, her memories and dreams. Although she seemed to appreciate the suggestion, as I said good-bye, I wondered whether she would actually follow through with it.

About six months later, I received a phone call from a young man who identified himself as Rose's oldest son, James. "My mother died last week," he said. "But she wanted you to know how much she appreciated your advice. All those years we were growing up, we never understood why she kept herself at a distance from us. Keeping that journal allowed her to be honest with us for the first time in her life. Our grandparents died when we were young, and we had no idea what they had been through—and how it had affected our mother."

The act of journaling had made a profound difference in Rose's life. By revealing the anguish of their family's past to her children, she exposed her true, vulnerable self, so that they were finally able to form an emotional connection with her. She and James, who was having difficulties with his marriage, had become especially close. He had moved into her house to help care for her in the last weeks before her death. "She looked so beautiful and peaceful just before she died," he said. "She didn't have anything to hide anymore. It was as if she cleansed herself of all the grief and anger she'd been carrying around all those years."

The pain of unresolved memories causes part of our psyche to engage in constantly blocking out the ancestral secret, even as another part is trying to unmask it. This doesn't make things easy for us. But try to think of this paradox as similar to the opposing forces at work when we try to break a bad habit or go on a diet: part of us still wants the forbidden food or behavior while the other part wants to be free. With an ancestral memory, it's *good* for you to break through to the forbidden memory.

We are divinely ordained in every cell, atom, and memory of our being to try to correct and reorganize ourselves whenever we fall out of harmony with cosmic rhythms. Ultimately, your psyche *will* work with you to reestablish your spiritual equilibrium. But until we come to terms with the past and how it continues to maintain its hold on us, or influence our karma, we remain spiritually restless, severed from the path of consciousness.

The key to freeing ourselves from the chains of unconscious, troubled memories that keep us from our path is the cultivation of an awareness of the individual links of those chains. When we can see these patterns reenacted in our lives, the chain begins to loosen. Thich Nhat Hanh has said, "We have to be able to recognize a habit when it manifests itself, because if we know how to recognize our habit, it will lose its energy and will not be able to push us anymore. . . . We have to practice in order to be able to transform this habit in us."

The focused-breath meditation practice that follows will help to alleviate the emotional pain of delving into your past and also make you more aware of your ancestral patterns. As you familiarize yourself with the practice, you will grow more adept at recognizing the role you may be playing in any traumatic, disharmonious, or stressful situations. Breath is a vital vehicle for recalling memory, and we will learn more about it as we progress.

### The Practice: Focused-Breath Meditation

Find a place in your home where you will not be disturbed by the telephone or any other distraction. Lie on your back on the floor with your eyes closed. Stretch your legs out (about eighteen inches apart), with your arms at your sides, palms facing up. Tuck your chin slightly into your chest, stretching out the back of your neck.

1. Inhale through your nose and direct the breath deeply into your abdomen. Now take time to become aware of areas of your body where you are holding on to stress. Do you notice tightness around your eyes? In your jaw? Your chest? Your belly? Bring your awareness into these areas, and spend a few minutes in each, observing the subtlest sensations and move-

ments. Now direct your breath into those places of tension where the discomfort of tremor, conflict, pain, numbness, or constriction are present. Exhale slowly through your nose. Repeat this practice three times.

2. Direct your next intake of breath into the area of stress with a definite intention to release this stress. Slowly exhale the breath, and feel the inner spaces expanding in and around the area of stress. Feel yourself becoming calmer and more relaxed.

3. Take a deep breath, and as you exhale, pay attention to the sense of peace permeating your body.

Repeat these steps five times.

Thus far, we have come to perceive the power of our own experience and that of our forebears. Now we will undertake to illuminate our understanding further by exploring sound medicine and spirit healing.

# Part Three

# SOUNDS OF
# THE COSMOS

# Chapter 9

## SOUND MEDICINE AND SPIRIT HEALING

*By means of the hymns one attains this world,*
*by holy chants the world is revealed by the*
*sages. With the syllable om as his sole support,*
*the wise attains that which is tranquil,*
*unaging, deathless, fearless—the Supreme.*
—*Prasna Upanishad* (5.7)

Years ago, I was lying on an operating table, about to have my eleventh surgery. The doctors who were going to cut open my abdomen to search for cancerous tumors were reluctant to administer general anesthesia because I'd already had so much during the previous operations. They were afraid I might react badly; that I might never again regain consciousness from the anesthesia-induced sleep. The best they could offer me was a local painkiller to numb the area. Wide awake and wondering how I would fare during this frightening ordeal, I tried to distract myself by gazing around the room. My gaze was drawn to one of the nurses, whose red hair, freckled complexion, and slight brogue told me that she must be Irish.

When she came over to check on me, I noted the name on her ID tag. "Kathleen, do you know the song 'Danny Boy'?" I asked her.

Her face lit up. "Oh, yes," she said. "It's my favorite."

"Would you mind singing it to me now? I've always loved it. I must have Irish karmic ancestry," I said jokingly.

She looked over at the surgeon, who nodded his permission. I'm sure he was ready to try anything that might distract me. As the local anesthetic took effect, the nurse massaged my head and began to sing in a lovely, lilting voice. My anxiety dissipated and I felt no pain at all as the surgeon made the first incision. The mood in the room seemed more upbeat. I suddenly realized that the entire surgical team was smiling and humming along as Kathleen repeated the hauntingly sweet ballad over and over.

Still conscious and watching them work, with my flesh draped over my stomach, I joined in the humming during the five-hour operation. "Here is your opportunity to transcend the pain," I told myself, as the strains of the familiar melody rose around me.

Ralph Spintge, M.D., a German anesthesiologist and one of the top researchers in the field, offered this summary of how music affects the body before and during surgical procedures:

> Physiological parameters like heart rate, arterial blood pressure, salivation, skin humidity, blood levels of stress hormones . . . show a significant decrease under anxiolytic [antianxiety] music compared with usual pharmacological premedication. . . . The subjective responses of the patients are most positive in about 97 percent [of 59,000]. These patients state that music is a real help to them to relax in the preoperative situation and during surgery in regional anesthesia.

That day, an intuitive sense had told me that music could comfort my spirit and minimize my pain. In the years that followed, as I absorbed myself in the study of the Vedas and developed a regular practice of chanting, I often recalled my experience in the operating room. It was the first time, although by no means the last, that I experienced the therapeutic properties of sound and music. I have also been told firsthand accounts of lifesaving miracles that healing sounds have accomplished. While I will never take such events for granted—because any form of healing is a gift from the universe that must be appreciated—these cases demonstrate to me the continuous marvel of life. The use of sound for spiritual, emotional, and physical healing traces its roots back to human prehistory.

Consider the idea that life itself emanates from sound. For what is sound but audible breath—the rhythm and melody of the One Spirit that dwells within all things? Sound vibration is a manifestation of life energy, and that energy, or *prana*, is the basis for self-healing. Indeed, sound is central to the very act of creation. Vedic lore tells us that the goddess Durga rode her lion, carried her *damaru* (a small, double-headed drum whose sound is associated with the element of space), and drummed the world into existence.

According to the *rishis*, the first emanation of creation emerged from *nada*, the inaudible cosmic vibrations known as the primordial sound. Through the transformation of this sound, the entire universe emerged, constantly resolving into other shapes and forms. The *Chandogya Upanishad* reveals cosmic sound as the Word: "The Word makes known heaven, earth, wind, space, the waters, fire, the celestials, humans, animals, grass, and trees."

Many other ancient cultures similarly trace the birth of the universe to sound and the spoken word. The Bible tells us that "God said, Let us make man in our image. . . ." (Gen. 1:26). According to the *Popul Vuh*, the creation story of the Mayan people of South America, the human race originated on earth through the power of sound: "Only by a miracle, by means of incantation were they created and made by the Creator." For the Aborigines of Australia, musical notes and words were the means by which their earliest ancestors "named" the world into being and provided a map for those who followed in their footsteps. In an ancient myth of the Aborigines, the Rainbow Serpent, Ngalijod, first created himself as a long, hollow log, *ubar*. This log produces a hypnotic vibration and is used as a musical instrument in sacred ceremonies. The hollow of the log is referred to as the womb of the Great Mother, and the sound or vibration is the energy that unites the tangible with the intangible world.

The reason that sound is fundamental to the creation story of so many cultures can perhaps best be understood through the Vedic tradition, in which the phenomenon of sound lies at the heart of daily spiritual practice. The *rishis*, who devoted themselves to meditation and contemplation of the Eternal, discerned that the universe is an ocean of vibration. They perceived that om, the infinite, "unstruck" sound, is the underlying resonant vibration of the universe, which can be heard in its unmanifest state during meditation. "The essence of word and sound is om," say the Upanishads. Elsewhere in the Vedic texts, om is described as "the most powerful one. Its power alone can bring enlightenment."

Centuries ago, the Vedic seers developed a complete system for sound as a spiritual and physical healing force, which they called *sangita*. The Sanskrit word for sound, music, and song, *sangita* embraces much more than just those forms of expression that are limited by human creativity. *Sangita* invokes the totality of the cosmic expressions of the celestials, which were conveyed to humankind by the *rishis*. This complex science of measures, rhythms, and melodies explains the causes and properties of the six seasons, the seven colors of the rainbow, the seven vital tissue layers of the body, and the rhythm of the mind.

The Vedic understanding of the universe as a vast vibratory field has more recently come under the scrutiny of contemporary scientists. One of the most compelling findings in support of this centuries-old idea has evolved from the observations of the natural phenomenon known as entrainment. This process causes the rhythmic vibrations of one object to affect a second object with a similar vibratory frequency, so that the second object begins to vibrate in resonance with the first.

You can visualize this principle if you think of two metronomes, placed side by side and beating at different rhythms. Now, imagine the metronomes becoming synchronous with each other so that eventually they beat at the same tempo. Christian Huygens, a seventeenth-century Dutch scientist, recorded another instance of entrainment, that of two clocks hung next to each other, whose pendulums began to swing at identical rhythms. Why does this synchronization occur? According to Fritjof Capra, author of *The Tao of Physics*, "Rhythmic patterns appear throughout the universe, from the very small to the very large. Atoms are patterns of probability waves, molecules are vibrating structures, and living organisms manifest multiple, interdependent patterns of fluctuations. Plants, animals, and human beings undergo cycles of activity and rest, and all their physiological functions oscillate in rhythms of various periodicities."

Such findings affirm what the *rishis* knew thousands of years ago: We are immersed in an ocean of sound energy. The entrainment that Huygens observed supports the Vedic truth that we can attune our rhythms to those of nature, the universe, the primordial sound wave, or the One Consciousness, which is infinite and all-pervasive. Our natural condition is to exist in harmony with this One Consciousness. Sound in its many manifestations can help us get beyond our misperception that reality is fragmented, and restore our sense of unity with the universe.

When we are ill, we fall into a state of disharmony with the cosmos. This idea was eloquently articulated by Hazrat Inayat Khan, a highly respected musician in India who came to the United States in the early part of the twentieth century to spread the teachings of Sufism to the West. Sufism is an esoteric Islamic sect that places such great importance on chanting and deep breathing that it refers to sound and music, *ghiza-I-ruh,* as "food for the soul." In his great masterpiece, *The Music of Life,* Inayat Khan wrote, ". . . if the body has lost its rhythm, something goes wrong with the mind; if the mind has lost its rhythm, the body goes wrong; if the heart has lost its rhythm, the mind is puzzled; and if the rhythm of the soul is lost, then all is wrong."

How does this work? According to Vedic principles, harmonious sounds collect in the various *pranas* of the body. The 72,000 or so *nadis* or channels that exist in the body are all sensitive to sound, and function through vibrations. Therefore, good sounds increase the vitality of these *nadis.* *Pranas* that flow through them also become more charged with vigor. When the *pranas* are healthy and filled with vitality, they stimulate healthy tissue and organ activity, so that we achieve good health. Vital *prana* and harmonious sound work hand in hand. They travel through the mind like a great wave, revitalizing the brain cells and inspiring the mind to produce fluent, clear, harmonious thoughts.

Like the Vedic seers, Sufis believe that the universe is filled with "vibrations . . . too fine to be either audible or visible to the material ears or eyes." They called this unheard, subtle sound the *saut-e sarmad.* "Those who are able to hear the *saut-e sarmad* and meditate on it are relieved from all worries, anxieties, sorrows, fears, and diseases; and the soul is freed from captivity in the senses and in the physical body," wrote Inayat Khan. "Yogis and ascetics blow *sing* [a horn] or *shanka* [a shell], which awakens in them this inner tone. . . . The bells and gongs in the churches and temples are meant to suggest to the thinker the same sacred sound, and thus lead him towards the inner life."

Sound as a healing force is a cornerstone of all the great spirit traditions. In this chapter, I will describe dramatic examples of how chanting mantras—an ancient and highly venerated Vedic practice—can have lifesaving and life-enhancing effects, especially for people in the midst of severe illness or crisis. You will learn to use singing bowls, drums, and other musical instruments in calming, curative techniques, whose efficacy has recently been recognized and proven by Western clinical research.

## CHANTS FOR HEALING: MANTRAS AS MEDICINE

Fred stood at the end of a long line of people waiting to talk to me after a workshop I gave in Boulder on sound and healing. By the time he reached me, the room had completely emptied out. Nevertheless, he spoke in a low, hesitant voice, as if he were nervous that he might be overheard. He said he was an English professor at a local college and a longtime yoga student, and he'd felt increasingly drawn to the Vedic teachings. But his interest in Ayurveda had taken on a sense of urgency recently, because he was HIV-positive and had developed a persistent cough.

Fred was very thin and pale, and had indeed coughed frequently throughout the workshop. "I was diagnosed three years ago, but I was asymptomatic until about six months ago. Then I got this cough that just wouldn't quit," he said.

The cough worsened, and soon afterward, he was diagnosed with PCP, Pneumocystis carinii pneumonia, a type of pneumonia that is a common AIDS-related infection. Since then, he had lost about ten pounds and his appetite, he couldn't concentrate, and he felt weak and lethargic. His doctor had urged him to begin taking a whole menu of medications, but Fred was resistant to the idea. He had just finished reading my book on Ayurvedic healing through diet and other therapies, and he wanted a regimen that would help him strengthen his system without drugs.

Fred needed to bolster his weakened immune system on both the physical and spiritual levels. I urged him to eliminate meat, chicken, and fish from his diet and to eat whole grains and root vegetables, especially beets, ginger, and daikon (a variety of radish), but to avoid other spicy or oily foods. In addition to his daily yoga practice, I suggested that he spend some time each day chanting a series of Vedic mantras, which I'd recorded on tape to help him entrain his internal vibrations with the vibrations of the universe. Thus, the instrument that is our own voice combines with Sanskrit words to create a powerful healing force that revives our intuition, consciousness, and inner wisdom and restores our natural state of balance.

Fred was a highly motivated, enthusiastic student and had a well-developed, resonant voice—although that is certainly not a requirement for chanting. Over the course of the next several weeks, I spoke to him often by phone, and within a month, he was reporting that he was feeling much stronger. He had gained a few pounds, and the PCP had cleared up.

Based on my own experience with a life-threatening disease, I sensed that Fred was stretching himself in too many directions with work, yoga, and other social commitments, and not allowing enough time for reflection and recharging his energies. I therefore proposed that he spend some time alone, somewhere far enough away from Denver where he would have no distractions and could truly focus on his health and healing.

Fred reacted to my proposal as if he'd just been offered a wonderful gift. His body and spirit were crying out for a respite, but he was so cut off from his intuitive self that he hadn't been able to recognize this need on his own. A friend lent him a house in the nearby Rocky Mountains, and Fred left for a monthlong retreat.

It didn't take long for him to adjust to the slow, simple routine that I had suggested he follow: He chanted for two hours a day, one session in the morning, one session in the afternoon. After the morning chanting session, he cooked a pot of *kichadi*, made of mung bean, ghee, and rice, which is very nourishing, easy to digest, and good for cleansing the digestive system (see appendix 3 for *kichadi* recipe). Next, he would take a quiet, contemplative walk, after which he would write in his journal, jotting down whatever came up for him, including his feelings about being gay and his unhappiness about the emotional distance between himself and his parents. He napped whenever he felt tired, ate when he was hungry, and sat still for many hours, simply listening to the rich and varied sounds of nature.

We spoke by phone almost every day, and I could hear from the sound of Fred's voice, and from what he was telling me, that both his health and his spirits were improving. By the time he returned to Boulder, he was feeling much stronger and calmer, and more energetic, and optimistic than he had in a very long time about the possibility of surviving with AIDS. From that day on, he made a point of chanting every day, because he had come to believe, as I do, that chanting the mantras was the foundation of his recovery.

A year after we met, Fred had his T-cell numbers tested to determine the strength of his immune system. (In HIV-positive and AIDS patients, T-cell counts can be drastically low, an indicator of a highly compromised immune system and the potential for worsening health, including opportunistic infections.) Although he was still experiencing occasional bouts of AIDS-related ailments, his T-cell count had risen significantly. The following year, his T-cell count was even higher, though there was still a trace of the virus in his system. By the third year, he was absolutely asymptomatic, and there was no longer any sign of the virus in his bloodstream. While this is common today among HIV patients taking antiviral therapy that includes protease inhibitors, it is virtually unheard of among patients, such as Fred, who are taking no antivirals at all.

Six years later, Fred feels so well that I sometimes think he has forgotten he is HIV-positive! He has participated in the Wise Earth programs in North Carolina and now teaches classes at a yoga school in his area. He also leads workshops on different aspects of *sadhana*, including sound and Ayurvedic diet. Although he believes he has benefited tremendously by following the principles of Ayurvedic nutrition, he is absolutely convinced that chanting has been the single most important factor in his recovery. He has told me that his chanting practice is as much a part of his daily routine as brushing his teeth and eating breakfast. In fact, chanting has become so integrated into his spiritual and emotional life that whenever he experiences a particularly stressful moment, one or another of the chants immediately comes to mind and the feelings of stress subside. I have heard similar stories from many of my students. Chanting has become so deeply ingrained in their own consciousness that during moments of crisis or distress they automatically think of the chants.

All Vedic mantras are powerful, but the seven chants that Fred initially learned are especially meaningful because they incorporate the primary truths that should be the focus of our spiritual life. I teach them to all my Wise Earth students for the betterment of their health, and I have included them below, along with a brief explanation of what each one means, so that you can begin your own chanting practice. Do not take these chants for granted or allow them to become part of the background din of your daily routine. After you have been reciting them for some time, come back to these pages and reread the words. Chant them as if you were learning them for the first time, so that you can recapture the original sense of discovery about the sounds of the words as you articulate each syllable.

1. A mantra for cleansing the mind of negative thoughts and promoting a state of spiritual and emotional tranquility.

> *Bhadram no apivataya manah*
> (Baa-drahm no ahpi-vah-tie-a mah-nah-ha)
> May my mind be turned toward auspiciousness.

2. A prayer to Lord Shiva in the form of Rudra, to achieve freedom from disease and evoke the spirit of healing.

> *Tryambakam yajamahe*
> *Sugandhim pushti vardanam*
> *Urvarukamiva bandhanan*
> *Mrityor mokshiya ma'mritata*
> *Om Shanti Shanti Shantih*
> (Tree-yam-bah-kai yah-jah-mah-hay
> Su-gan-dim push-tee var-dah-nam
> Urvah-roo-kah-mee-vah ban-dhah-naan
> Mrit-yor-muk-shee-yah mah-amree-tah-aatah)
> *Om Shanti Shanti Shanti*
> We worship the fragrant three-eyed One
> Who confers ever-increasing prosperity.
> Let us be saved from the hold of death.
> Like a cucumber freed from its hold.
> Let us not turn away from liberation.

3. A prayer for self-knowledge and clarity, for global peace and harmony; to inspire universal truth and gain enlightenment.

> *Asato ma sad gamaya*
> *Tamaso ma jyotir gamaya*
> *Mrtyorma amritam gamaya*
> *Om Shanti Shanti Shantih*
> (Asah-tow-mah sad gah-mah-yah
> Tah-mah-so mah jyo-teer gah-mah-yah
> Mrit-yor-mah amrit-ahm gah-mah-yah)
> *Om Shanti Shanti Shanti*
> Lead me from unreal to real (through knowledge),
> From darkness (or ignorance) to light (knowledge),
> From death (limitations) to immortality
>     (liberation).

4. A prayer upon awakening for remembering our divinity; to maintain awareness of the sanctity of our limbs, by which we connect to the external world.

> *Karagre vasate Laksmih karamule Sarasvati*
> *Karamadhye tu Govindah prabhate karandarsanam*
> *Om Shanti Shanti Shantih*
> (Kah-rah-gray vah-say-tay laksh-me-he
> Kah-rah-moo-lay sah-ras-vah-tee
> Kah-rah-madh-yay too go-vin-dah-ha
> Prah-bhah-tay kah-rah-dar-shah-nam)
> *Om Shanti Shanti Shanti*
> On the tip of my fingers is Goddess Lakshmi,
> On the base of my fingers is Goddess Saraswati,
> In the middle of my fingers is Lord Govinda.
> In this manner, I look at my palms.

5. A prayer for self-knowledge, and recognition that all things come from the One; to evoke the spirit of wholeness in all things.

*Purnamadah purnamidam purnat*
*Purnamudachyate*
*Purṇasya purnamadaya*
*Purnamevavashishyate*
*Om Shanti Shanti Shantih*
(Poor-nah-mah-daf poor-nah-me-dam poor-nahat
Poor-nah-moo-datch-yah-tay
Poor-nas-yah poor-nah-mah-dah-yah
Poor-nah-may-vah-vah-shish-yah-tay)
*Om Shanti Shanti Shanti*
That is whole; this is whole.
From the whole, this whole came.
Remove this whole from that whole,
What remains is still whole.

6. A prayer to the Divine for peace and harmony with our teachers; to invoke peace within the self and to dissolve mistrust of our self and fear of authority figures.

*Saha navavatu*
*Saha nau bhunaktu*
*Saha viryam karavavahai*
*Tejasvinavadhitamastu ma vidvishavahi*
*Om Shanti Shanti Shantih*
(Sah-ha nah-vah-vah-tu
Sah-ha now bhuh-nak-tu
Sah-ha veer-yam kah-rah-vah-vah-hai
Tey-jas-veena-vadhee-tah-mas-tu mah vid-vee-sha-vah-hai-ee)
*Om Shanti Shanti Shanti*

May He protect us both.

May He nourish us.

May we acquire the capacity (to study and understand the scriptures).

May our studies be brilliant.

May we not cavil at each other.


7. A prayer of gratitude to the Giver of Consciousness for food, life force, and all things.

*Brahmarpanam Brahma havih*
*Brahmagnau Brahmana hutam*
*Brahmaiva tena gantavyam*
*Brahmakarma samadhina*
*Om Shanti Shanti Shantih*
(Bhram-haar-pah-nam
Bhrah-mah hah-ve-he
Bhram-haag-now bhrah-mah-nah hu-tam
Bhram-ayva tena gan-tav-yam
Bhrah-mah-kar-ma samaah-dhee-nah)
*Om Shanti Shanti Shanti*
Brahman is the offering.
Brahman is the oblation.
Poured out by Brahman into the fire of Brahman.
Brahman is to be attained by the one who contemplates the action of Brahman.
(Brahman refers to Pure Consciousness.)


Not long ago I met Anna, a fourteen-year-old girl who had been diagnosed with anorexia. Anna said that her reason for not eating was that voices in her head were ordering her not to touch a morsel of food, or else she would be severely punished. I taught her parents the various food *sadhanas* that you will learn in greater detail in the next section, because many people with eating disorders have responded positively to them.

Anna, however, did not improve as we had hoped. She steadfastly refused to eat anything but the most minute portions of food and continued to lose weight at an alarming rate. As I meditated one day, I realized that she needed to be bathed in the sounds of Vedic chants. I recorded a powerful chant for her that evokes the Divine Mother's presence— *Lalita Sahasranama,* a thousand names of the Mother. Anna's parents later described to me her reaction the first time they played the tape in her presence: She suddenly became very quiet, and her expression became fixed, almost as if she were in a trance. As soon as the tape ended, she asked her mother to play it again. "I love the voice. I love the music," she said.

She listened to the tape repeatedly throughout the next week. Then, she announced, "The voices are gone. I don't hear them anymore. All I hear is the voice of the chants." Anna is now eating normally and is on her way to recovery.

We should not underestimate the power of such chants to balance our internal bodily functions and to harmonize our inner selves with our universe. As David Simon, M.D., points out in his book, *The Wisdom of Healing,* the word enchantment "refers to the magic of sound that leads to oneness; enchantment literally means 'one through chanting.' " Simon also refers to the physiological effects of chanting, noting that chants are chemically metabolized into brain chemicals known as opiates; they are as powerful as narcotic drugs without being damaging to one's health. Indeed, these opiates—the most well-known type is the endorphin—often promote healing in the body. Such is the power of sound: it can heal us and teach us to heal ourselves.

When I perform my daily chanting *sadhana*, I identify with the eloquent words of Rabindranath Tagore, the renowned Indian writer and Nobel Prize winner who wrote:

> *When Thou commandest me to sing . . . all that is harsh and*
> *dissonant in my life melts into one sweet harmony . . .*

Resting in the vibrations of my practice of sound, I feel as if the Mother takes pleasure in my singing. I can feel my voice merge with her energy. I become the sound, and the sound becomes all that is. The energy of the sound takes my mind and consciousness as far as the sound waves themselves travel. They restore and heal me daily.

## MUSIC FOR HEALING

Raga was the first and most advanced system of music known to the earth and is said to have come directly from Shiva, who taught this eternal form of music to the *rishis*. According to Vedic thinking, raga emulates the mystic rhythms of cosmic sound. A complex group of sounds and musical scales are used to evoke a particular emotional state.

Ravi Shankar, one of India's best-known classical musicians, eloquently expressed this idea in his autobiography, *My Music—My Life:* "Our tradition teaches that sound is God—*Nada Brahma*. That is, musical sound and the musical experience are preparatory steps to the realization of the self. We view music as a kind of spiritual discipline that raises one's inner being to divine peacefulness and bliss. . . . The highest aim of our music is to reveal the essence of the universe it reflects, and the ragas are among the means by which this essence can be apprehended."

The Vedic text *Sangita Darpana* informs us that the ragas represent the full gamut of human experience. The five primary forms of raga sprang from the five heads of Shiva: four ragas came from the four directions, and the fifth raga came from the head that was turned toward the heavens. A sixth raga emerged from Parvati, Shiva's consort.

Each of the six primary ragas represents a season and is traditionally performed at the appropriate time of the year. The ragas and their corresponding seasons are:

> *hindle*—spring
> *dipak*—summer
> *megha*—early fall
> *bhairava*—autumn
> *sri*—early winter
> *malkauns*—late winter

The *rishis* gave us this definition for raga: "That which colors the spirit is a raga." According to Vedic thought, every raga has existed since the time of transmission from Shiva; thus, musicians who are said to have composed ragas, in actuality discovered a particular musical piece that was already known to the universe. Ragas have been used for healing throughout the centuries by Indian physicians, and many stories are told about the power of raga to change the course of nature, enchant wild animals, and cure plagues:

- During the medieval period (the eleventh century to the eighteenth C.E.), the *"Mradang* Raga" and the *"Pakhavaj* Raga" were played to make the elephants dance. Deer hunters played the *"Todi* Raga," and their intoxicated prey would willingly approach them.
- Tansen, a great Indian composer of the sixteenth century, was a court musician for Emperor Akbar. Tansen composed

and sang the "*Megha* Raga" (raga of the clouds), consisting of mainly guttural sounds. While he was singing, the heavens opened with torrential rains to drive away the drought and famine. This same raga is said to have cured pestilence during Emperor Akbar's reign.

• Tansen also composed the now-extinct mystic "Raga *Dipak*" (raga of light). So powerful was Tansen's rendition of this raga that nature raged out of control. The winds began to howl, and fire destroyed the emperor's palace. No singer or composer has since dared to perform this raga.

• In his book *Nada Brahma,* the late Joachim-Ernst Berendt, one of Europe's preeminent jazz musicians and composers, carefully examined and explicated the idea that the world is sound. Berendt wrote, "It is said that some [great musicians and saint-musicians] could light fires or the oil lamps by singing one raga; or bring rain, melt stones, cause flowers to blossom, and attract ferocious wild animals—even snakes and tigers—to a peaceful, quiet circle in a forest around a singing musician."

The Vedic seers and other spiritual leaders of the world's wisdom traditions intuitively understood and embraced the healing potential of chanting. Within the Judeo-Christian tradition, we have only to read the Book of Samuel, in the Old Testament, which tells the story of King Saul, who was plagued by "an evil spirit from the Lord." A young shepherd by the name of David, famous for his musicianship, was summoned to play for the king. David "took a harp and played with his hand so Saul was refreshed and was well, and the evil spirit departed from him." (1 Sam. 16:23)

Alfred Tomatis is a French physician who has been called "the Einstein of sound" because of his groundbreaking research and clinical work in the field of healing sound and hearing. In an 1986 interview that was published in *Music-*

*works 35, The Canadian Journal of Sound Exploration,* Tomatis talks of being summoned in the late 1960s for a consultation at a Benedictine monastery in the south of France, where many of the monks were suffering from a mysterious ailment that left them enervated and exhausted. Tomatis described their condition thusly: "Seventy of the ninety monks were slumping in their cells like wet dishrags." After taking their medical histories, he arrived at a simple yet startling conclusion as to the source of the problem. The monks had been accustomed to singing Gregorian chants six to eight hours a day. But because of the reforms authorized by Vatican II in the mid-sixties, the number of hours the brothers spent chanting had been greatly curtailed. Tomatis theorized that the chanting had energized the monks by "awakening the field of [their] consciousness." He urged them to resume their previous chanting schedule. Within five months, the monks were all fully recovered from their puzzling malaise.

Tomatis characterized the Gregorian chants, which require that the singer take long, slow breaths, as "fantastic energy food." The monks were nourishing their bodies and spirits with every note they sang. Is it any wonder, then, that they felt so tired and sapped of vitality when deprived of their accustomed source of energy?

Some years ago, I visited a man in a hospital named Jeff. An architect who was dying of a brain tumor, Jeff was so ill that he couldn't tolerate any food or medication. He weighed only seventy pounds. I held his hand carefully, because sometimes a person that fragile cannot bear even to be touched, and began to chant. He had looked so wan and sad when I first came into his room, but as I sang, he began to smile. "Chant again," he kept telling me, each time I stopped.

I chanted the same mantra over and over again for about an hour. When I finally left the room, Jeff was smiling, and I could feel that his spirits had risen considerably. At his wife's request, I made a tape for him to play in his hospital room. She called me about a week later to report that he had started to eat, and that he was able to keep the food down.

Jeff listened to the tape every day for a month, for many hours, and was able to eat enough that he gained twenty pounds. His doctor could give him no further treatment to stop the progression of the cancer but felt that Jeff was strong enough to be discharged from the hospital. Jeff's house, which he had designed himself, was perched on a cliff overlooking a verdant plain that stretched toward the Pacific Ocean. Jeff's wife, Laura, told me that every morning she and Jeff would sit out on the deck and chant the mantras they had learned from the three tapes I had given them. Toward the end of his life, Jeff was in considerable physical pain, but his mind and spirit were at ease. He died two years after I'd visited him in the hospital, and after his death, Laura told me that those were the two happiest years of their marriage. In the last moments of his life, she said, he asked her to play all three tapes very loudly, all at the same time. Then he asked her to turn down the volume and said, "Tell Bri. Maya that her voice will always be with me."

I was deeply moved when Laura told me that those were among Jeff's last words to her. I feel blessed to have been included in the dying thoughts of this dear man, and grateful to the Divine Mother whose guidance allowed me to enrich his final months and moments.

Each of us holds a unique inner melody that responds to song, rhythm, and music. However, as we grow up and are consumed by our everyday routines, we tend to move away from this profound source of healing. You may look to revive this precious pastime—the medicine of the soul—which costs so little. Music restores the body's immunity and brings us into alliance with our spirit rhythms. Practice regularly to recall your inner melody and resonate with universal harmony.

## BRACING THE SPIRIT WITH NATURE'S RICH MELODIES

I live in a small hut in the Smoky Mountains, surrounded by lush green meadows and pastures. A large herd of cows grazes in the nearby fields, and I often watch them from my porch as I sing the Vedic chants and play my frame drum and Himalayan singing bowls. When I begin to chant, the cows stop chewing their cud and join in a chorus with me. The farmer who owns the herd is convinced that since my arrival in this valley five years ago, the cows produce double the amount of milk, and the milk tastes noticeably sweeter. I have also noticed that the deer and the bucks regularly emerge into the open pasture, stand in one spot as though transfixed, and listen to my chanting. The crows also seem to want to emulate my sounds, trying to produce a more melodious sound than their usual *ka ka*.

The music of nature exists to remind all life-forms of their profound connection to the primordial sound. We can discern the music of the celestial sphere and our own inner sound by listening to nature's elements and her animals. Each form of natural sound has a specific bearing on the health of every creature. The gurgling of a brook enhances our sensual vibrancy. The fluttering sound of a bird's wings ignites delicate emotions within the heart. The swishing sounds of golden corn or wheat swaying in the breeze encourages *prana* to flow freely, awakening the deep resonance of our soul.

The more deeply based in nature the sound is, the finer its

harmonic resonance. Whether we are talking about the trickling of a stream, the whooshing of the wind, the clapping of
thunder, the plopping of fat raindrops, the chirping of birds,
the splashing of waves, or the silence of a still afternoon,
every natural sound serves to enhance our internal melody.

Even those sounds that generally give rise to fear—like the
roar of a tiger or the hissing of a snake—produce a harmonic
resonance within our body, because they are a dynamic part
of the universe's sound. If our mind is clouded by fear, we
may not be able to recognize the harmonic response that all
natural sounds evoke within us. Once we have conquered
our fear, however, we are more likely to experience the grand
lift of spirit in the presence of nature's awesome sounds.

Cathy, a family friend and professional chef, has a deep
love for animals. She cares for a large, thriving family of
goats, pigs, dogs, cats, horses, ducks, and geese on her organic farm in North Carolina. Her animal haven started years
ago when she began to take in, and care for, abused animals.
One such animal was Henry, a potbellied pig. Henry was so
severely malnourished that Cathy created a space for him
inside her house and cooked him sumptuous meals. Soon
Henry regained his vitality and took to following Cathy
wherever she went on the farm.

Henry loves food more than anything else in the world—
or so I thought until the day I sat down on Cathy's porch and
began to chant *Om Namah Shivaya*. Henry, who had been
feasting on yet another mammoth meal, galloped outside
and planted himself in front of me. As he wagged his tail,
keeping rhythm with the beat, I called for Cathy to come
join me. She added her voice to mine, and the louder we
chanted, the more vigorously Henry shook his tail. Inspired
by his passion, Cathy and I started dancing in time to our
chanting. Henry jumped right in, gleefully leaping around in
circles. Ever since then, Henry has been an enthusiastic

dancer who wags his tail whenever he sees me coming. His favorite chant remains *Om Namah Shivaya*.

You only have to listen to nature in order to experience the harmonies and rhythms of the universe. Perhaps you only need to step outside into your yard or a city park. If you cannot travel to the countryside often, here are some examples to remind you of the sounds of the seasons.

### The Practice: Harmonizing Inner Rhythms with Nature's Sound

In spring: the gurgling of the streams; the *bhrung, bhrung, bhrung* of the earth.

In summer: the stillness of the morning air; the *shwee, shwee, shwee* of the wind in the trees.

In early fall: the trickling of the raindrops; the *plop, plop, plop* of water into mud.

In autumn: the rustling of the leaves; the *shoo, shoo, shoo* of the harvest.

In early winter: the *hrum, hrum, hrum* from the scurrying and preparation for winter.

In late winter: the *krunck, krunck, krunck* from crackling branches under the snow.

Seize every chance to fill your heart and open your spirit to the inner universe within, wherein you will discover all of nature.

### The Practice: Nature's Meditation

Sit in a meditative posture during the mellow time of dusk. Visualize yourself on top of a mountain and listen to the music of the galaxies. See a butterfly. Listen to the fluttering sound of its wings and recapture the gentleness of your heart. You are standing on the shores of the ocean. Revive your energy from the splashing sound of the waves. A flock of squawking seagulls fly overhead.

Find yourself enjoying the quiet *aah* of the full moon and feel your *shakti-prana* move within you. It's winter, a deer is running through the underbrush. You can hear the crackling of the branches under the snow.

Now, you are sitting by a gurgling brook. Feel your *shiva* and *shakti* energies merging within and without. The light has turned golden. It is dusk. You are walking in a wheat field, listening to the rustling of autumnal leaves. Follow the quiet flow of your breath as you revel in your own sonorous spirit of being. Know that the center of the universe is within you.

## FEASTING THE SPIRIT WITH SONG

We all are inherently musicians who play the sacred rhythms of life and spirit. We need only to find the sound practice that suits us best. Drumming is an especially excellent *sadhana* for women because the original drummers of the universe were the goddesses. Drumming awakens the *shakti* energy and nourishes the womb, as master drummer Layne Redmond documents in her inspiring history, *When the Drummers Were Women.* A *Phardhans* folk song of India eloquently expresses this very idea: "My Singer, from the earthen drum, what sweet music you bring, from the earthen drum of my body."

Like the goddess Durga who played the rattle drum, the Greek goddess Cybele whose instrument was the hoop or frame drum, or the Egyptian goddess Sekhmet, who also carried the frame drum, you may reclaim your birthright as a sacred musician. Even if you are not ready to drum and make music yourself, you may choose to listen to the ancient, rhythmic sounds, and wrap yourself in their magnificent harmonies.

Aside from the voice, the first musical instrument known

to the earth was the divine flute. Depicted as the musical instrument of the cowherd god, Krishna, the flute is said to be the most powerful instrument because it is an extension of the human voice. Vedic lore says that through playing his divine flute, Krishna enraptured the hearts of a vast community of *gopis*, female cowherds, and led them into absolute consciousness.

I frequently use Himalayan singing bowls (often known as Tibetan singing bowls, although they originated in the Vedic lands)—which have an uncanny vibratory power—for healing rituals. You can also play these bowls, as you chant. Bowl sounds mimic the energetic waves of the mind. Listening to the otherworldly sounds produced by the bowls is among the most effective ways I know to clear the mind, and I use them almost every day in my own personal practice. I invariably begin my meditation by playing my bowl, circling its rim with a mallet twelve or more times, so that I feel as if I am being bathed in the vibrations. I typically use the singing bowls to work with women who are confronting traumas in the present or the past, such as an abusive relationship or an abortion. The bowl-centered meditations and ceremonies we develop enable women to be released from their fear, guilt, anger, or anxiety. For example, a woman, dressed all in white, the color of the compassionate goddess, Saraswati, might position herself in the squatting posture (see pages 104–105) as she plays the singing bowl while utilizing a particular breath practice for the *shakti-prana*. We evoke Saraswati to restore our regenerative and creative energies. I might also mix herbs for her, placing a mixture of Ayurvedic botanicals into a smaller bowl within my bowl; the sound vibrations render the herbs extremely potent, from an energetic perspective.

I use other instruments as well, including a particular type of xylophone that is supported by three small gourds; a round frame drum, about ten inches in diameter, that has a flat skin stretched across the top; a *dholak*, which is a traditional North Indian drum; and a small kettledrum called a *damaru*. Many of the tones they produce are specific to the seven chakras. These instruments are still widely used in the major forms of Vedic worship by singers who accompany dancers with their chants and songs.

I encourage my students to buy bowls, drums, or bells for their own use at home. You should be able to buy your own singing bowl in stores that specialize in Himilayan, Tibetan, or other Eastern cultural artifacts. You can also order bowls, bells, and other such instruments from the stores and catalogs in the resources section on page 398.

To play your singing bowl, you should sit cross-legged on the floor or brace yourself against the wall. Or, if you choose to sit in an upright chair, place the bowl in your lap, although it will not then have the same resonance as when it's sitting on the floor or ground. The ideal way to play singing bowls is to place them on the earth; the resonant tones are deeper and last much longer. You will, however, need to place a doughnut-shaped pad around the bottom of the bowl, so that the bowl sits near to the ground but does not move around while you play it.

It was said of Brahma, the Creator: "He meditated a hundred thousand years, and the result of his meditation was the creation of sound and music." Those who embrace the path of meditation are enhancing their practice through varieties of sound and music, including those they create themselves with their voices and with all manner of beautiful instruments. They are creating rituals of meaning and substance that help them to connect with the Divine Mother, and to heal themselves on deepening levels of consciousness. I invite you to join this *sadhana* of sound, music, and voice, the oldest and most profound form of healing known to humankind.

## MUSICAL HEALING
## BY AYURVEDIC TYPE

Each one of us has a unique connection to sound and music, a relationship that is linked to the physical and spiritual elements of which we are made. The ancient Ayurvedic medicine and science of health and healing describes three body types—*vata*, *pitta*, and *kapha*—that govern all of our physiological and psychological functions, and thus comprise each individual's constitution. For a discussion about the Ayurvedic system for determining your metabolic type and conditions relating to each type, refer to the metabolic type chart on page 276. Once you have determined your particular *dosha*, or metabolic type, you can follow the guidelines below to select the kind of music that is best suited to you.

Whatever your *dosha*, you may choose from Vedic chants, Indian ragas, invocations of native cultures, European classical music, or any other form of rhythmic sound that appeals to you. Here is a brief description of the musical tones and instruments best suited to your metabolic type:

**Music for *Vata* Type:** Soft music with low, mellow tones.
**Instruments:** vocals; stringed instruments such as sitar, vina, and tambouri (three of India's oldest stringed instruments); guitar, mandolin, bass, and violin; wind instruments such as chimes, didgeridoo (one of the oldest-known wind instruments in the world, dating back some 40,000 years to the Aboriginal culture), Incan panpipes; all drums and

percussion instruments; Himalayan singing bowls; keyboard instruments such as piano and harmonium.

**Music for *Pitta* Type:** Soft music with rhythmic middle tones.

**Instruments:** vocals; reed instruments such as flute, clarinet, and saxophone; mouth organ; stringed instruments such as violin, dulcimer, and mandolin; keyboard instruments such as piano and harmonium; all types of percussion instruments including gentle drums; Himalayan singing bowls; wind instruments such as the accordion and Scottish bagpipes.

**Music for *Kapha* Type:** Energizing music with higher tones and solid bass.

**Instruments:** vocals; all types of drums, such as the Indian *dholak* and tabla, African congo, and water drum; all types of keyboard instruments such as electric keyboard, piano, and harmonium; percussion instruments such as Himalayan bowls, bells, and chimes; wind instruments such as didgeridoo, Incan panpipes, and accordion.

# Chapter 10

## THE INNER SOUND OF THE HUMAN VOICE

*All that God does shall win our praise.*
*We magnify His name with hymns,*
*Seeking beneficence from the Mighty.*
—*Rig Veda* (1.42.10)

Each one of us possesses a unique inner sound, a melody informed by the memories of our individual journey through the cosmos. Through cultivating our inner sound, we can experience our deepest spiritual healing. In this chapter, I will tell you how I came to discover my own inner sound and help you to find yours, which is an important step on the path of practice.

*Sadhana* holds a paradoxical truth: In order to awaken our inner sound, we engage in spiritual practices that facilitate the discovery of our inner silence, a kind of dynamic stillness. Twenty-one years after my journey with cancer, I returned to the Himalayas to enter a five-month period of silence. I extracted myself from the world, even from my teachings of *sadhana*. My intention was to complete my surrender to the Divine. Through meditation, I also inquired into the nature of my own inner vibratory world of sound, and its relationship to the primordial sound that supports all of life. As I sat in the lap of the sacred, I reclaimed the sacred in myself.

My sitting was done in a small flat, across from the Agni Temple in Katmandu, Nepal. Throughout the five months that I spent there, I marveled at the exquisite vibrations of the Himalayas, where one can still feel the presence of the gods and seers. But in that holy land, the dissonance of human poverty, grief, and corruption also resound, particularly in the cities at the feet of these celestial mountains. My powers of awareness grew rapidly as I lived there in the silence.

I spent many hours in meditation. I also went on long and vigorous walks through the marketplaces, fields, hills, and temples. One day, I went to visit a Krishna temple in the foothills. I trekked across green rice fields, which were alive with the spirit of Krishna and the *gopis*, the young female cowherds whom he entranced by his rapturous presence.

The shimmering light of the noonday sun seemed to dance in concert with the wind sweeping across the vast fields. I heard a faint melody reverberating through the grass—the song of Krishna's flute! The blades of grain took on the dancing posture of the slender Krishna, and soon there were hundreds of Krishnas bending and swaying before me. The grazing cows, their lotus eyes transfixed in a steady gaze, seemed to behold the same vision and hear the same song.

In the ensuing days, that melody took form and shape and grew more resonant within me. It began with the musical refrain of Krishna's flute and quickly escalated into a symphony of high-pitched stringed instruments. By the fifth day, it crescendoed into gentle, repetitive staccato invocations of the *bija* mantras, which sounded extraordinarily poignant, as though they were being chanted by a thousand androgynous voices. (The melody and style in which I have since taught the *bija* mantras came as a direct result of what I heard during this retreat.)

The sounds were symphonic, larger than life, but predominantly without volume. They filled my head, yet they were gentle, almost a whisper at times. They appeared to have arisen from within my mind, enveloping my entire being. I was swathed and nurtured by these celestial melodies for days. Still, today, this same musical refrain will often appear in my mind, my own inner song that comes from the memory of my entire history. I know this particular melody is my very own unique inner song.

As this musical silence within me grew louder, a wondrous peacefulness pervaded my spirit. That tranquility brought forth a deep longing that no finite, mortal pleasure could possibly fill, and I found myself reflecting on my past. The words of Kalidasa (one of India's greatest Sanskrit poets who wrote in the fourth century) came to mind: "How the fragment of melody or the fragrance of a flower will evoke forgotten memories, filling the soul with sadness, as though vague remembrances from other lives are passing over the spirit." This sadness was not a longing to go back, but a recognition that I was navigating yet another turn in the river that was my life.

Entering silence, I also entered into my heart—what the Vedas would call "the cave of the heart"—and recognized the seamless union that prevails between the self and the Divine. In that solitude, God spoke within me and reaffirmed that healing and wholeness are possible when we discover the inner sound that lies within our hearts.

When I emerged from my silence, I felt joy and lightness but also a physical ache. The pain was a natural response to witnessing old memories of many lifetimes. The observance of silence awakens our inner sound, unearths ancestral memories, and empties our hearts of wounded memories so that we can heal.

Silence is the path to the center of our inner world. As we grow into silence, we go beyond imagination, intellectual fluctuations, and individual being. The realm we enter is formless and wordless. It is the state of enlightenment that the Vedas call *samadhi*—complete meditative absorption that lies beyond the spiritual states of contemplation, concentration, and meditation. In *samadhi* we are immersed in the state of complete inner silence. We enter the nonstate of undifferentiated consciousness.

We must practice inner silence to understand the essence of the *sadhana* of sound. Only silence can ultimately sustain the inner song. Only in silence can we find the center of the universe within ourselves. The voice of the Divine is our inner sound, aroused through silence. As Tagore said so eloquently, "If thou speaketh not, my Lord, I shall fill my heart with thy silence."

Our deepest wounds and bonds are inevitably revealed when we examine our hearts. While sitting in silence, I was finally able to relinquish my ties to my father, realizing that my heart would not be whole until I finally ceased to mourn his absence. By freeing myself of this grief, I felt a shift throughout my being and a new consciousness of my inner vibratory field that has sustained me ever since.

Cultivating your inner song is not something I can teach you with a simple set of how-to instructions. Instead, I teach my students how to enter that same deep silence, preferably while in extended retreat. Do not begin to meditate with the intention of uncovering your inner song. Rather, from the intention of entering silence completely, keep your mind and heart open to your inner ear. Silence is the container of sound, and in time, your unique sound—be it a series of tones, a melody, the fragment of a chant—will naturally arise. Later in this chapter, I will talk about specific mantras that are linked to the seven chakras. You can use these practices to tap into the vast potential of your voice to retrieve the sounds you were born with, sounds as uniquely yours as your fingerprints. You may use some of these methods to discover your inner sound, but it is often found arising in that silence, with no particular technique other than an opening consciousness that often comes from the absence of speech and human interaction.

## THE SOUNDS OF SILENCE

When you allow your inner sound to arise during your practice of silence, do not decide in advance what sounds will come or what form they will take. Be open in heart and mind to what comes to you. In the case of one woman, the sounds that arose were strongly associated with memories, and conveyed an important message that she would not otherwise have heard.

Marion, an eighty-year-old Danish woman, had lived in the United States for many years. Although generally in very good health, she kept falling down and breaking her hip, so that finally, she had to have hip-replacement surgery. While in the hospital, she was given a book about meditation. She found the subject so interesting that she decided to take a two-week, intensive, silent Vipassana meditation course at a well-known yoga center, as soon as she was recovered enough to travel.

Soon after she returned from the yoga center, she attended a workshop I was giving on sound *sadhanas*. During one of the breaks, she hurried up to the front of the room, shook my hand, and said, "I thought perhaps you could help me, because for a long time, I've felt tired of living. But I have a very strong constitution. Maybe I keep falling because I'm hoping that one of these days I won't ever get up again."

You can imagine how distressing it was to hear this wonderfully bright, articulate person matter-of-factly express such sad emotions. A former United Nations attaché whose intellect and vigor had not been diminished by age, she was obviously a powerhouse. "You can't go until your time is right. Your mind is too powerful, so don't keep falling down and breaking your hips because that's going to be too painful," I said firmly. "Now why did you come to this particular workshop?"

"Because I've been feeling so empty and lonely after the Vipassana meditation," she confided.

"All that silence is exactly what brought you to the sound," I reassured her. I asked her to tell me more about the meditation experience.

"It was the most wretched thing I've ever done," she said unequivocally. "The first day I was fidgety and antsy. I couldn't sit, so I left and I walked around the grounds."

"What was your mind telling you?"

"It was very angry. I kept hearing a voice that said, 'I just broke my hip, I don't want to sit, it hurts my back. This is not for me.' I kept feeling that I didn't want to live."

I nodded my head in sympathy and agreement. All those days of undirected silent meditation were probably too demanding a regimen for an elderly woman who was already having doubts about the meaning of her life.

"The next day I decided to try sitting again. What kept coming into my mind was that I hadn't been back to Copenhagen in ten years, and how much I miss it." In meditation, what had come to Marion most powerfully were the sounds of her native land.

"So you gained at least one gem of remembrance from sitting in silence," I said. "Tell me a little about Copenhagen."

"Have you ever been there in the spring? I miss the sounds of the city, and the smell of the wildflowers . . . a sea of wildflowers . . . no place is more beautiful than Copenhagen in the springtime. The streams sparkle with crystal waters because the snow has just melted."

"Why have you stayed away so long?" I asked.

"The family situation is very difficult. This one is ill, that one is drinking, this one is fighting with that one, and all of my relatives get insulted if I don't spend time with each and every one of them. And when I do go to visit, they get upset if I don't take sides in their arguments. There's so much conflict, so many obligations. It's terribly hurtful and draining."

It was clear to me that she needed to reconnect with her roots—with the familiar sensory experiences that had nourished her as a child and were part of her heritage. The silence of meditation, painful though it had been, had helped her discover the wounds in her heart and spirit. The loneliness she had found lodged there had led her to sound, and its remarkable healing powers.

"Marion, get on a plane, and go back home," I instructed her. "Spend the spring in Denmark. That is what you're lonely for—the smells and sounds of home. Take good care of yourself, even it makes you feel selfish! See the people you want to see, ignore the others. Make this trip for yourself and nobody else."

Tears filled her blue eyes. I could feel her spirit lighten, as if she had been longing to hear the very words I had spoken, words of permission that she had not been able to give to herself. Throughout the rest of the workshop, I could hear Marion's sweet voice, with its lilting Scandinavian accent, chanting the mantras, resonating in harmony with the vibrations of her soul.

I received a lovely letter from her a couple of months later in which she described her trip to Denmark. Following my advice, she had limited her time with family members and friends. She had spent hours walking around the city and traveling into the surrounding countryside, taking in the sights as if through the fresh eyes of a tourist. She visited castles, climbing the stairs to the turrets, and strolled along riverbanks that she remembered from childhood. She even went horseback riding at a favorite farm where her family had spent several summer holidays. She felt wonderful, she said, rejuvenated and refreshed. "No more falling, Bri. Maya," she wrote. "Certainly not on purpose!"

## CREATING YOUR OWN SILENT RETREAT

There is no silence other than the silence of the mind. Given all the pressures and demands we face each day, how do we make time in our lives to enter the profound inner silence that unites us with the universal greater consciousness? A daily meditation practice is the foundation upon which we build a quiet mind and equanimity that helps us in everyday life. But as I discovered during my stay in Nepal, a retreat into silence can reveal opportunities for healing, self-awareness, and deeper spiritual awareness that are normally hidden by the clatter of daily life. In order to approach that state of tranquility through extended silence, I periodically set aside time—a week to ten days, if possible—to engage in a silent retreat. You may want to begin with a morning or evening, or a weekend.

Although I am a monk, I play many roles—spiritual teacher, healer, author, lecturer, gardener, and student, to name a few. In short, like you, I have a very full life that requires some planning and rearranging so that I can withdraw into silence. I begin my preparations by tidying up my living space. I clean my altars, respond to the many inquiries for spiritual and health assistance, put away my files, sort through loose papers that may be lying around, and prepare for my frequent travels. Silence is about resting the mind as much as resting the mouth. So I want to eliminate anything that will distract my thoughts, anything left undone or unfinished to which my mind can attach.

Once I enter into silence, I sit in meditation for six or

seven hours at a stretch. When my body gets tired, however, I stand up and stretch. When my belly feels hungry, I prepare myself the simplest of meals—a pot of *kichadi*, a delicious mixture of grain and beans (see recipe on page 374), and perhaps some greens that I pick from my garden. I minimize physical activity, although I do take a short walk every day, because if my mind is preoccupied with a thought or feeling, the walking meditation will help to dissolve it.

I look at the deer grazing in the fields and the hawks flying overhead. I notice the green grass, the buds coming up in the fields, the river flowing lower than normal this year. I take in the sights and sounds of nature all around me, but I do not hold on to the perceptions. My mind observes, then moves on. I leave the river where it is, I leave the fields where they are, I leave the cows as they are. I do not take them with me when I return to sit in my cabin.

My mind becomes immersed in the realm of consciousness that is thought without thoughts. Sometimes I see visions or lights, other times I experience absolute tranquility. There is no pushing or doing. I am simply there, simply present.

How do you make room in your own busy life for a retreat? If your schedule is as full as those of the women and men I meet during my travels, chances are you would be hard-pressed to find time to spend a day in silence, let alone a week, especially if you are a parent. If you have a responsibility to your family and your husband's schedule does not allow for him to care for the children so that you can spend some hours alone, in silence, try to find a community of like-minded women within your larger community who are willing to trade for one day (or even an afternoon) a month.

Once you have emptied your calendar of all your responsibilities, you may be tempted to read, write letters, or pay bills. Instead, see how it feels to take yourself on a picnic in the country or at a park, or spend a long time soaking in a bath. Practice *sadhanas*: meditate, do breathing exercises, play the drums, grind spices, take a hike into nature and do some yoga poses. Practice being with yourself in silence. Notice and detach. Begin to heal your heart.

## THE MYSTIC SOUND WITHIN YOU

As you uncover your inner sound, you also recognize the importance of giving voice to that sound. The Vedic ancients revealed that the vibration of cosmic sound is contained within our deepest self through the medium of the human voice. The origin of speech, the *Rig Veda* tells us, may be traced back to the Goddess Vac, who is called the Mother of the Vedas. Vac is depicted as having four *pada* (feet), or aspects, one of which is the force of rhythmic speech. The *rishis* also inform us that the rhythmic speech of the human voice was the first life-generating sound *sadhana*. Saraswati, the river goddess, absorbed Vac's qualities and imparted her knowledge of speech, art, literature, and music to the celestial musicians and dancers. These divinities taught the "act of song" to the great sages—Bharata, Hanuman, Narada, and others— who advocated that we humans use rhythmic speech and music to transcend the physical and mental planes.

Bharata tells us that the human voice was the first musical instrument in the universe. Tala, an ancient sequence of sounds that symbolizes the evolutionary cycles of birth, growth, transformation, dissolution, and death, replicates the tempo of the human voice. The ragas of Indian classical music are derived from tala, which was created around a single axial note to emulate the variations-on-a-single-note theme of human speech. Its free-flowing form has a nourishing and calming effect on the mind, because its music reflects the transcendent vibrations of human sound.

It is said in the Vedas that the ultimate journey of every soul in the universe is to gain liberation through self-knowledge from the cycles of rebirths and to recognize that individually, separately, and together we are One with Pure Consciousness. I took my vows as a *brahmacharini* in the ancient Advaita Vedanta tradition of my ancestors in preparation for that infinite and final freedom. But you do not have to choose a monastic life in order to nourish and repair the sanctity of the heart. You need only safeguard your inner sound and walk the path that belongs to you.

As I have emphasized, the way to your inner sound is first to sit in silence. You may initially enter into this process through the practice of *shanti* mudra, the hand gesture for peace and tranquility, which will deepen and replenish your inner silence. This simple practice can be done anywhere and at any time.

### The Practice: *Shanti* Mudra for Inner Silence

Facing north, sit in the yoga mudra posture or in a meditative pose. Rest your hands in your lap and close your eyes.

Relax your hands and connect the tips of the thumb and index finger to form a circle. Keeping them in this relaxed position, rest the hands on your knees, palms up. Breathe normally and hold the *shanti* mudra for five minutes.

Open your eyes. Maintaining the mudra position, gently stretch the arms out in front of you. Simultaneously rotate each arm outward to draw circles (approximately eighteen inches in diameter) in the air. Repeat these circles seven times.

Relax your hands and place them in your lap. Release the mudra and sit for a few moments in silence.

In my own experience, the longer I remained in silence, the stronger my personal sound became. When I later began to chant the Vedic mantras, my inner song grew richer, and *kundalini-shakti* began her ascent within me, as I related earlier. As your personal sound begins to rise within you, the sacred power of your voice blossoms. To recover all that is held within your journey—that is, your whole cosmic anatomy—you must let loose your voice from the depths of your being. Give yourself permission to express all your natural urges to make noise, even those you were taught to suppress for fear of offending others. Moan, groan, giggle, laugh, snore, belch, gurgle, chuckle, scream, cry, sob, whisper, wail, hum, sing, mutter, or babble to your heart's content.

Pay attention to your sounds as you release them, and remain attentive to the miracle of the mystic sound within you. Goddess Vac's cardinal rule of sound is: Never stifle the natural expressions of your inner sound. A hymn from the *Rig Veda* expresses regret at those whose speech, sight, and hearing do not reflect Vac's sonic wisdom. Create an affirmation of your own as a way to remember the sanctity of your sound. Keep it in the foreground of your mind every time you use your voice. Here is an example:

> *My voice is my most sacred power.*
> *I use it only to express my inner truth.*

Each one of our inner sounds, when nurtured and expressed, can direct us toward the natural vibrational balance of body, mind, and spirit that gives us clarity and purpose in our daily lives. Consider these Vedic principles regarding the way in which sound affects us on physiologic and spiritual levels:

- Harmonious sounds gather in the various *pranas* of the body.
- The 72,000 or so *nadis* (the nerve channels through which

*prana* flows) that exist in the body are all sound/vibration sensitive. They function strictly through vibrational energy. Therefore, good sounds increase the vitality of these *nadis*. *Pranas* that are flowing through them also become more charged with vigor.

• When the *pranas* are healthy and filled with energy and vitality, they stimulate healthy tissue and organ activity so that good health is achieved and maintained.

• Vital *prana* and harmonious sound work hand in hand. They travel through the mind like a great wave, revitalizing cells of the brain and inspiring the mind to produce fluent, clear, harmonious thoughts.

We have many ways to tap into the power of sound to stimulate and balance *prana* throughout the body, but using our voice to express our inner song (to chant) is the most potent. Yet the human voice is our most misunderstood and misused possession. We take it for granted, using—and abusing—it for the most mundane, trivial, and hurtful communications, forgetting to honor it as the divine instrument of cosmic sound within us.

The seers emulated the primordial sound in order to fashion the first human expression, called *sruti*, the cosmic revelation as heard by the *rishis*. *Sruti* is also referred to as the Word. The song of *Sama Veda* informs us that, "Verily, if there were no Word, there would be no knowledge neither of right or wrong, nor of truth and untruth, nor of the pleasing and unpleasing. The Word makes all this known." This original Word informed Vedic ritual speech, mantras, chants, and music, which all carry the cosmic rhythms and memory of the universe's entire experience. The Vedic seers declared the spoken word, *sruti,* as their most significant contribution to humanity. Most ancient people left their imprint on history through the medium of precious materials—gold, silver, bronze, onyx, and granite. While time has eroded these monuments, the Vedic tradition's rich legacy of the spoken word, recited daily by an unbroken chain of generations, still lives on.

The voice as a divine human instrument is our most powerful tool for healing. It expresses our individuality and unique creativity, our inner rhythm and memory. The Vedas tell us that both breath and light arise from the cosmic sound. Thus, when we use our personal sound as the raw expression of inner power and harmony—by chanting or reciting the *bija* mantras, the intrinsic sounds of the body's chakras—we entrain our inner rhythms with those of the cosmos and harness our intrinsic ability to become conscious.

## CHAKRAS AND SPIRIT RHYTHMS

The Vedic healing system, which enables us to balance and harmonize our *pranic* energies, centers around the seven chakras. Sound interventions can be used to specifically address and overcome blockages in each of these centers. A complete explanation of the chakras and their relationship to psycho-spiritual issues and specific healing sounds follows.

## THE SEVEN STAGES OF LIFE

Each chakra or energy center has a specific purpose and physical and spiritual area of influence. We are meant to develop each chakra, and energy therein, as we grow, to fulfill our assignment in life, to uncover our deepest identity, and to connect with the One Spirit. One by one, from the root to the crown chakra, we learn to utilize, incorporate, and then

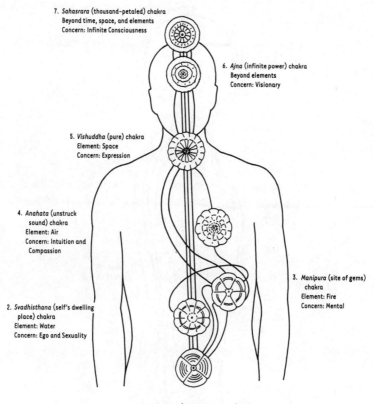

7. *Sahasrara* (thousand-petaled) chakra
Beyond time, space, and elements
Concern: Infinite Consciousness

6. *Ajna* (infinite power) chakra
Beyond elements
Concern: Visionary

5. *Vishuddha* (pure) chakra
Element: Space
Concern: Expression

4. *Anahata* (unstruck
sound) chakra
Element: Air
Concern: Intuition and
Compassion

3. *Manipura* (site of gems)
chakra
Element: Fire
Concern: Mental

2. *Svadhisthana* (self's dwelling
place) chakra
Element: Water
Concern: Ego and Sexuality

1. *Muladhara* (foundation, or root) chakra
Element: Earth
Concern: Survival

*Example A: Seven chakras unfolding kundalini energy: the projectile movement of the chakras' energies. Each chakra, rooted in the sushumna, a column of energy in the spine, emanates its own energy and flows into the energy of the other chakras.*

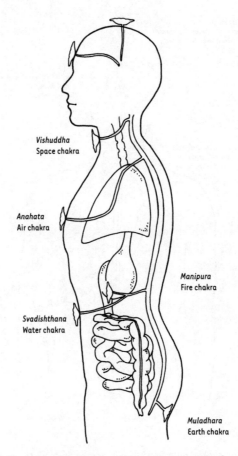

*Vishuddha*
Space chakra

*Anahata*
Air chakra

*Manipura*
Fire chakra

*Svadishthana*
Water chakra

*Muladhara*
Earth chakra

*Example B: The source of the first five chakras' energy emerging from the central channel within the spine and emanating outward.*

transcend the particular energies and lessons inherent in each chakra. Each chakra corresponds to a stage of life. As we work through each one, we prepare ourselves for the next stage of life.

The first five chakras relate to the five physical elements of creation, so they can be more easily understood than the highest two. The sixth and seventh chakras are beyond the realm of sound and consciousness.

In the first stage of life, the survival stage (birth to fourteen years), we tend to live mainly from the first chakra, called *muladhara* (root center) in Sanskrit. Pervaded by the dominant element of earth, the first chakra provides the foundational strength necessary to sustain a healthy life. Located at the base of the spine, in the perineum (between the anus and genitals), this chakra gives us great stability when it is in a state of balance. It is affected by our relationship to our family of origin, since during the first fourteen years of life, we are meant to be guided by our parents, teachers, and elders.

The *muladhara*, or root chakra, is associated with survival, which is crucial to existence but can be limiting. As long as we remain fixated only on survival, we cannot evolve to our higher spiritual purpose. We must come to understand survival as merely a means to an end.

As we move into the second, or ego stage of life (fifteen to twenty-eight years), we begin to experience the energy of the next chakra. Located in the sacrum, the second chakra, or *svadhisthana* (self-place), carries within its vibratory field the primal feminine force of procreation, *shakti-prana*. Representing the water element of the universe and located near the genital region, this chakra reveals the early stages of our evolution. Until we are able to reclaim the power of our inner sound, the energy of this chakra generally reflects the murky, unresolved conditions of the elemental human affairs to which it relates: money, sex, and power.

As we grow into the second chakra, our sensory perceptions develop, and we begin to experience our individuality and sexuality. We often get caught within the dark waters of deception and false perception that may be our karmic inheritance. Many people become stuck within second chakra terrain in their pursuit of gratification through sexual encounters, relationships, or the pursuit of money and power. It is said that we require many rebirths to transcend this region, with its seductive urges. A life of indulgence and irreverence makes it difficult to move on to the next plateau, yet once this difficult crossing has been achieved, we become familiar with the vibration of our ascending consciousness.

Growing into the third stage of life, the mental stage (twenty-nine to forty-two years), we may expect to experience a definitive shift from a sensorial existence to the terrain of the third chakra, *manipura* (full of radiance), which rules the mind. Centrally positioned in the region of the navel and solar plexus, *manipura* is pervaded by the fire element and is the catalytic force that keeps the elements of the first and second chakras in check. The condition of *tejas*, the light of pure consciousness within the body, and the practice of *tapas*, the observance of yogic disciplines to induce inner vitality, both find their source in this chakra. The third chakra marks a quantum leap in our mental and material progress as well as in our spiritual growth. The mind-oriented activities in the fields of academia, science, and technology are rooted in the interplay of the mental fires of the third chakra.

The addictive nature of the mental concepts that reside in *manipura*, however, make it extremely difficult to move from the third to the fourth chakra and, correspondingly, from the third to the fourth stage of life. Pressing against the heart chakra, the fire of the lower three chakras can make our physical and emotional rhythms go awry, which in turn negatively influences *ojas*, the body's immunological force. For that reason, the evolution to the fourth, or heart, chakra is considered to be one of the most arduous of human accomplishments.

In the fourth, intuitive stage of our lives (forty-three to fifty-six years), we receive the sacred opportunity to ascend into the powerful vibratory field of the heart chakra, the seat of individual consciousness. In doing so, we unwittingly enter the terrain of spiritual maturity. From this point, the human journey quickens its stride, resonating harmonically with the higher rhythms of the spirit.

The fourth chakra, *anahata* (unstruck or soundless sound), resides slightly to the right of our biological heart, in the center of the chest. Epicenter of the cosmic vibrational forces, the heart chakra is pervaded by the air element. Reclaiming the vibrations of the fourth chakra marks a profound leap in our evolutionary growth, as our powers of spiritual consciousness begin to flourish and the sonic energy of the heart is awakened along with our intuition. Mystics have reported feeling powerful physical sensations in the area of the heart during their most ecstatic states of divine union. Just as the fourth chakra serves as the gateway between the more basic survival-oriented impulses of the lower three chakras and the more rarefied spiritual aspirations of the highest three, the fourth stage of life represents a major transition in our inner orientation: from obsession with the self to compassion for others.

Once the fourth stage has been accomplished, ascendance into the fifth chakra is almost guaranteed. By this time, the transcendent rhythms of the spirit have gained tremendous momentum, generating the upward force that moves directly into the fifth stage of life (fifty-seven to seventy years). This "inner song" stage corresponds to the fifth chakra, *vishuddha* (purified), the cradle of primordial sound. Located at the base of the throat and associated with the element of space and with our voice, *vishuddha* is the key vibratory center through which we can recover our personal inner sound.

The fifth stage gives us the power of voice. Until we ascend to this resonant space within, we inhibit our self-expression and creativity. In the West, the power of the voice has been lost to many and, as a result, we have lost our spiritual way, our spiritual values, or dharma.

As we grow into fifth-chakra awareness, we learn to express our inner sound by recovering our unique stillness in harmony with creation and cosmic rhythms. During this stage, human consciousness comes alive in our *buddhi*, or innermost intuition, making possible the soul's emergence back into the Divine.

As we move into the sixth or visionary stage of life, we begin to experience levels of consciousness that are beyond the five senses and earth elements. Unlike the previous states, we can come into the sixth stage at any age, although the age guideline of seventy-one to eighty-four is generally given. Attaining the sixth chakra depends solely on our own inner awakening. This can happen at any time, once we have become aware of our ability to be conscious, although generally our chances of awakening increase with maturity.

The sixth, or *ajna* (command), chakra is located near the medulla oblongata at the base of the brain (the so-called "third eye"). It represents the core of consciousness in each of us. This chakra is said to be the home of the *ahamkara* (memory and ego sense). Once we are able to dissolve the ego sense that wrongly perceives us as separate from the unitive consciousness, we can begin to merge with this consciousness, while still in a material, tangible form.

The seventh chakra is located just above the crown of the head, near the pineal gland, outside the physical body. Its Sanskrit name, *sahasrara,* means "thousand-petaled," indicating infinite potential. Reaching the seventh, infinite-consciousness stage of life, we have reconciled the perceptions of the "divided reality" and have the opportunity to enter into a union with the One Spirit. The physical age range of eighty-four to ninety-eight is only an approximate or metaphoric guideline. Ageless human consciousness is a state of being that the *rishis* call *sat-chit-ananda*: ever existing, ever conscious, ever complete. This state of consciousness occurs when we recognize the self as stripped of all "time-space" distinctions and qualifications—to be identical to pure consciousness. In this ineffable state, we completely transcend the material plane of names and forms, space and time. We merge with pure consciousness and are complete in our self-knowledge.

Chakras work primarily through the matrix of our spirit. As wholesome foods feed the physical body and metabolic biorhythms, and healthy breath-practices nourish the anatomy and rhythms of our astral body, the harmonious vibrations of chakra activity nurture our causal or spirit rhythms. The chakras function through the vibrations of cosmic sound. When we develop our spiritual sound and rhythms, we transcend the many restrictions of our physical and subtle bodies and begin to live in accord with our authentic nature and the cosmos. We are able to move beyond all conflicts, both external and within the mind, becoming one with every creature. Our mind, intuition, and body are strengthened through the primordial sounds associated with the chakras.

Over thousands of years, the seers have developed a complex system that relates the primordial sound of *om*, which is organic to the human heart and affects the operations of all the chakras. As centers of consciousness within the body, each chakra has its own sacred syllable. The seven chakras also correspond to the seven notes of the Vedic musical scale called *saptak*, and the seven colors of the rainbow that ties the life force of earth to heaven. They also correspond to seven bodily tissues and seven apertures in the head, all of which mirror a cosmic anatomy in the human body.

The cosmic vibrations within the chakras may remain dormant through countless rebirths, or they may open gradually over a number of lifetimes. The *sadhanas* we undertake enable us to gradually become aware of the chakras' vibrational powers and awaken our kundalini. As this *pranic* energy begins to ascend through the ladder of consciousness, or chakras, it arouses our spiritual rhythms and intuition, stimulates our cosmic and ancestral memories, and allows us to see the unity of our multidimensional existence in the energy, vibration, and light of the cosmos.

## RESONATING WITH THE VIBRATION OF EACH CHAKRA

Each of the seven chakras has a corresponding *bija* mantra, although only six of them carry distinguishable sounds. The crown chakra, which relates to inner consciousness, is the abode of unwavering silence; its *bija* sound is called *visarga*, a particular breathing sound that is heard internally. The vibrations of all the *bija* mantras reverberate within the crown chakra. Once cultivated, these vibrations evoke the grace of the guarding deities of the chakras. When the deities are awakened, the sacred mantra of each chakra reveals its spirit to you.

## Bija Mantras

| Sound | Chakra | Color | God Deity | Goddess Deity |
|-------|--------|-------|-----------|---------------|
| — | crown (7) | — | Guru | Mahashakti |
| Om | third eye (6) | gold | Shiva/Shakti | Hakini |
| Ham | throat (5) | gold | Panchavaktra | Shakini |
| Yam | heart (4) | gold | Ishana Shiva | Kakini |
| Ram | navel (3) | gold | Braddha Rudra | Lakini |
| Vam | genitals (2) | gold | Vishnu | Rakini |
| Lam | root (1) | gold | Bala Brahma | Dakini |

## YOGA MUDRA: POSTURE OF MEDITATION FOR CHAKRA WORK

The yoga mudra posture creates a strong foundation in the root of your body and stimulates the energy of all the chakras. This posture brings awareness to the perineum, which is located in a small triangular area between the anus and genitals. To identify the perineum, sit in an erect, meditative posture. As you focus on your pelvic floor, inhale and contract your anal muscles. Slowly exhale and release the contraction. Repeat three times. Each time you contract your pelvic floor, narrow your focus on the location of the perineum.

Yoga mudra keeps the head, neck, and trunk erect, which creates an unobstructed passage in the spinal column so that the subtle breath can flow in a spiral rhythm through the chakras. As the ascending energy merges into *shakti-prana*, it can catapult us into the multidimensional realm of greater understanding.

Yoga mudra is also called the lotus pose. Rooted in the mud of earthly existence, the lotus transforms the mire of life into the purity and tranquility of an exquisite flower, which holds the cosmic memory of consciousness. This posture, which encompasses both stability and fluidity, evokes the subtle *pranic* rhythm held in the lotus plant. When we achieve dexterity in this posture, we become profoundly still, like Shiva, universal consciousness; and animated, like Mahashakti, energizing consciousness.

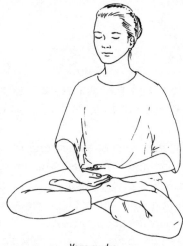

*Yoga mudra*

### The Practice: Yoga Mudra Posture

Place a yoga mat or folded blanket on the floor and face east or north. You may also support yourself in the posture by sitting on a pillow. Rest your right foot on your left thigh, and pull your left foot through to rest on your right thigh. If you have difficulty achieving this posture, you may use the easier *sukhasana* posture by simply folding your legs without resting your feet on your thighs. If you are unable to perform either yoga mudra or *sukhasana*, sit upright in a chair or in any comfortable posture to do your chakra practice. Keep your spine straight but relaxed, by tilting your chin slightly forward. Rest your hands in your lap.

Be careful not to force your body into yoga mudra. Your posture should always feel comfortable before you sustain it. You can start by holding the posture for three to five minutes to build flexibility and work toward holding it for about twenty minutes. As you continue this practice, your body will become increasingly flexible.

When you feel comfortable in either yoga mudra or *sukhasana* pose, begin the lotus-meditation practice (see below). I suggest that you spend a month or more working on this posture before going on to the chakra-vibration work. You will then be prepared to ascend through the vibratory fields of the chakras, where you will experience the vibrations akin to the *bija* mantra of each chakra.

### The Practice: Resounding *Bija* Mantras

Sit in yoga mudra or in *sukhasana* pose, either early in the morning or just before sunset. Bring your attention inward to your perineum. Repeat each *bija* mantra clearly as you ascend the chakras, starting with the root chakra. Observe this practice for about seven minutes every day for seven weeks, before progressing to the chakra-visualization practice.

- Learn the *bija* sounds by repeating them in the following sequence: *om, ham, yam, ram, vam, lam.*
- Starting with the *bija* sound of the root chakra *(lam)*, chant each mantra once as you visualize climbing the ladder of chakras up the spine. (See drawing of chakra positions along the spine on p. 245.)
- Pause for a moment after repeating each *bija* mantra.

- Now recite all six *bija* sounds in sequence. Repeat nine times.
- As you repeat the mantras, focus on allowing the chanting to become seamless so that the each sequence of sounds merges into the next, without beginning or end.

I conducted a *satsanga* for chanting class some years ago at a yoga school run by one of my students, and ended my presentation by inviting everyone present to join me in reciting the *bija* mantras. We chanted together for about ten minutes, and the energy in the room created by the chorus of seventy-some voices was palpable. The following day, I met individually with several of the yoga students who had asked to consult with me about various health or emotional issues. One young woman, Ruthie, was experiencing early menopause and wanted to discuss Ayurvedic remedies for her symptoms. But the first words out of her mouth had nothing to do with hot flashes or night sweats. "I so much enjoyed the chanting last evening," she said as soon as she sat down. "I've been practicing chanting for several years, and the changes in my life have been profound. I'm a writer, and my second novel is being published next month, but I honestly believe that I never would have written either book if I hadn't started chanting."

She went on to tell me that she was the youngest of three children, none of whom had been given much encouragement to express their feelings or opinions. Her father was a career army officer who tyrannized his family in much the same way he ruled over his troops. Her mother was a recovering alcoholic, now sober five years, whose drunken episodes had often kept the children awake at night. "But we never told anyone, not friends or our teachers or any of our relatives. No matter what was happening at home, we knew to keep it a secret."

Ruthie was an avid reader who used books as an escape from the difficulties of her family life. From the days of her earliest childhood, she dreamed of writing fiction. But instead of enrolling in a postgraduate creative-writing program as several of her college professors had urged her to do, she moved to New York and took a job in advertising. She received several promotions and became an account executive with a great deal of responsibility. "I was making very good money, was well thought of in the company, but I was miserable," she said. "I'd have to force myself out of bed every morning because I couldn't face coming up with one more ad campaign or writing one more line of copy for a product that didn't matter to me."

One evening, a friend "dragged me, under protest, to a yoga class conducted by one of your students. I lay down on the mat, fully expecting to hate the experience. But I found the poses calming and challenging, and I especially loved that the teacher encouraged us to hum during many of the poses. As soon as she started us chanting, I was hooked."

Ruthie became a regular at the yoga school, often attending classes two or sometimes three times a week. One Sunday, she attended a workshop where I was demonstrating the *bija* mantras and how they relate to the chakras. After the session, Ruthie told me, "When you had us repeatedly sing out *ham* for the throat chakra, I became aware of a tightness in that area. I kept choking up and coughing, as if something were stuck there, so that the sound couldn't come through."

That afternoon, Ruthie decided to begin psychotherapy and to continue her chanting practice. What was "stuck" in her throat, she came to understand, were all the secrets she'd had to keep as a child—secrets that continued to haunt her because, unconsciously, she still feared her father's anger and recriminations. "As I explored all the forbidden subjects that

I'd never allowed myself to talk about, it slowly dawned on me that my ongoing loyalty to our family's code of silence had kept me from doing the one thing I wanted most in life, which was to write fiction. My excuse all those years had been that I had nothing worth saying. In fact, I had lots of stories to tell, but I couldn't let them out, even if they were disguised as fiction. The prohibition against speaking honestly still loomed too large in my imagination."

This realization became the key that unlocked Ruthie's creative potential. She started to keep a journal in which she gave herself permission to write whatever she was feeling or thinking, and out of the pages of that journal came the idea for her first novel.

"Today, when I sing out *ham*, I no longer feel the tension in my throat. I feel free to express myself, and that freedom has given me the life I've always wanted," she said.

At my request, she sent me copies of both books, and I was particularly struck by the integrity and authenticity of her narrative voice. Through the power of the *bija* mantras, she had found and was able to translate her inner sound into written words that spoke her truth.

### The Practice: *Bija*-Mantra Sounding—Expanding Your Vocal Power

When you repeat the *bija* mantras, you gradually cleanse and harmonize your inner vibrations and bring them into alliance with your personal sound. Find a tranquil space in the early morning, and sit facing the rising sun. Practice the following exercise for about seven minutes every day for seven weeks.

To warm up, start your practice by reciting seven rounds of *bija* mantras, as presented earlier:

*Om, Ham, Yam, Ram, Vam, Lam*

Then recite three rounds of the second progression, as follows:

*Om Ha Ha Ham*
*Om Ya Ya Yam*
*Om Ra Ra Ram*
*Om Va Va Vam*
*Om La La Lam*

Finally, recite three rounds of the third progression that follows:

*Ha Ha Ham*
*Ya Ya Yam*
*Ra Ra Ram*
*Va Va Vam*
*La La Lam*

Sit in silence for a few minutes, becoming aware of the vibrations that linger in the surrounding space after you finish chanting. You may feel your body swaying slightly. Let the mantra sounds continue to resonate in your mind and body, noting any changes in your mood or physical state.

As you continue to practice the *bija* sounds, you will find that certain sounds linger in your consciousness throughout the day, long after you get up from the sounding practice. You may suddenly realize that you are humming a particular sequence of sounds that you had been chanting early that morning. You may feel a different momentum in your stride as you move about. Perhaps you will begin to hear the distant flight of a bird. You may stop in the middle of your workday and realize that the melody in your head is resonating with the pulse of your heart. Suddenly, at the most unexpected time, you may burst into a song or a dance.

One of the most amazing stories I have heard about the power of these mystical sounds involved a family friend, Angela. In her Land Rover, en route to a ski resort not far from her home, Angela was negotiating the twists and turns of highway I-40, a winding road that cuts through the foothills of the Smoky Mountains. She had driven the highway many times before and knew to be careful—especially in bad weather, because there was no shoulder, just a sheer drop off the side of the mountain. On this particular day, she hit a patch of ice and went into a skid. Her vehicle spun around and shot across the road so that it seemed to be headed straight over the side of the cliff.

Angela has been studying meditation at the Wise Earth School for many years, and had recently begun studying chanting with me. (Chanting is now an intrinsic part of her practice.) Throughout the drive, she had been silently chanting the *bija* mantras, as she often did during the course of her day. As the van went out of control, she suddenly began to sing the mantras aloud. Her reaction was totally involuntary. In a matter of seconds, the van came to a complete stop.

Angela believes that her life was saved that day by the numinous grace of the Divine Mother, because there is no logical explanation for why the van did not fly off the edge of the road. Nothing about her chanting changed her physical reactions or reality as she tried to steer clear of danger. By instinctively surrendering herself to the vibrations of the mantras, she is certain that she invoked the deities that safeguarded her soul and body through this brush with mortality.

## AWAKENING THE UNMANIFEST VIBRATIONS OF YOUR CHAKRAS

To arouse the vibrations of your inner song and bring them into alliance with spirit, the ancients devised a powerful and expanded system of *bija* sounds relating each chakra to its source in the cosmic sound. Here, each *bija* syllable is pronounced with a nasalized sound, indicated in Sanskrit by a *bindu*, a dot above the "m" of the hum. This *bindu* represents the echo, or final refrain, of the sound *om*. The *bindu* is the seed at the center of om, signifying the immanent power of the Divine.

*Bindu* is the symbolic state of consciousness, the highest state of meditation wherein the *buddhi*'s power is collected to a single-pointed focus. Georg Feuerstein, Ph.D, succinctly describes the meaning of the *bindu* in his book *The Shambhala Guide to Yoga* when he says that "the dot symbolizes the sheer concentrated potency of sound before it bursts into manifestation."

### The Practice: *Bija*-Sound Meditation

The key to this sound-meditation practice is in the pronunciation of the *bija* syllable *hrim*, which permeates each chakra. Pronounce this as it appears, and then add a nasalized hum to the "m" that ends the syllable. I suggest spending up to five minutes daily on this sound. Practice this sound daily, just before sunrise or just after sunset. The whole practice should take up to four weeks. The more you practice, the more entrenched this vibration will be within you. Here is the *bija* sound that encompasses all seven chakras:

*Hrim*
(Hreem)

Repeat *hrim* slowly and feel your inner reverberation in each of the seven chakras. Pronounce the sound clearly while pausing for a brief second between each sound. Allow the mind to rest within the sound of *hrim*, and listen as your inner song comes alive.

## THE LOTUS MANDALA

The seers gave us the mandala, an intricate, circular-shaped design comprised of triangles within circles within yet more circles, as a way to focus the mind in meditation. The mandala has many variations, but the blossoming lotus is a classical mandala image that is linked to the chakras. Each chakra is characterized by a color of the rainbow that corresponds to its element. For the purpose of this practice, we will concentrate on the color of gold—the origin of the rainbow colors and the gold of consciousness that transcends all colors. Gold is also the natural hue of the *bija* mantras. Meditating on the light of the lotus mandala in each chakra invokes the deity of each chakra. The lotus mandala symbolizes unified consciousness, joining the circle of heart energy and consciousness.

### The Practice: Visualizing the Lotus Mandala

Sit in yoga mudra or in *sukhasana*, and visualize the central column of your spine lit from within. Visualize a blooming yellow lotus with a golden core in your root chakra. Climb to the next rung of the ladder, and visualize the sacrum chakra as a sky blue lotus with a golden center. Take another step up to the solar plexus chakra and visualize a pink lotus with a golden heart. Another rung of the ladder, in your heart chakra, is a dove gray lotus with a golden center. As you ascend yet another rung, you enter the throat chakra, symbolized by a smoky green lotus with a golden core. Next, entering the hallowed space of the "third eye," you visualize a translucent white lotus with a shimmering golden heart. At the summit of the ladder is your crown chakra, beyond color, form, and element. Here, the pristine, crystal lotus with its golden core reflects the myriad rainbow colors brightly glowing from each of the chakras below.

These chakra *sadhanas* allow us to enjoy the miracle of merging into the deities' energies. Each one of us holds the capacity to shimmer in the golden light as we are illuminated from within. I suggest that you spend at least three months with this practice. Over time, it will unleash profound joy and pleasure within you as you reach the crown chakra. Returning to the root chakra, you will begin to feel more deeply connected with your spiritual center. The practice, as a whole, will greatly enhance your energy, as well as your emotional and spiritual clarity. The *Maitri Upanishad* put it this way: "Words cannot describe the joy of the spirit whose spirit is cleansed in deep contemplation—who is one with his/her own Spirit. Only those who experience this joy know what it is."

## WORDS THAT HARM, WORDS THAT HEAL

*Ahimsa,* a Vedic term that describes an awareness of nonviolence toward self, nature, and life, is the most important exercise we can put into practice in our daily lives. The attitude of *ahimsa* should inform all aspects of our behavior and speech, because the hurt we incur through negative thought and speech—both of which have a damaging, dissonant effect on us and everything around us—is the most grievous act of aggression we can commit. Every battle or war or fight, whether personal or political, sprang from someone's disharmonious thought, followed by the verbal articulation of that thought.

The *rishis* caution us to guide our thoughts by using our words carefully, and urge us to always speak in accord with what we think. In essence, our words must flow in harmony with our thoughts, or we will create an inner conflict caused by the discrepancy between what we think and what we say. How often do you find yourself thinking one thing and saying another? Imagine that you meet a friend on the street and notice that she is wearing a short, tight-fitting skirt. You think, *That skirt is much too tight on her, and she's too old to be wearing something that short.* Yet you greet her with a kiss and say, "You look great in that skirt!"

I am not suggesting that in such a case you say aloud what you are thinking, because it would be hurtful, but you also should not tell her a lie. Try, as a beginning practice, to find something you truly like about her and make a point of mentioning that. The deeper practice is about curbing all such negative thoughts. I have developed a simple exercise in keeping with the practice of what the *rishis* called *vac tapasya* to help evoke healthy, harmonious thoughts and to bring forward positive, pleasant words. The *Rig Veda* concurs: "Speech yields its milk to him who is able to milk speech."

### The Practice: *Vac Tapasya*

Spend fifteen minutes every day allowing your mind to run free. Notice whatever negative, hurtful thoughts come up. Keep a notepad close to you and write down those thoughts and the person or situations they concern. Record your thought processes as they occur, without whitewashing or censoring them. Let yourself be angry, judgmental, or unkind, but above all, be honest. Repeat each negative thought aloud. For example: "Mary is so demanding. I can't bear to have dinner with her." Then repeat the Vedic attitude: "I know that every negative thought reflects my own inner condition."

Now take responsibility for your feelings from which the negative thought sprang: "I am being intolerant of Mary. It will not be pleasant for Mary if I see her with this attitude."

As a general rule in *vac tapasya*, always consider your words carefully before you speak them aloud. Do not use an angry, accusatory, or aggressive tone. If you feel pressured to respond or speak in a way that you think may be hurtful to another person, use your notebook to tell this person your raw, unedited feelings in the form of a letter that you do not send. Let the letter sit for a week. Then, before you read it, make one small change. Replace the name of the person to whom it is addressed with your own name. This may help you understand that the letter has less to do with the person with whom you are angry, and is more about your hurt feelings, which stem from your negative thoughts and feelings about your own life.

During the deep quietude of my Himalayan retreat, I became aware that silence is the invisible content of primordial sound. I discovered, as well, that by practicing the *sadhanas* of sound we gain access to the vibrations of the universe—vibrations that can heal our spirits, minds, and bodies. The human voice is the primary and most potent instrument for effecting these cures. When we chant, hum, sing, or speak kindly and thoughtfully, we resonate with and express our inner song—the unique sound of our soul. I was compelled by the vital force of my life to walk this particular path of practice, so that my heart could become full, and free of burdens. I invite you to undertake your own journey along the pathways of sound and silence, so that your heart may become fully open, your wounds may be healed, and you may recover your unique inner song, as I did. The *Tejabindu Upanishad* says, "Let us meditate on the radiant Self, the Ultimate Reality known to the sages in *samadhi*." The *sadhana* of sound can lead you to *samadhi*, which is the true essence of yoga—a state that transcends consciousness so that we achieve a sense of cosmic union with the Divine.

*Part Four*

# FEEDING
# THE SOUL

# Chapter 11

## HEALTHY FOOD, HEALTHY SPIRIT

*May the universe never abuse food.*
*Breath is food. The body eats foods.*
*The body rests on breath.*
*Breath rests on the body.*
*Food is resting on food.*
*The one who knows this*
*becomes rich in food and great in fame.*
—*Taittiriya Upanishad* (11.7)

Peggy describes herself as "a compulsive doer," a whirlwind of activity who draws people to her with her contagious enthusiasm for life. She is a pediatrician, as well a practitioner of yoga for over twenty-five years, and she manages to find the time to run her own yoga studio in San Francisco. Serious in her commitment to *sadhana*, she wakes up early every morning so that she can do yoga, meditate, and chant. Over the course of the last several years, she has also spent several weeks studying breath practices with me.

Peggy has never had any health problems and, in all the time I have known her, she has never complained of fatigue, in spite of her very demanding schedule. So I was surprised when she called one day to inquire about a workshop on breath and mentioned that she had been feeling much less energetic lately. She was also having memory lapses and a couple of times had even forgotten to show up to teach a class. She was also feeling spaced out and fidgety. "But I'm forty-eight, approaching menopause, so doesn't it make sense that I should be slowing down?"

I realize that fluctuating hormone levels during the peri-menopausal period may cause memory loss and other symptoms such as Peggy described. But knowing her as I do, I also suspected that she had become too rigid and austere in her practice. I could sense her surprise when I said, "You don't need another class on breath just now. You need to focus on food *sadhana*. You can start by eating a good breakfast every day."

Peggy's response was that she didn't have time for breakfast because she meditated before work for three hours. I urged her to shorten her meditation to one hour. "The mind has to be fed through meditation, but your physical self needs feeding, too," I said. "Your life is very busy and hectic, and you are punishing your body by not nourishing yourself."

As part of her food *sadhana*, I asked Peggy to buy a cast-iron pot and to cook whole oats for breakfast, because oats are particularly good for improving memory. I also recommended that she be sure not to skip lunch, which might include steamed vegetables such as asparagus or acorn squash, depending on the season, and a tablespoon of ghee. A typical dinner could be brown rice and mung dhal, a delicious dish made of mung beans that is high in protein and very healthy (see recipe on page 381).

Peggy has been a vegetarian for many years, but now I was asking her to eat three meals a day, at the same time each day, and in a mindful manner (i.e., comfortably seated, paying attention to each mouthful that she swallowed, instead of swallowing a handful of nuts and dried fruit as she rushed off to her next appointment or class).

I saw Peggy about two months later when I was giving a talk in San Francisco. She had never looked better: her skin, which tended to be dry, was clear and glowing; her hair was thick and lustrous; her face even seemed to look less lined.

More important, she was no longer having memory problems and her vitality was restored to its normal level.

Peggy's story is a powerful testament to the practice of food *sadhana*. Each and every physical thing in the universe is composed of the same five elements: earth, water, fire, air, and space. We humans are formed from the same ingredients as a tree or a squirrel, a grain of sand or a drop of rain. The five elements in our foods nurture the five elements in our bodies. Put differently, the elements that nourish us are the same elements that are within us. When we recognize this integral connection—that we are sustained by the five elements of nature—we understand that each bite of food is a blessing from Mother Nature. This realization is the beginning of *sadhana*, the foundation from which we start to build a spiritual life.

The sacred sutra of *annam* says that food for humans is that which grows on the earth; it is all plant and mineral life (with the exception of some animal milk). The seven stages of a fruitful plant are identical to the seven stages of a fruitful human life. The life cycle of a plant begins with a good seed, one that retains its essential nature from the well of universal memory and has not been tampered with or genetically manipulated. The seed successively transforms to sprout, young plant, mature plant, flowering plant, fruitful plant, and then returns back to the earth as seed. At every stage, the plant may be harvested and prepared as food. After it has been ingested, and a human being is physically and spiritually nourished, the waste and roughage are restored to the earth. There, peacefully huddled in the womb of the Mother, the seed waits for its moment in time, then pierces through the earth to fulfill its cosmic destiny.

## FOOD IS MEMORY

According to Ayurveda, the body consists of seven vital tissues: plasma, blood, muscle, fat, bone, marrow, and reproductive tissue. These vital tissues, which are formed from the same elements, energy, and memory that make up plant life, are sustained by nature's food and rhythms. The purpose and intention of nature's food is to fulfill and revitalize the memories of the vital tissues. Formed from the same substance of cosmic memories, the plant seed and the human body are eternally intertwined. Neither the seed nor the body can exist without each other. Hold a good seed in your hand, and know that it unfolds the entire universe from within itself.

The plant is our most ancient ancestor. All life was born from this sacred creation. As it emerged into its manifested state, the plant absorbed the universe's first memory, that of *yajna*, or divine sacrifice. The Vedic seers believe that the universe is founded on the act of sacrifice, and plants unflinchingly adhere to this standard. While animals roam, birds fly, fish swim, and all the rest of life moves about, plants are rooted steadfastly in the earth. The tiger lily doesn't hop about the pond looking for a better view. The peppermint doesn't come up in spring and say, "I don't like the temperature, I'm going back down." The poplar doesn't covet what other beings have, saying, "That sunflower has a better position than I."

Plants bend before the tides of the seasons and yield their food to all creatures. Season after season, they dazzle us with their beauty, bringing forth exquisite flowers, fruits, fragrances, colors, and joyous sustenance. In winter, they retreat into the earth to replenish the cosmic memory of their seed. In spring, they push through the dense soil to reveal another tender sprout.

The *rishis* tell us that our most significant task as human beings is to take nothing from life for ourselves, but rather to give of ourselves to life. If we were to align our lives with those of plants and emulate their memory of random, selfless acts of giving, we would know that the most divine action we can perform is one of sacrifice, as executed by every tree, plant, shrub, grass, and herb.

According to the Vedic concept of *dana* or "open-handedness," giving something back to Mother Nature is one of the virtues that leads most directly to personal consciousness. Taking in nature's food, as we were intended, fosters in us compassion, selflessness, service, and the ability to give of ourselves. The more we give, the greater our gifts become and the greater is that which comes back to us. The more altruistic we become, the more conscious we become. So important is the spirit of "open-handedness" that the seers devised *dana* mudra as a way to cultivate this extraordinary virtue.

### The Practice: *Dana* Mudra

Extend your right hand with fingers pointing downward and the palm of the hand facing outward. Close your eyes and feel a shift in the back of your neck and in the *anahata* (heart) chakra. Hold the posture for a few minutes and then release it. Practice this mudra whenever you experience difficulty in being generous or in asking for what you need. The paradox is that by giving, you get back so much more than you invest.

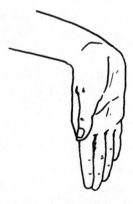

Dana *mudra*

## FOOD: MOTHER-ESSENCE
## OF HEALING

Each season brings forth the foods that best serve our needs during that particular time of the year. Together, the seasons produce the six tastes of natural foods necessary for human survival. When you eat the earth's food in harmony with her seasons and your metabolic type, or *dosha*, you fortify and strengthen your physical and spiritual bodies.

The Ayurvedic idea of *rasa*, a Sanskrit word that means "taste" but also "sap, juice, elixir, essence" as well as "love, feeling, and esthetic sentiment," teaches that taste is a vital part of the process of nutrition. The complex chain of reactions that creates taste begins with the five-sensory perception of taste, which leads to the mental reception of it by the brain cells, which beckon the appetite. The seers describe appetite as the total intelligence of the body acting in accord with its external surroundings. Thus, food is desired, ingested, digested, and returned to the earth in a natural, harmonious cycle.

*Rasa* is the mother-essence of healing. It gives us the ability to "taste" the entire world, making it possible to fulfill all of our desires. These tastes refer to all the impressions that we experience, not only by the tongue, but by all the sense organs—the nose, eyes, ears, and skin. We may "taste" the emotions of joy or sorrow, fear or courage, just as we may "taste" music—a form of sonic taste that reaches the most profound depths of our being.

According to the principle of *rasa*, there are six essential natural tastes: sweet, salty, sour, pungent, bitter, and astringent. The six tastes originate from the water element, the foundation that sustains all of life. Without water, there can be no taste, and without taste, we cannot remember our union with Mother Nature. When natural, earth-based taste is tampered with, it loses its ability to transmit the vibrations that our system needs to replenish our physical and spiritual rhythms. All six of nature's tastes are necessary for our immunologic and spiritual functions.

Each of the six tastes sustains good health in our diet when eaten in accord with its season. The extent to which you consume each taste largely depends on your metabolic type, or *dosha*. Before you can understand how to balance the six tastes to best suit your dietary needs, you must first be able to identify your *dosha*, which you can do in the next exercise (also see appendix 1, Your Metabolic Type).

## YOUR AYURVEDIC CONSTITUTION

Knowing your metabolic type will help you maintain your health and preserve balance in your life. It will also help you diagnose any ailments or diseases, and help to prevent those that are common to your metabolic type. The proportion to which the *doshas*, *vata*, *pitta*, and *kapha* exist within you makes your constitution different from someone else's. Once you are born, your type or constitution remains constant throughout your lifetime. The condition or energy of your *doshas* can change, however, owing to disharmonious factors in your lifestyle and environment. The practices of *sadhana* can help restore the *doshas* to a state of harmony and help maintain your health even in the face of challenges and stress.

Although each of us is endowed with our primary spiritual sound or rhythm, our physical, daily rhythms fall into three distinct metabolic types: quick and irregular *(vata)*, fast and decisive *(pitta)*, and slow and methodical *(kapha)*.

To determine your metabolic type, spend a few minutes answering the questions in the chart on the next page. Be honest with yourself; there are no right or wrong answers to these questions. Remember that your evaluation will be colored by the qualities of your present lifestyle. Six months after you have been observing the *sadhanas* you're learning in this book, take the quiz again. Your answers at that time will be more in keeping with your true constitutional nature.

## DETERMINING YOUR METABOLIC TYPE

**Directions:** Review all three categories of the Metabolic Quiz set out below and answer "yes" to the questions that you feel most accurately reflect you. The category that yields five or more affirmative answers indicates your dominant metabolic type. Ask a spouse, parent, or friend to double-check your assessment so that your scores will be as accurate as possible. For example, if your scores are 5 for *vata*, 3 for *pitta*, and 2 for *kapha*, then your Ayurvedic metabolic type is predominantly *vata*. As you progress in your knowledge of Ayurveda, you may find it helpful to be aware of your secondary type. In the example just given, for instance, you would categorize yourself as *vata-pitta*.

## Metabolic Type: *Vata*

- Do you get flustered easily during most activities?
- Do you have a very short attention span?
- Do you learn quickly and forget quickly?
- Do you have difficulty putting on weight?
- Do you love to make "slurpy" sounds while eating?
- Do you feel close to people in physical or emotional pain?
- Do you sleep poorly?
- Do you have flighty and fearful dreams?
- Do you tend to be a loner?

If you answered five or more of these queries in the affirmative, your rhythms are quick and irregular.

**Metabolic Type:** *Pitta*

- Do you excel in doing more than one activity at the same time?
- Do you tend to remain completely focused on your tasks?
- Do you learn quickly and forget slowly?
- Do you gain weight easily and lose it easily?
- Do you get ravenously hungry and love to eat?
- Do you like to be around successful people?
- Do you sleep lightly and moderately?
- Do you have violent, fiery dreams on occasion?
- Do you tend to be ambitious?

If you answered five or more of these queries in the affirmative, your rhythms are fast and decisive.

**Metabolic Type:** *Kapha*

- Do you get easily flustered when doing more than one thing at a time?
- Do you have excellent endurance?
- Do you learn slowly and forget slowly?
- Do you gain weight easily?
- Do you crave crunchy foods?
- Do you love to help people in physical or emotional need?
- Do you sleep long and deeply?
- Do you have watery, sensual dreams?
- Do you become possessive on occasion?

If you answered five or more of these queries in the affirmative, your rhythms are slow and methodical.

## THE SIX TASTES AND THEIR EFFECTS

Each *dosha* is primarily nourished by three tastes—the three that are not of its own nature (see below). For example, *kapha* types do best when they include pungent, bitter, and astringent tastes in their diets. I am not suggesting that *kaphas* cannot eat grains and fruits, which are mostly sweet, but that they must be mindful of the quality and quantity of sweet tastes. *Pitta* is nourished by primarily sweet, bitter, and astringent tastes; *vata* by sweet, salty, and sour tastes. The box that follows describes the qualities of each of the six tastes, listed according to their predominance in the universe.

1. **Sweet** is the dominant taste of all forms of sustenance because almost all foods contain some degree of sweetness. Water and earth elements produce the sweet taste, which includes all carbohydrates, sugars, fats, and amino acids. The primary element of life, which is water, is considered sweet, as are milk and all sugars. Sweet increases bodily tissues, nurtures the body, and relieves hunger. Our diets should therefore be proportionately high in good-quality "sweet" foods, including grains, root vegetables, and fruits. I am *not* recommending that you eat foods made of refined or simple sugars or white flour, which have no nutritive value and are *not* "natural" foods. Sweet is most beneficial for the *pitta* type.

2. **Pungent,** formed from the elements of air and fire, helps stimulate appetite and maintains metabolism and the balance of secretions in the body. This taste is most benefi-

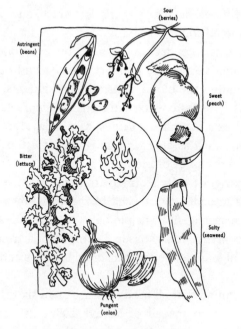

*The six tastes of nature*

cial for the *kapha* type and includes foods such as garlic, ginger, kale, mustard, tomatoes, and peppers.

3. **Salty** is most beneficial for the *vata* type, although it may be used in small quantities by all types as it helps to cleanse bodily tissues and activate digestion. The third most dominant taste, it is formed from the elements of water and fire and is found in all salts and seaweeds. Most watery vegetables, such as tomatoes, zucchini, and cucumber, are naturally high in saline.

4. **Sour** is formed from earth and fire elements and helps digestion and the elimination of wastes from the body. This taste may be used in small quantities by everyone, although it is most beneficial for the *vata* type. Most fruits are considered sour, with some sweetness. All organic acids and

fermented foods, such as yogurt, soy sauce, and pickles, are also considered sour.

5. **Bitter** is intended to be used by everyone in small quantity, and is especially good for the *pitta* and *kapha* types. Bitter detoxifies the blood, controls skin ailments, and tones the organs. This taste is formed from the elements of air and space and exists in all medicines, alkaloids, glycosides, and bitter foods such as aloe vera, arugula, radicchio, dandelion greens, and the spice turmeric.

6. **Astringent** taste, formed from the elements of earth and air, is intended to be used in medicinal measure by all types. The astringent principle helps to reduce bodily secretion and constrict bodily tissue. Examples of astringent foods are those high in tannin, such as dried legumes and bark teas.

Keep in mind that all foods consist of all six tastes, just as each of us is composed of all five elements and all three *doshas*. The science of Ayurvedic medicine, which is based on the study of the *doshas*, teaches that the six tastes should be enjoyed proportionately. As a general rule:

• sweet taste should be the most dominant taste in our main meal of the day.
• pungent, salty, and sour tastes should be used moderately as secondary tastes, depending on the season.
• Bitter and astringent tastes are always used as minor or accent tastes, and should also be increased or decreased according to the particular season.

When we do not balance the tastes in our diet, we disturb the body's tissue memory. This disruption causes the cells to become distorted so that they transmute themselves into what we call disease.

I learned this fundamental truth firsthand years ago when I was in the process of eliminating processed foods, white sugar, and commercial dairy products from my diet. Instead I chose to eat wholesome organic foods. My vital tissues were able to reclaim their memory of health, natural strength, and resilience.

One day I strayed from my new regimen and ate an Indian sweet dessert that was packed with refined sugar and commercial dairy. Within just a few hours, I had developed a raging fever. That night, I had a nightmare—a vision of thousands of slaughtered cows. I understood the terrible dream to be a sign that my vital tissues had gone into shock, a protest against the "polluted fodder" I had introduced into my body. The dessert contained sour milk, refined white sugar, and hydrogenated oil, also sour. The ingredients were thus mostly sweet and sour, a completely unbalanced food, no matter what the season. My reaction was a profound reminder from the universe that my body had become sensitized to junk food, and that I could never again eat unwholesome foods. Since then, I cook as much as possible for myself, even when I travel. I never eat out, unless I can be sure that the food has been prepared by a conscious, nature-loving person in a wholesome atmosphere.

I have heard many similar stories from my students and others who practice the food *sadhanas*. Rina, for example, is a singer, who was recently recording a selection of Vedic chants with me. She arrived at the music studio one morning looking so pale that I instantly knew she did not felt well. The night before, she had gone to a Christmas party and eaten a plateful of eggplant parmigiana. Because she had been practicing food *sadhanas* for the past year, her body had become sensitized to unwholesome foods and had reacted to the intake of a low-quality dairy product combined with a vegetable from the nightshade family. She had become so nauseated that she had to leave the party and had been awake most of the night vomiting and suffering severe stomach cramps.

Because we were on a tight schedule at the studio, Rina was determined to perform that day. But she had neither the breath nor the stamina to hold the notes. "I'll never eat that kind of food again," she told me, having learned a difficult but important lesson about honoring the needs of her body and vital tissues. Wholesome food brings forth your cosmic memories, attunes you to the rhythms of nature, and enables you to rediscover your sacred inner self.

Barbara, who attended one of my workshops several years ago, was attractive but very thin. In her mid-thirties, she had a friendly smile and a quick laugh. Despite her apparent cheerfulness, Barbara carried a deep sadness behind her eyes, and the skin muscles of her face and neck indicated a long-term eating disorder. She fidgeted uneasily in her seat throughout the lecture, as though she felt buffeted by her churning emotions. I had hoped that Barbara would stay after the workshop to speak with me, but she was among the first to leave. But when I left the building some time later, Barbara was waiting for me on the steps. "I just wanted to say goodbye," she said, smiling.

"Are you sure that's all you wanted to say to me?" I asked.

Her smile faded as she shook her head. She cleared her throat, as if she were about to speak, but no words came out. Taking her by the hand, I led her back into the lobby of the building and found us a place to sit in the stairwell. After several moments of silence, Barbara began to tell me her story. She had been sexually abused as a teenager and had been in and out of counseling for twenty years. She thought she had healed her wounds but still could not sustain an intimate relationship with a man.

When she chose to be celibate, she began eating compulsively and gained fifteen pounds within a few weeks. Unhappy about the extra weight, she got into the habit of forcing herself to vomit up whatever she had just eaten. So began her three-year battle with bulimia. She was desperate to stop, she said, her eyes brimming with tears. Was there anything I could do to help her break the pattern of bingeing and purging?

I offered Barbara a tissue and then explained to her the effect of ancestral memories on our bodies and on our relationship to food. I asked her to delve into her family's history because I suspected that she would find other instances of sexual abuse besides her own and gave her several exercises to recover ancestral memories. I also provided her with specific food *sadhanas* and dietary recommendations: whole grains (including bulgur, barley, brown rice, millet, and buckwheat) and fresh organic vegetables. I especially wanted her to eat root vegetables, sweet potatoes, radishes, and parsnips to fortify her lower body, because I sensed that the tissues of her reproductive organs were still suffering from the memory of the abuse. Lots of fresh fruits would increase her vitality and sense of joy. I also recommended that she eat nuts so that she would have something crunchy to chew away the negative memories. I also suggested she buy herself bouquets of lemon balm and lavender and keep potted herbs and flowers in her bedroom so she could inhale more of life's fragrance.

Barbara dutifully noted down all of my suggestions and I asked her to keep me informed of her progress. I hugged her warmly, feeling the faintness of her heartbeat. Even as we said good-bye, I knew that she would not write to me. I wondered whether she would have the impetus to delve into her ancestral past and find the source of her impaired ancestral memories.

Many years later, I was shopping in a health-food store

in Soho, a neighborhood in downtown Manhattan, when someone tapped me on the shoulder. I turned to face a woman whose hair was cropped short and dyed green. "You don't remember me, do you?" she asked with a giggle. I probably would not have recognized her if not for her infectious laugh.

Barbara had undergone a rebirth. She was glowing with health. Her eyes were bright and her manner was easy and open. She quickly updated me, saying that I had helped her to become conscious of her food choices, so that she was able to eat normally again and cure herself of the bulimia. By embracing a wholesome approach to food, one that honored nature's way, she had also found the inner strength to uncover her painful ancestral memories. She had resolved her issues about men, she said, smiling. As if on cue, her much younger boyfriend appeared, also sporting a colorful hairdo, carrying a basketful of organic fruits and vegetables. We were introduced, and then they went off to finish their shopping.

Barbara chose to embrace these healing practices and therefore benefited from the life-giving, memory-laden foods that nature intended her to eat. As you reorient your palate to those tastes and foods that are most healthful for you as an individual, you begin to feel more balanced and you are less vulnerable to disease. I invite you now to learn more about how to practice specific food *sadhanas*. While at first it may seem that they take more effort and time than you are accustomed to giving to food preparation, the rewards are plentiful, and the doing itself soon becomes a source of satisfaction. It is an effective and pleasurable path of practice.

# DEVELOPING EVERYDAY AWARENESS THROUGH FOOD *SADHANA*

According to the Vedic seers, food is the only medium that carries *ojas, prana,* and *tejas* (the three primordial states of the universe) into our vital tissues. As such, food is the primary vehicle by which the universe transmits memory, energy, and vibration to all species. Food is said to be the Mother-Essence of healing—it is *rasa*, the taste of life.

Not only do food *sadhanas* impart *rasa*, they also nourish and influence our life force and internal sound. Every bite we eat, every motion and sound we make in the spirit of *sadhana* invokes the vibration, energy, and memory of the universe. Pounding the husk off whole grains with a large mortar and pestle invokes the energy of the heart. It strengthens its rhythmic beat and awakens the heart's cellular memory, purpose, and compassion. Sifting grains and beans in a straw basket to remove the husks and stones creates a soothing sound that helps to restore the resilience and fluidity of *prana*. The *shwee, shwee, shwee* of sifting grain winnows out discordant thoughts. The sound and movement of cutting vegetables along their growth or life lines to emphasize their anatomical forms sharpens the senses.

For the best healing effect of *sadhana*, however, we must also reclaim the kitchen from the dissonance of the complexities of modern life. Fruits, vegetables, teas—all foods, and especially those that are used for medicinal purposes, such as herbs, are highly susceptible to energy and vibrational fields. Electric current can shatter the *tanmatra* (energy quanta)—the memory of the food. The noise generated by refrigerators, food processors, stoves, and other appliances can actually mutate the quantum energy structure of food. I am talking not only about audible dissonance, but also what we do not hear—the vibrations that shrivel the food's cosmic memory, causing the food to forget its purpose.

As I began simplifying my life many years ago in New York City, I first got rid of my blender, juicer, and television. A year later, I was ready to get rid of the larger items, including my vacuum cleaner and refrigerator. Today, I live very simply in a log cabin that was built in 1900. A wood furnace provides me with heat in the winter. I use an old bathtub, water-fed by a spring that comes from the top of Mount Pisgah. I have no washing machine, no refrigerator, no electrical appliances at all. I often wash my clothes in a stream on a scrub board and line-dry them in the sun. Most of my diet consists of food I have grown in my organic garden. I supplement my food with whole grains and dried beans that I buy from my local health-food store or at the farmer's market.

I realize that you may not be ready for these very extreme measures, so let me assure you that you do not need to unplug all of your appliances and give them away. Try this compromise: gradually reduce your dependency on your juicer, mixer, and can opener. Use a hand grinder instead of your electric blender. At some point, consider getting a smaller refrigerator, so that you can store food for only a limited period. Many people use their refrigerators as a storage space for bottles of ketchup, mayonnaise, mustard, and soda. You should eventually eliminate these items from your diet because many of these foods are packed with chemical preservatives and complex mixtures of ingredients that convert into destructive acids when they enter the digestive system. Don't overcrowd your refrigerator with leftovers. These should be used by the next day at the latest. Refrigerated, stale foods are considered by Ayurvedic medicine to be *tamasic*; they cause us to become lethargic and sluggish and in some people, they induce nightmares.

Even worse than the effects of appliances is the chemical and genetic manipulation of food by means of additives, irradiation, genetic engineering, and freezing. These processes alter food at the very core of its memory. Insecticides and chemical fertilizers endanger the environment and distort the memory core of the food. But genetic manipulation deliberately alters the food's memory and essence, so that the food forgets what it is supposed to do when we ingest it. We are nourished not only by the vitamins, minerals, and enzymes in food, but also by its resonant field of memories that communicate with our tissues. When that memory is tampered with, the resulting food does not satisfy our physical or spiritual needs. We overeat in a futile attempt to assuage our real hunger.

Our well-being depends on the sacred memory, energy, and vibration of the foods we eat as well as the air we breathe and the sounds we hear. We would do well to remember, every time we opt for food that is convenient, fast, or modern, that we may be undermining the divine source of *sadhana*. When we eat food that has been *artificially* transmuted, our inner rhythms start to malfunction, alienating us from our cosmic source.

Nature has provided us with her clay, wood, fire, stone, minerals, metals, leaves, and straw. All of these can be made into or used as peaceful instruments that provide us with healthful sustenance. Throughout history, farmers recognized these truths and worked the earth reverently. Even in times of bitter harvest, they recognized the cyclical rhythms of nature and continued to be grateful for what they received.

As we put the food *sadhanas* into practice, we recover a mindfulness of our world. Our instruments of perception— the mind and the senses—grow ever more acute; our spirit becomes imbued with joy, light, and love. Our inner rhythms merge into harmony, our mind becomes peaceful, our intuition blooms, and we are granted the possibility of complete healing.

You may recall the story I told in chapter 5 about Joanie, who had been suffering from serious claustrophobia, anxiety, and manic-depression. Joanie credits her recovery to her practice of breath *sadhanas*, as well as the food *sadhanas* she introduced into her life. She had never been much of an eater and didn't like to cook, especially during her worst bouts of depression. Sometimes, even making a green salad or boiling a pot of pasta had felt like too much of an effort for her.

Her unhealthy diet of fast-food hamburgers, luncheon-meat sandwiches, cookies, and ice cream was exacerbating her illness, so I encouraged her to gradually incorporate a seasonal variety of whole grains, fresh vegetables, and fruits into her diet. As her emotional health improved, Joanie discovered that she actually enjoyed preparing food. She began experimenting with different vegetables and spices, taking pleasure in the different colors and aromas and tactile sensations.

Cooking became a healing practice for her marriage, too: She and her husband started shopping together on weekends at a nearby farmer's market that offered plentiful organic, locally grown produce. He happily joined her in the kitchen, helping her sift the grains and knead the dough for chapati. Joanie told me that she particularly grew to love the taste of chapati and *dhal*, so much so that she made them every day for about three months. She had an image of the golden *dhal* filling up the pit in her stomach. She knew that this was a metaphor for the hole in her life. It was as if the chapati and *dhal* were neutralizing the "sinking feeling" she had lived with for so many years. She also loved cutting vegetables along their life lines; with every cut, she could feel her focus growing sharper and her memory of positive feelings beginning to strengthen. Her husband told me that the *sadhana* of cutting vegetables and fruits had helped Joanie to cut through the dense fog of depression that had almost destroyed her joy and enthusiasm for life.

### The Practice: Cutting Vegetables

• Be conscious of the *prana* of all life. Cut vegetables, herbs, and fruits along their life lines. Conscious cutting makes for a sharper *buddhi*.

• Do not overcook vegetables. Allow them to maintain their unique flavors and vivid colors.

There are eight distinct types of vegetables. To maintain the integrity of food and to adhere to the spirit of *sadhana*, each food must be cut in accord with its shape and *pranic* force (or life or growth line). These are the many noble ways you may cut each type of vegetable. (Follow the same rules for cutting fruits.)

1. Elongated root—carrots, daikon, parsnips
   • Shavings: Scrape vegetable in thin or thick pieces.
   • Matchsticks: Cut diagonally in pieces of $1/8''$ thickness, then stack slices and cut in half.
   • Half-rounds: Slice in half lengthwise, then cut in half to desired thickness.
   • Log-cut: Slice into $2''$ pieces, then cut each piece vertically and slice lengthwise in $1/2''$ to $1/4''$ thickness.

2. Round root/earthbound—turnips, potatoes, rutabagas, winter squash
   • Cubes: Slice vertically into three pieces, cut each piece into vertical logs, then cut into cubes of desired size.

3. Stalked and tightly flowered—cauliflower, broccoli
   • Florets: Remove flower and place facedown on cutting

board. Cut into stem *toward* the flower and gently separate flowers with your hands.

- Half-moon stems: Slice lengthwise along center of stem, place facedown on cutting board, and cut diagonally or in half-moons at thickness of 1/4". (If broccoli skin is thick, peel it off before cutting.)

4. Variegated—peppers, okra
   - First, cut peppers vertically along their life line or growth line, then cross-cut against the grain to desired size.
   - Cut okra diagonally in thin pieces.

5. Expanded—leafy greens such as collard, kale, mustard, and lettuce
   - Diagonal slice: Fold leaf lengthwise along the spine and remove stem. Open leaves and pile twelve pieces on top of each other, then fold over along the spine and slice thinly on the diagonal. Cut stems on the diagonal into thin pieces.

6. Multi-layered—onion, cabbage
   - Crescents: Cut in half lengthwise along center grain. Lay each half facedown on cutting board and slice lengthwise in crescents of desired thickness.
   - Minced: Cut in half lengthwise along center grain. Place each half facedown on cutting board and slice lengthwise, then cross-cut against the grain to desired size.

7. Elongated/bunched—plantain and banana
   - See above instructions for elongated root.

8. Podded/stringed—peas, string beans, snow peas, pole beans, sugar snap peas
   - Open pod along life line. Remove string by snapping it off at the end and pulling downward to remove string before cooking. These may also be cooked whole.

Think of yourself as a multidimensional artist. Your kitchen is your dimensionless field of infinite play—the room to which you retreat to revel in color, sound, texture, and movement. The myriad aromas, sounds, tastes, and textures of nature's foods enliven every one of our cells and memories. The nose becomes a direct means to consciousness; the eyes become the gateway to divine light; the ears, the pathway to inner harmony. The tongue absorbs a kaleidoscope of flavors; the sense of touch allows us to experience the temperatures and textures of the universe. All of these experiences have the power to bring our inner rhythms into harmony, making us more aware of the essences of life.

When looking around my own kitchen, I savor the delightful profusion of sensory stimuli with which I am surrounded: the smell of roasted sesame seeds as I grind them with my mortar and pestle; the aroma of cumin seeds roasting in ghee; the soothing *shhh* sound as I pour the seeds into the cooked *dhal*. I never tire of smelling the fragrant summer *masala*—fennel, coriander, cumin, and ginger, all ground together; of hearing the hiss of mustard seeds popping in a hot skillet; of inhaling the aroma of saffron and cardamom boiling in milk; of noticing that the pale yellow color of the herbed milk resembles the first light of dawn.

My kitchen holds ample evidence of nature's bounty. A *tali*, an intricately decorated Indian brass tray, is laid out with spring greens and herbs fresh out of my garden: violet-flowered oregano, white-flowered arugula, dandelion leaves and spring mustard, the season's first cilantro leaves, licorice, and mint. In the autumn, lemon cucumbers, broccoli, collards, and acorn squash overflow the straw baskets in which I store them.

My shelves are lined with glass jars filled with yellow mung beans, red *aduki* beans, black rice, white basmati rice, golden-orange corn, varieties of ivory-, tan-, and buff-colored rices, and speckled North Carolina beans. An open cabinet displays jars of tea leaves such as lavender, rose petal, rose hip, hawthorn berry, dried orange peel, licorice root, and raspberry leaves. On one windowsill are drying trays that hold a variety of beans, okra, and pumpkin seeds. Bunches of mint, thyme, marjoram, Indian basil, parsley, cilantro, comfrey, and tansy hang in front of a bay window, drying for use during the winter months. Two wind chimes also hang by the window and provide me with echoes of celestial music whenever a breeze blows.

An earthenware fire-pot, camphor cubes, and *dhup* (pine kindling) are set on a shelf in my kitchen. A small statue of Ganesha, the elephant-headed god, sits next to the fire pot. Before every meal, I put pieces of camphor and pine into the pot, along with a tiny amount of whatever meal I have prepared and I light a fire and say my prayers before eating.

## THE KITCHEN AS SACRED SPACE

The kitchen environment and the rituals of spice grinding can create a kind of sacred space. In one instance, it may have been the key to healing for a young girl with a serious eating disorder. By age nine, Sita had developed an aversion to food. Her parents tried all kinds of therapies but could not get her to eat, and the poor child was wasting away because she refused to eat almost every food she was offered. Determined not to allow her daughter to die of malnutrition, her mother, Lucy, attended one of my food *sadhana* workshops. She remained after the program to seek my help.

I advised her not to force the child to eat, but rather, to introduce the daily practice of grinding spices into their home. Lucy was clearly dubious. After all the expert advice, psychological interventions, and carefully constructed menus, my suggestion seemed ridiculously simple and beside the point. But the practice sounded so easy, and she was willing to try anything to save her daughter's health. She dutifully bought a *suribachi* (a circular Japanese bowl traditionally used for grinding spices).

The next day, while Sita was drawing at the kitchen table, Lucy followed the instructions I had given at the workshop for making *masala*. She dry-roasted a variety of seeds, including mustard, coriander, cumin, fennel, and cardamom. Then she ground and mixed them in the *suribachi*. Sita sat with her head bent over the table, coloring away, appearing not to notice what Lucy was doing. Lucy repeated the roasting and grinding the next day. Sita again showed little interest except occasionally to look up from her book and glance over at her mother. The following day, when Lucy announced that she was going into the kitchen to grind spices, Sita immediately jumped up from the couch where she had been watching television and said, "Can I help? I love the smell."

Sita dragged a chair over to the stove so she could stir the seeds in the skillet. Then she helped Lucy separate the roasted spices into several small dishes so that they could be poured one by one into the *suribachi*. Soon Sita was happily absorbed in grinding the seeds. "Which smell do you like the best?" Lucy asked her. "Let me try them all," said Sita. "Then I'll tell you."

She hummed a little tune to herself as she and her mother took turns grinding the spices. Sita grinned when she got to the cardamom. "This is the one I really love," she said.

"Would you like to taste that smell, Sita?" Lucy asked. Sita nodded, so Lucy warmed up some milk and added the ground cardamom for her. While Lucy watched in stunned silence, holding her breath, Sita drank the entire cup of milk—the first milk she'd had in months. That moment marked the beginning of Sita's return to health. Her interest in food was gradually rekindled, and over the course of the next several months she overcame her resistance to eating. When I last heard from Lucy, she said that Sita had been totally cured of her eating disorder and often helps her mother prepare their meals. She has taken charge of grinding the spices every afternoon, and her very favorite food is Cream of Wheat with cardamom, cinnamon, and raisins.

Sita's story is a testament to the simple practice of *sadhana*, which awakened in her a profound memory of taste and restored her appetite for life. The *Taittiriya Upanishad* tells us:

> *The essence of all things here is the Earth.*
> *The essence of Earth is water.*
> *The essence of water is plants.*
> *The essence of plants is a person.*

Let's take this text one step further and ask ourselves: What is the essence of a person? I believe it is the fundamental nature that is uniquely ours and connects us to the universe. We are all on a lifelong quest for consciousness, which emerges from the cultivation of awareness—the inner knowing that depends entirely on the harmonious relationship we develop with nature. The practice of food *sadhana* restores our cognitive memory and our ability to heal ourselves of physical disease and emotional wounds. Open your heart to Mother Nature's wisdom, feast at her table, and you will never go hungry.

## Chapter 12

# FOOD *SADHANAS*: VEDIC NUTRITION AND PRACTICE

*O our mother the Earth, O our father the Sky,*
*Your children are we, and with tired backs*
*We bring you the gifts that you love.*
*Then weave for us a garment of brightness . . .*
*May the fringes be the falling rain,*
*May the border be the standing rainbow.*
—A Tewa Pueblo Prayer

Food *sadhana* practices are sacred rites that will help develop your awareness of food and your ability to rediscover all of nature's wholesome rhythms.

Whatever your present health condition, constitution, or karma, you can improve it through the reverent practices of *sadhana*. The food *sadhanas* will be most important in this effort. The practices and dietary recommendations in this chapter are derived from the healing food regimen I developed during and after my cancer journey. They are also informed by the experiences of the hundreds of people whom I have guided into recovery from illness. Because I feel it's important for people to experience the tranquil energetic effects of my kitchen, I often consult with them about their health in the space where I do my food preparation.

Our food, our body, and nature are all one entity. The flesh of our body is made of the same elements as the flesh of a melon. Our bodily fluids are composed of the same elements as the milk of a coconut. Our hands and legs are like the limbs of a tree; the leaves of a tree are like our lungs, and its bark is like our skin. When we treat the earth's food irreverently, it bleeds. When rivers are polluted, they choke. And when a forest is clear-cut, it dies. But when we live in reverence with the earth, we also honor our individual bodies.

## RECLAIMING OUR LIMBS OF *SADHANA*

Hands are considered our most precious organs of action. In Vedic thought, hands and feet are said to be the conduits of the five elements: space, air, fire, water, and earth. One of the five elements courses through each finger. (See below.)

thumb—space
forefinger—air
middle finger—fire
ring finger—water
little finger—earth

*The hand of* sadhana *representing the five elements*

When we use our limbs in accord with the sacred laws of nature, every action worships and praises the omniscient divinity in all things. When we feed our young children, we are sharing with them all the maternal energies of the universe. In Vedic tradition, we eat with our hands because the five elements within them begin to transform the food and make it digestible even before it reaches the mouth. Likewise, when we clasp our hands in prayer, we activate the elements within our hands, stimulating a surge of heightened consciousness throughout the body.

The ancient Vedic tradition of eating food with the hands is derived from mudra practice. Gathering the fingertips of the right hand as they touch the food stimulates the five elements and invites the fire of digestion to bring forth its digestive juices. In Vedic thought, the right hand beckons the solar energy of the universe, inviting it to enter or be received by the body. The left hand (used for cleaning the body) beckons the lunar energy of the universe, inviting energy of completion or closure of the body. The *sadhana* of feeding yourself from hand to mouth enhances your vital memory and inner balance.

Part of food *sadhana* is learning the sacred art of using your hands for food preparation and eating. This is an important step in reclaiming your healing energies. Massage your hands when you wash grains and legumes. Knead your energies into your dough. Roll out and pat breads flat with your hands. Tear leafy greens with your fingers. Warm your hands by mashing potatoes with them. At the end of the day, celebrate your hands by anointing them with a soothing oil or lotion.

Be conscious of how you use your hands when you wash yourself after awakening. Offer gratitude to the Divine with them. Cradle both the young and the elderly in your arms. Bring your hands close to your heart in prayer. In this harmonious exchange, the living breath of the earth's precious food infuses your entire being and stimulates the vibrations of your heart.

When we clasp our hands, we stimulate *prana* that circulates through the heart, which increases its vitality and brings a sense of resolve and clarity. The act of prayer helps to heal the heart, not only of the trespasses of the present life, but also of the wounds incurred through timeless rebirths. When you bring your hands together, you are transforming all five elements back into their source of *tejas*, the state of the universe's subtle fire and energy. You immediately feel the support of the Divine whether or not a desired result is forthcoming.

Reciting the following Vedic prayer each morning can help you to remember the sanctity of your hands and your connection to the healing energies of our universe:

> *Karagre vasate Lakshmi karamule Sarasvati*
> *Karamadhye tu Govindah prabhate karandarsanam*
> (Kah-rah-gray vah-say-tay laksh-me-he
> kah-rah-moo-lay sah-ras-vah-tee
> Kah-rah-madh-yay too go-vin-dah-ha
> prah-bhah-tay kah-rah-dar-shah-nam)
> On the tip of my fingers is Goddess Lakshmi,
> On the base of my fingers is Goddess Saraswati,
> In the middle of my fingers is Lord Govinda.
> In this manner, I look at my palms.

In the Vedic pantheon of celestials, Lakshmi symbolizes the energy of wealth; Saraswati, the energy of inspiration and wisdom; and Govinda, the energy of Divine Love.

## SEAT OF SADHANA: HEALING POSTURES

The way we sit is as important as the way we use our hands. Yogic tradition has given us numerous postures that are specifically designed to help us harness the earth's memory, energy, and vibration, as well as strengthen the primordial female and male energies: Shakti in women and Shiva in men. For the food *sadhana* practices, instructions for the single most important postures for both women and men are set out below.

## SQUATTING POSTURE: A WOMAN'S SEAT

The squatting posture—one of the postures of the Divine Mother—invokes the cosmic memory of the maternal instinct. In chapter 4, squatting was used to help you remember your *shakti* energy and to bring you into direct communion with the Mother. Women since the beginning of time have effortlessly assumed the squatting posture to perform their daily tasks and rituals. This practice has for the most part been abandoned by modern women.

When we move into a squatting posture, we inhale the breath of the earth into us. As women, our most powerful *shakti* energies collect below our belly. It is as important to receive and revive our *apana* breath by absorbing the earth's magnetic forces through our lower channel as it is to rejuvenate *prana* through nasal inhalation. Since no other posture can rejuvenate us in this way, try to squat whenever possible!

Squatting enables us to receive the earth's energies through our lower aperture. The magnetic force of the earth draws the *apana*, or descending air, downward, bringing it into a state of fullness. As a result, a deep warmth is fueled in the belly, keeping the tissues and organs of the lower body in harmony with the earth's vibrations. When the *apana* air is recharged in this natural way, it strengthens and moves *prana* throughout the entire body.

The food *sadhanas*, in particular, afford ample opportunity for squatting. I have a table in my kitchen that is just a foot or so off the ground, so that I can prepare food while squatting—in the ideal posture for these *sadhanas*. However, many women (and men) initially find the posture too difficult to maintain. If you feel awkward in the pose, you may, of course, assume any comfortable position when you practice the food *sadhanas*. When we squat while planting the good seed, reaping the harvest, grinding spices, pounding grain, kneading dough, cutting vegetables, preparing a meal, feasting on nature's banquet, and releasing our bodily waste back to the earth, we are acting in accord with natural cycles. The posture also helps to increase self-esteem and overcome depression. You may wish to reread the instructions on how to assume the squatting posture by turning to page 105.

## DIAMOND POSTURE: AWAKENING MASCULINE PRIMORDIAL ENERGY

The diamond posture, or *vajra asana*, takes its name from *vajra*, the thunderbolt of Indra, the mythological Vedic ruler of the universe, said to safeguard all creation. Indra dispels all omens, spells, and other negative vibrations with his thunderbolt. This posture helps to garner the centrifugal energy locked within our root chakra. It also helps to awaken the Shiva energies within us, unlocking and dissipating all negative vibrations held in the body. Assuming the diamond position redirects the *prana* to flow in the vibrational pattern of the thunderbolt. This posture directs tremendous strength to the bodily fires (and, in particular, the digestive fire) and also helps to safeguard the body's sexual energy and vitality. It is especially good for women during menstrual cycles and pregnancy.

The diamond posture also strengthens the body's immunity and its vibrational field. It revives the reproductive organs and helps *prana* ascend into consciousness. It relieves indigestion, constipation, stomachaches, and ulcers. The diamond posture also stimulates the digestive fire, increases circulation, tones the small and large intestines, and strengthens the prostate gland. It is a specific posture for men.

### The Practice: Diamond Posture in Practice

Find a clean, uncluttered space on the floor or ground and face north. Sit on your heels, with your knees close together. Spread the heels slightly apart to accommodate the buttocks comfortably between them. If you find it uncomfortable to sit on your heels, place a pillow between your calves and your thighs, so you are seated on the pillow.

Place your hands on your knees and relax your arms. Gently tilt your chin downward, toward the chest. Then as you lift the chin to face directly forward, bring awareness to your spine. Keep your back straight and relaxed.

Breathe deeply into the pelvic floor and lock your breath, tightening your anal muscles. Hold the breath for thirty seconds or so, then release it. Maintain the posture and breathe normally. Assume this or the squatting posture as much as possible during your food *sadhana* practices.

## CREATING A *SADHANA* SPACE

As I mentioned in the previous chapter, after I became cancer-free, I was inspired to reconfigure my living space in order to create a more wholesome atmosphere in which to develop my *sadhana* practices. I cleaned out my apartment

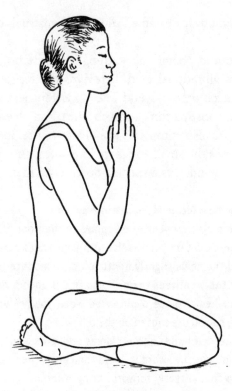

Vajra asana—*diamond posture*

on Horatio Street, built an altar adorned with sacred Hindu images, and transformed my kitchen. In addition to discarding all the electrical appliances, I replaced the fluorescent light with a gentler bulb. I gave away all of my frozen and canned foods, as well as the old boxes of grains, beans, and spices that I'd stored in my cupboard for too many months to count.

Although I couldn't duplicate the earthen walls or wood-burning stove of my family's simple kitchen in Guyana, I could outfit my kitchen with clay and wooden bowls and utensils, a rolling pin and board, some straw baskets, a bam-boo sieve, a strainer, a food steamer, a few stainless steel and enamel pots and pans, a pressure cooker, and a large mortar and pestle. Today, the kitchen is still my favorite space in my little cabin in the North Carolina woods, because it is there that I am most reminded of my family and childhood home.

Space is essential to our happiness. Our surroundings can help heal us. When our energies are aligned with the cosmic rhythms, we are able to create a living environment that speaks to our deepest needs. Lucilla is an excellent example of this healing practice.

A Brazilian who had lived in the United States for many years, Lucilla came to see me just after she had been diagnosed with breast cancer. Her oncologist had recommended that she undergo a mastectomy, but Lucilla, who was then thirty-five, was determined to find an alternative to the operation. She was willing to try just about anything short of surgery, she said, as she followed me into my kitchen, where I had just finished preparing a *masala*. I asked her to tell me a little bit about her life.

She had no children and spent her free time gardening and doing volunteer work at a senior citizens' residence. She loved her husband, Paul, very much, but she often felt very unhappy, lonely, and neglected. He was a carpenter, who "builds for everyone else but me," she said, without trying to hide her resentment. "I've been after him for ten years to fix my kitchen cabinets because they're falling apart, but he hasn't found the time."

My first thought was that Lucilla's breast cancer was a remarkable example of divine synchronicity. I did not believe it was a coincidence that she developed cancer in her chest area, given that her husband was ignoring the chests in her kitchen.

"He's even too busy to take care of me now that I have cancer," she went on. "He doesn't have time to take me to the doctor, so my sister comes with me to the appointments. I'm glad she's around, but shouldn't my husband be there with me?"

It was obvious that her health would improve markedly if she were able to get her husband's attention. She was suffering terribly because she didn't feel loved or cared for, and in conjunction with whatever other therapies I suggested, her feelings of abandonment also had to be addressed. "Trust me, Lucilla. This is a very simple situation," I said. "You need to hire someone to fix the kitchen cabinets."

She was visibly stunned by my suggestion, having come to me for a serious discussion about breast cancer, not home renovations.

"Bear with me," I said. "You may not realize that you have a core issue of feeling neglected by Paul. Get the cabinets fixed, because that will speak to your need to be cared for. I want you to hire a young, good-looking carpenter, someone who looks like Brad Pitt. Perhaps that will open his eyes." Lucilla burst out laughing, and I could see her energy shifting.

"Don't tell him anything about it. Don't ask his permission. Do it on your own. Hire and pay the man yourself. Have him come in and make you the best set of kitchen cabinets you could imagine," I instructed her. "Paul will have to notice what's going on, and maybe then you two can begin to communicate about your needs. Tell him that he has to support you emotionally during this difficult time, that your home needs to be tended to, that you need him to recognize your existence. At the very least, you'll have the kitchen you want."

"But what if he gets angry?" she asked.

"Then you respond calmly. Say to him, 'How many years have I been asking you to do this? And by the way, here I am, fighting this cancer by myself.'"

The grin on Lucilla's face told me the idea appealed to her. I had one more piece of advice: "Don't think of this as getting back at Paul, but rather that you want to bring a young man's gentle energy of repair into your kitchen."

Before she left that day, I taught her how to make the *kichadi* and told her to follow a very *sattvic* diet, which included whole grains, barley soup, long-grain brown rice, and bitter vegetables like dandelion leaves. (The dandelion leaves are good for a *pitta* condition—the anger and neglect which had caused the inflammation in the breast—because bitter reduces *pitta*.) I made her a packet of teas—raspberry, rose flower, hibiscus, and red clover—to rebalance her hormonal functions and address her cancerous condition.

Lucilla was almost dancing with excitement at the prospect of finding someone to take care of her external environment while she attended to her internal environment. She wasted no time hiring a handsome, young carpenter named George, who started to build her a beautiful set of oak cabinets. The plan had its desired effect. Even Paul could not ignore the fact that major renovations were taking place in his very own kitchen.

Over the course of several conversations, Lucilla was able to make him understand how much she missed his active presence in their marriage and how badly she needed his support, especially at this time. Rather than reacting with anger, as she had feared, he apologized for neglecting her and told her how embarrassed and remorseful he felt. Paul agreed that George should finish the job. He also began coming home earlier and insisted on accompanying her to all her medical appointments.

Lucilla's health crisis also had a positive resolution. She strictly followed the diet I had outlined, and after six months her doctor, astonished, told her that the cancer had totally disappeared. My advice to her had one other, totally unexpected result. Paul was so impressed with George's craftsmanship that he hired him as a partner to share his workload so that he could spend more time with Lucilla.

I am not suggesting that you, or anyone else with cancer, ignore your doctor's recommendations. Lucilla's story is intended to be an example to you of the importance of a wholesome environment, wholesome communication, and wholesome foods in your health. I myself am a living example of the help Western surgery can provide, since it gave me time to find the path of practice that would ultimately heal me entirely. The food, breath, and sound *sadhanas* can be used together with any Western medical regimen, and will help those treatments be more effective.

## PREPARING A *SADHANA* KITCHEN

The first step on Lucilla's path of practice was to find the means to make her kitchen a comfortable, hospitable environment for preparing and eating food. You, too, must begin your food *sadhana* by acknowledging the importance of the kitchen as the living hearth of your home, and its floor as a symbol of the earth's surface. Your kitchen is a sacred space. Keep it clean and uncluttered. Observe a few minutes of silence before you enter it. Spread a colorful cotton cloth on the floor for seated *sadhanas*.

Simplify your kitchen by getting rid of all the utensils that you do not use. Take some time to inspect your cabinets. Identify the pots, pans, serving dishes, plates, and flatware that you have not used for a year or more. Give them to a charity or to someone you know who can use them. In my own kitchen, twenty years ago, I found two electric coffee-grinders, a bamboo steamer, an electric face-steamer, a blender, and an assortment of stainless-steel pots and saucepans that I hadn't used in years. I put them all in a big carton and donated them to the Salvation Army.

Choose a few good-quality stainless-steel and enamel pots and pans, as well as several cast-iron skillets and a stainless-steel pressure cooker. I recommend that you use cooking utensils made of a variety of materials, because they all lend different energies to the food. For example, stainless steel conducts heat without interfering with the energies of the food. Enamel pots and pans are even more protective of the energy. Stainless steel, enamel, and glassware tend to lend a cooling energy to foods, whereas earthenware, ceramics, copper, and cast iron add a more warming energy.

You will also need some wooden bowls and ladles, a ceramic hand-grater for your ginger and garlic, and most important, a grinding stone and mortar and pestle for your spices. Every *sadhana* kitchen must have a sharp knife. A Vedic adage says that if we mindfully cut each vegetable, fruit, and herb, our knives, senses, and mind will remain forever sharp.

Honor the sanctity of the kitchen with a clean body and a peaceful mind. Invite children, family, and friends to join you in the kitchen for your *sadhana* activities. You may discover, as Leona, one of my students, did, that sometimes even those who profess not to be interested in cooking can be lured into lending a hand.

Leona was preparing a large pot of kasha varneshkes, a traditional Eastern European Jewish dish made of bow tie–shaped noodles and buckwheat groats mixed with vegetable broth and fried onions, to bring to a friend's house for dinner. Her mother, who had been visiting her in Manhattan overnight, was about to leave for her home in Connecticut, but she was tempted into the kitchen by the delectably nutty aroma of the roasted buckwheat and the sizzle of the onions frying in ghee.

"Let me stir the onions," she said, gently pushing Leona away from the stove. As she continued stirring with one hand, she used the other to dip a spoon into the pot of buckwheat and noodles for a quick taste check. "This needs a bit more salt," she said. "Maybe some pepper, too."

As Leona later described the scene to me, her mother stayed at the stove, alternately stirring, tasting, and spicing, until she declared the dish ready to be served. "She had her coat on the whole time because she was literally on her way out the door," Leona said, still smiling at the memory. "But kasha varneshkes is real Jewish comfort food, and the smell of it was just too familiar and irresistible. Now that she's widowed, my mother keeps telling me how much she hates to cook, but you certainly would have thought otherwise that day."

## BE AWARE OF QUANTITY

The quantity of food you eat plays as important a role in maintaining good health as the quality of food. Generally, eat enough food to satisfy your system, without having a feeling of heaviness afterward. Ayurveda recommends filling half of the stomach with solid food, one quarter with liquid, and leaving the remaining quarter empty to ease digestion.

A simple way to determine the appropriate amount of solid food to be taken at each meal is to cup both hands together and measure the amount of food that would fill this "cup" to the brim. A single cupped handful of liquid is the ideal ration of liquid at each meal. The "cup" of your hands is referred to as *anjali* and is the perfect measure for your particular stomach. The smaller your hands, the less food and drink you need to sustain yourself.

When you are doing hard physical work, you will want to eat a larger amount of food. When you are exerting very little energy throughout the day, you will want to reduce the quantity of food proportionately. During illness or the seasonal junctions (see appendix 2), we reduce our food intake to one-third the size of a normal meal. Decreasing the amount of food allows the digestive system to reorganize itself by reducing its workload, so the body is nourished without unduly disturbing *agni*, the fire of digestion. The appropriate quantity of food allows *apana*, the breath responsible for evacuation of wastes from the body, and *prana* to move downward, while *agni* is encouraged to rekindle.

## CHOOSING WHOLESOME QUALITY FOOD

The Ayurvedic sage Charaka taught that, "For food to be digested in a timely manner, thus promoting energy, healthy complexion, strength, and longevity, it must not only be imbibed in proper measure, but must also be of wholesome quality." Here are some ways to ensure good quality in our food.

- Remain alert to the smell, color, touch, and taste of foods.
- Use foods that are seasonally and organically grown.
- Encourage the resurgence of organic community spirit by supporting your local farmers as much as possible.
- Avoid using foods with preservatives or those that have been genetically engineered or altered in any way.
- Discard all old spices, frozen foods, and commercially canned foods.
- Use only organic or certified raw milk and dairy products. *Pitta* types who are allergic to cow's milk may use soy milk instead. *Vata* types may use rice or almond milk. *Kapha* types may use rice, soy, or goat's milk.
- Use pure ghee made from sweet butter, not from vegetable oil (see ghee recipe on page 329).
- Do not use hydrogenated or commercial brands of oils. Use only naturally processed oils available at health-food stores.
- Use pure, spring, well, or rainwater. (In parts of the country where acid rain is prevalent, avoid using rainwater.)
- Whenever sugar is called for in a recipe, use only natural brown sugar, jaggery (unrefined Indian palm sugar), Sucanat

(specially processed brown sugar made from the juice of sugar-cane), raw honey, or pure maple syrup. Never use white sugar or commercial brands of brown sugar or sugar substitutes.

• Use Ayurvedic rock salt. Sea salt may be substituted if rock salt is unavailable. Do not use commercial salt, iodized salt, or salt substitutes.

• Use fresh organic fruits that have not been waxed or sprayed with chemical pesticides, and dried fruits that have not been sulfurized or treated with processed sugars or chemicals.

• Use organic fruit juices.

Wholesome foods can be purchased from health-food stores and/or through Ayurvedic resources, some of which are listed in appendix 4.


## HARMONY IN EATING

Eating is a wonderful act of *sadhana*. As noted earlier, when we touch nature's food with our hands, it brings the universe's fire through our fingers into the food, and then joins it with the fire of digestion, *agni*. If we are aware of awakening the fire within ourselves, we digest the food more smoothly. It is said in the Vedas that only when the digestive system is awry can disease arise in the body.

Like most people do today, I remember all too well juggling a hectic schedule during the years I spent in New York City before I was diagnosed with cancer. I skipped breakfast, ate a less-than-nutritious lunch on the run, and sat down to dinner at nine o'clock. How could proper digestion occur when we force the system to put up with such abuse year after year? No wonder, then, that we have such a high incidence of cancer and heart disease in Western society, when we refuse to observe the integrity of our physiology by nourishing our bodies and souls with dignity and respect. Here are some simple guidelines to help you honor the *sadhana* of food and facilitate digestion:

- Maintain a consistent mealtime schedule.
- Be mindful of your conversations during meals. While it is best to observe silence during meals, you may choose to engage in calm, soothing conversations.
- Experience the joy of eating with your own hands— from hand to mouth.
- Chew your food well and be aware of its smells, tastes, textures, and the sounds it makes while you are ingesting it.
- Be attentive to your digestion during meals. Never eat when you are upset. Wholesome foods turn sour in our digestive tracts from negative emotions.
- Allow a few hours to pass between meals and bedtime.
- Sit on your heels for fifteen minutes after meals, or take a gentle walk to encourage proper digestion.
- Never eat and run. Never eat while standing up or lying down.

## OFFERING FOOD TO MOTHER EARTH

Many traditions share the custom of offering a small portion of cooked food to the divine giver of all nourishment before the meal is served or tasted. The first portion is given to the universe as a token of gratitude. We feed the gods and goddesses before we feed ourselves. In my tradition, a small fire is lit in an earthen or brass pot, which is kept on a stand or altar in the kitchen, and the food is offered into the fire.

The offering may be accompanied by any form of prayer you choose. The traditional Jewish prayer before a meal, for example, offers thanks to God "who brings forth bread from the earth." Catholics often ask for a blessing from the Lord for "these your gifts, which we are about to receive from your bounty." No matter what your faith or spiritual tradition, prayer encourages confidence, joy, and fearlessness as it brings you within the protection of divine forces. The following is a Vedic prayer from the *Bhagavad Gita* to Brahman, the Infinite One (see page 216 for phonetic pronunciation).

*Brahmarpanam brahma havih*
*Brahmagnau brahmana hutam*
*Brahmaiva tena gantavyam*
*Brahmakarma samadhina*
*Om Shanti Shanti Shantih*

Brahman is the offering.
Brahman is the oblation.
Poured out by Brahman into the fire of Brahman.
Brahman is to be attained by the one who contemplates the
    action of Brahman.
(Brahman refers to Pure Consciousness.)

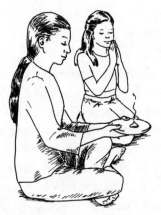

*Offering food to the fire*

## SADHANA OF THE SEED

Spice grinding is more than just a way to make *masala*. It is meditation in motion—a practice that helps us grow into maturity and splendor. The spice-grinding stone that my grandmother bequeathed to my mother was so important that she carried it with her (one of few possessions) when she fled from Guyana during the civil war.

The grinding stone and mortar and pestle are ancient symbols of the power of male and female energies. The mortar or base is Parashakti, the primordial feminine power that brought forth manifestation. The pestle is the lingam, or Parashiva, the masculine force that represents all-pervasive Consciousness. When we grind our spices, we bring our feminine and masculine forces into a state of balance.

Perhaps for this reason, the grinding stone and mortar and pestle have been used by so many cultures throughout time. Shapes and materials vary worldwide with many versions still in use today: the *suribachi* and *surikogi* (unglazed pottery bowl and a wooden pestle) in Japan; the earthenware mortar and pestle in Thailand; the large fluted stone mortar and pestle used in Mexico and Peru; and the porcelain apothecary-style mortar and pestle used in England and in much of Europe. No Vedic kitchen is complete without at least one mortar and pestle. The most popular type is called *sil batta*. *Sil* is the flat stone base, and *batta* is the handheld stone roller which is worked back and forth across the base.

Stone supports the earth, lending her strength and security. We use stones to build dams, barriers, bridges, and the foundations of our homes—all structures that give stability to our lives. As Saint Francis of Assisi wrote in one of his sonnets, "When you build your dream in life, build on it slowly, stone by stone." The grinding stone you choose becomes a symbol of your stability and purpose. Look for a base stone that represents who you are, and a hand stone that fits comfortably in your palm. Wash the stones with a nontoxic detergent and use a scrub brush to remove loose dirt and pieces of sediment. If possible, place them in the sun to dry; otherwise, wipe them off well with a cloth made of natural fibers. After the rocks are thoroughly dried, rub them with sunflower oil, wipe off excess oil, and leave them in the sun for an hour. Wash well after each use.

Charlie, a yoga teacher and longtime student of mine who healed himself into remission from the HIV virus by bringing these practices of breath, sound, and food into his life, has attracted a thriving community around him as a result of teaching *sadhanas* to his students. They enjoy trekking with Charlie into the nearby mountains to find grinding blocks and hand stones straight from the earth.

Hand tools remain unparalleled for grinding spices in the spirit of *sadhana*. Since the invention of mechanical grinding tools, the fragrance has been retained, but the vital connection of hand on stone or hand on clay has been lost. The rhythms of stone grinding on stone, and earth on earth, renews our cellular memories of our connection with the earth and enhances the energy of *rasa*. Spices recall our ancestral pasts. The aroma of each spice also triggers a cosmic memory and a particular rhythm of nature.

Spice grinding is such an ancient, universal ritual that it can serve as a bridge between generations. Aaron, for example, was having trouble communicating with his mother, who had breast cancer. An only child, he had never been close to her, but now he wanted to support her and didn't know how.

I had noticed that during one of my workshops he had particularly enjoyed grinding spice. So when he confided his concern to me, I said, "You love using the *suribachi*. Bring it with you when you next go to see her, and ask her to help you make a *masala*."

Aaron shook his head and said, "She's a modern woman. She wouldn't be interested in anything as old-fashioned as spice grinding."

Aaron is a computer whiz—a brilliant, impatient young man who tends to make snap judgments and assumptions about people. Knowing this, I said, "You'd be surprised. Your mother probably has more connection to *sadhana* than you do." I suggested he bring her a gift of a *suribachi*, along with some bags of cinnamon, cardamom, clove, and coriander. I also told him to buy a *katori*, a round, covered Indian spice container, made of wood or stainless steel, with seven little compartments in which to store the ground spices.

He was so convinced that his mother would have no use for the spices or the *katori* that he kept after me to offer some words of spiritual wisdom that he could carry with him when he went to see her. Aaron is stubborn, but I can be stubborn, too. "Grind spices with her," I said firmly. "And if you need something solid to grasp on to, what could be more perfect than a *suribachi*?"

For lack of a better solution, Aaron accepted my suggestion. As he later wrote me, "Much to my surprise, my mother was receptive to my suggestion that she practice *sadhana* to reawaken her healing memories. She began to taste the difference in her food from hand-grinding her spices, and said she felt a new surge of energy from the brief practices we did together." Indeed, she was so taken with the beauty of the gift that she presented him with her mother's mortar and pestle, "in gratitude for my *sadhana* sharings with her."

## MAKING *MASALA*

The *masala* recipes that follow change with each season. *Masalas* are used to enhance the flavor of cooked foods, and as a rejuvenating tonic for the body. They may be used with any cooked food except for desserts, and are particularly good with grains, vegetables, and beans. As you make *masalas* over time, you will gain in confidence and self-expression. Soon you will want to create your own *masala* combinations from the many spice seeds available to you. Inquire into the spices of your own ancestry. Use them to make *masalas* that will stimulate your ancestral memories.

Begin by roasting fresh seeds. Roasting helps renew the energy and memory of the seeds. Using a cast-iron skillet, roast one type of seed at a time for two to three minutes, over a moderate flame, until they begin to crackle or pop. Be careful not to burn the seeds.

Then sit on the kitchen floor, preferably in the squatting or diamond posture, if you can comfortably do so, and place a mortar and pestle on the ground. Grind the seeds one kind at a time, in a clockwise motion. Allow yourself to become immersed in the circular movement of your arm. Be mindful of the blissful aroma and sonorous resonance of each spice as it is ground. Acknowledge, as well, the inner tranquility you feel as you grind away the cares and fears of the day. Be aware of the rich taste this *sadhana* gives to your food.

Use a grinding stone and roller (*sil* and *batta*) for ingredients such as cinnamon sticks, cloves, fresh ginger, garlic or turmeric root, fresh or dried chilies, and dried tomatoes or tamarind, which are difficult to grind with a mortar and pestle. When grinding fresh roots or dried fruits, use a quarter palmful of water as you grind to help blend the ingredients. Wet *masala* must be used at once and cannot be stored. The quantities provided in each recipe will last a family of two people about one week.

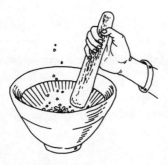

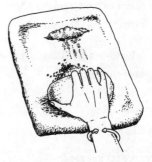

*Grinding spice seeds in a suribachi*      *Grinding spice seeds with a sil and batta*

### The Practice: Making Seasonal *Masalas*

SPRING *MASALA*

*1 tablespoon cumin seeds*
*2 tablespoons coriander seeds*
*1 tablespoon yellow mustard seeds*
*1 teaspoon black peppercorns*
*1 teaspoon cardamom seeds*

SUMMER *MASALA*

*2 tablespoons coriander seeds*
*1 tablespoon fennel seeds*
*1 tablespoon cardamom seeds*
*1 tablespoon poppy seeds*
*10 clove buds*
*1 teaspoon saffron thistles*

Grind the saffron thistles along with the fennel seeds. Do not roast them.

## EARLY FALL MASALA

2 tablespoons ajwain (or celery seeds)
1 tablespoon black mustard seeds
1 tablespoon white peppercorns
1 teaspoon freshly ground ginger
$1/2$ teaspoon grated nutmeg

Roast and grind the spice seeds before adding the ginger powder and grated nutmeg.

## AUTUMN MASALA

$1/2$ cup sesame seeds
1 teaspoon freshly ground cayenne pepper
1 teaspoon sea salt

Roast and grind the sesame seeds before adding the cayenne and salt.

## EARLY WINTER MASALA

2 tablespoons cumin seeds
2 tablespoons caraway seeds
1 teaspoon black mustard seeds
1 teaspoon turmeric powder
1 teaspoon garlic powder

Roast and grind the seeds before adding the spice powders.

## LATE WINTER MASALA (WET)

3 cloves garlic
1 fresh gingerroot (2" piece)
2 tablespoons coriander seeds

*4 dried red chilies*

*1 teaspoon turmeric*

Peel the garlic and ginger, roast the coriander seeds, and grind all the ingredients together on a grinding stone. Use a half palmful of water to meld the ground ingredients. Add turmeric powder toward the end of grinding.

## SADHANA OF THE GRAIN

Humans are bound together by grain, the earth's most sacred food and the foundation of every known culture. Rice fortified the Asians, millet sustained Africans, quinoa gave strength to the Incas. Wheat nourished the Europeans, buckwheat sustained the Eastern Europeans. Corn nurtured the indigenous people of the Americas.

Grain was given life by Gaja, the eternal elephant, who carries the memory of plants and herbs. This memory lives on in all the elephants on earth. In order for us to retain the memories of our foods, the elephant must also thrive. If the elephant becomes extinct, grains, fruits, vegetables, and herbs may still exist, but we will not be able to gain access to their cosmic memories, since the elephant is the keeper of this block of cosmic memory. When we eat such foods, they will lack vital nourishment, and the human race, too, will be weakened and eventually become extinct.

We must begin to see all plants and the *sadhana* practices that sustain them as reaching as far as the galaxies and stars. These practices are not only about composting, sowing, and then reaping the bounty of nature, they are also about recognizing the divine life carried by each seed and grain, life they give to us as sustenance and memory.

So revered is grain in my culture that when the harvest is especially abundant, even the gods can become jealous. At such times the elders would hop around the fields and shout, "Bad rice, bad rice!" to distract the gods' attention from the bounty. The grain of my ancestors can be cooked in hundreds of ways and is one of the most important offerings during religious ceremonies.

Rice is the first food an Indian bride offers to her husband at her nuptials. It is also the first solid food an Indian mother offers to her infant. The Chinese word for rice is the same word as food. A common greeting in China is, "Have you had rice today?" Japanese mothers encourage their children to eat all the rice in their bowls by calling each grain a little Buddha. In Thailand the dinner bell is tolled accompanied by the exclamation, "Eat rice!"

### The Practice: Washing Grains

Begin your *sadhana* of the grain by massaging your hands with the grains as you wash them, rubbing them between your palms. Feel the energy of the sun and wind carried in the seed-memory, soaking into your being. Feel the stimulating touch and vibrancy of your hands as you wash the grains. After you cook the grains, savor their rich taste.

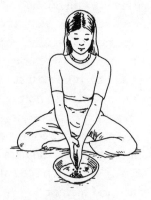

Washing grain

### The Practice: Cracking Whole Grains

Crack whole grains—including rice, wheat, corn, rye, and buckwheat—by pounding them in a large mortar with a pestle. Revel in the glorious sound of the pounding. Feel the rhythm of your heart moving into harmony with the rhythms of your breath. Be mindful of the healing effects of the cracked grain as you hear, smell, and eat it.

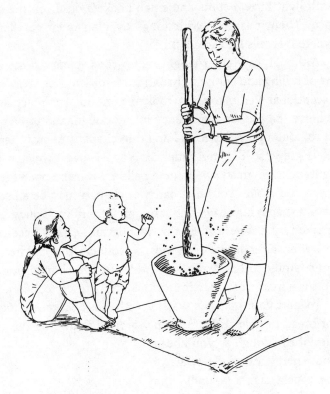

*A family pounding grain in large stone mortar*

## SADHANA OF THE BREAD

Chapati is the most popular of all Vedic breads. This simple recipe is traditionally made from *atta*, a finely milled wheat flour, although barley, buckwheat, spelt, soy, or corn flours may also be used in equal quantity. The chapati is baked on a hot griddle, called a *tava*, until it is three-fourths cooked, with light brown spots and small pockets of air on the surface. Then it is held with tongs over an open gas flame, where it swells into a balloon.

Although my father taught me to cook, I learned the fine art of rolling and cooking chapati from my mother, who is an exceptional Vedic cook. It took me months of practice to achieve the proper consistency in my dough, and to be able to roll out a perfectly round and thin chapati. As my chapati skills grew, so did my patience. Now, I love to watch the light, delicate bread swell into a balloon over the open fire of my wood stove. Your first batch of chapati may be all sorts of odd shapes and sizes, and it might not puff up. You will be amazed by how effortless this wonderful *sadhana* becomes, however, after just a few tries. Encourage the children in your family to help knead and roll out the chapati dough. This is a marvelous practice for the family to do together.

To start your *sadhana*, wash your hands and knead dough for bread or chapati from freshly ground flour. Feel the texture of the dough as you knead your energy into it. Be aware of the touch, sights, sounds, and smell of the bread as it passes through all the phases of its preparation. Then marvel at its delicious taste.

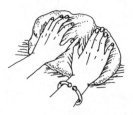

*Kneading dough*

### The Practice: Making Chapati

CHAPATI | Serves 4

*2 cups whole wheat flour*
*³/₄ cup warm water*

Pour the flour into a large mixing bowl and work it with your fingertips. Add half the water and knead the dough for 5 minutes. Add the remaining water and continue to knead for an additional 5 minutes. Cover with a clean damp cloth and let stand for 2 hours. Then divide the dough into 10 small pieces.

Lightly flour a clean table surface and, using a rolling pin, carefully roll out each piece into a thin, round patty. Preheat an iron skillet or traditional *tava*, and cook the flatbread for about 1 minute on each side over medium heat. Do not use any oil on the skillet. Remove with tongs and place the chapati directly over an open flame until it swells. Disregard this step if an open flame is not available.

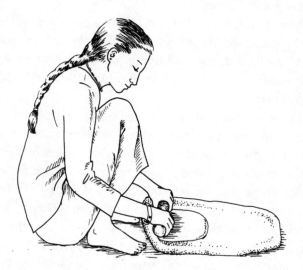

*Rolling chapati*

## SADHANA OF THE CHUTNEY

Chutneys are said to be the re-creation of the Divine Mother's love and fertility. They are a celebration of the creativity, joy, and freshness of the human spirit. Chutney making is a lavish *sadhana*. It celebrates the perennial youthfulness of your spirit and replenishes your body's vitality. Although chutneys can be made all year long, we can take special delight in this *sadhana* during the summer months, when we enjoy an abundance of fresh fruits.

According to Indian tradition, before a young man marries, his mother will put the prospective bride's homemaking skills to the test by asking her to make some chutney. If the bride makes a good chutney, she has proven that she will be a good wife and mother. The happy mother proclaims, "A bride who makes a fine chutney has a good womb for bearing my grandchildren."

To make a fine chutney, you must achieve a delicate, yet happy, union of ingredients, artfully blended in texture, color, smell, and taste. Chutney making is one of India's most ancient arts, said to foster creativity, youthfulness, and fertility in the maker.

Margie, a twenty-seven-year-old organic farmer who lives in my community, had been trying to get pregnant for three years. Her doctor could find no physical reason for her lack of success and suggested she try to conceive with the aid of fertility drugs. Maggie refused and instead turned to me for help. I suspected that the root of her infertility lay in her extremely heavy workload. She seemed constantly on the move from one activity to the next. If she wasn't involved in one of the many farm chores, she was busy gardening or baking bread, canning fresh fruits and vegetables, or selling her handmade goods at her little roadside store.

Such labor-intensive work can make it difficult for the sperm to unite with the ovum, because the *ojas*, the body's energy, is fatigued. I sensed just from looking at Maggie that her estrogen and progesterone, both of which are necessary for conception and pregnancy, were greatly reduced. Lowered levels of estrogen result in less fertility. Her face also had a weathered and tough look that was inappropriate to her age, and her body was losing its feminine softness.

I needed to help Maggie find a way to relax and take better care of herself, because she was greatly stressed by not getting pregnant. "I'm running out of time," she repeatedly told me. When I reminded her that she was only twenty-seven, she said, "But I feel like I'm fifty."

I explained to her that she had to take a step back, pace herself, and stop working so hard. Maggie nodded her assent. She very much wanted to be a mother and would do whatever I recommended, but I knew that in spite of her great intentions, she would have a difficult time just sitting still. So I showed her how to make chutney from the fruits of her orchard as a meditative practice to relieve her anxiety, and engage and gratify all of her senses.

What I really wanted to tell her was to indulge herself by soaking in long, hot aromatherapy baths; to spend more time with her husband; and to schedule quiet dinners with her husband where they wouldn't dwell on all the problems of running their business. But I knew that she would never permit herself such luxuries, and she needed a form of self-nurturance that was agreeable to her rhythms—a simple *sadhana* that suited her driven personality but would still encourage her body to make time for menstruation and ovulation.

Maggie took my advice and hired a high-school girl to help in the farm store, so that she was relieved at least of that responsibility. That summer, she made many bottles of fine fruit chutneys. When autumn came, Maggie knocked at my door and announced that she was pregnant. "If it's a girl, I'm naming her after you," she declared. "Better yet," I teased her, "why don't you call her Chutney!"

Fresh chutneys are ground daily in large stone mortars in most Indian households. They accent the simplest to the most lavish meals. In South India, chutney is often served as a main dish. There are literally hundreds of delicious combinations, from the traditional sweet mango or coconut chutneys to the hot, piquant ginger, lemon, tamarind, and chili mixtures. The more extravagant preparations are made from fresh and dried fruits such as mangoes, peaches, plums, cherries, dates, and currants, and are spiced with *masalas* and fresh herbs, marinated in ghee or jaggery (unprocessed brown sugar). No Vedic meal is complete without a dab of this luscious concoction.

As your artistry develops, you may try your hand at creating your own chutney recipes by combining various fruits, spices, and herbs. The following is the Wise Earth School's classic mango chutney recipe:

### The Practice: The Art of Making Mango Chutney

MANGO CHUTNEY | Serves 12

$^1/_2$ *cup water*

*1 tablespoon lemon balm herb*

*3 ripe mangoes*

*1 cup dates*

*1 tablespoon grated fresh ginger*

$^1/_2$ *cup moist raisins*

*2 tablespoons ghee (see recipe on page 329)*

*1 teaspoon cinnamon powder*

*1 teaspoon cardamom powder*

$^1/_2$ *teaspoon clove powder*

Bring a half cup of water to a boil, and remove from heat. Place a table-spoon of dried lemon balm herb into the water, cover, and allow to stand for 10 minutes. Strain the tea and set aside. Wash and peel mangoes and cut them into chunks, discarding the large seeds. Place the mango pieces in a large bowl. Remove the seeds from dates, cut into fine pieces, and, along with the fresh grated ginger, add to the mango along with the raisins.

Warm the ghee in a skillet and add the spice powders, keep over heat until the ghee begins to bubble. Remove from heat and pour into the mango mixture. Using a tea strainer, pour the lemon balm decoction into the chutney. Use your clean hands to mix the chutney. Pour into a clean glass jar and store in a cool place. Fresh chutneys need to be used within a week to avoid spoilage.

## SADHANA OF THE MILK: FIRST FOOD ON EARTH

The Upanishads and many other religious scriptures mention milk as a sacred food for human beings. The Old Testament, for example, refers to the Israelites' Promised Land as the "land flowing with milk and honey." In my culture, the cow is considered the most auspicious animal by virtue of the milk she provides. Called "go" in Sanskrit, the cow bears the same name as Lord Krishna, who is also called Gopala, the Lord who protects both the sacred scriptures and the earth's sacred cow.

Ayurveda considers milk to be the first and most complete food on earth. Milk was traditionally collected well after the delivery of the cow's calf, so that it could be properly di-gested by the humans. From this salubrious food come butter-milk, butter, yogurt, and ghee. But milk is *sattvic*, peaceful, only when its quality remains pure and unadulterated.

Milk has been used widely but not wisely throughout the ages. Because of the corruption prevalent in today's animal husbandry industry, we are in danger of losing this first food of the earth. The cruel treatment of animals as well as the arsenal of poisons, chemicals, hormones, and rendered protein used in the cows' feed all contribute to the misery of this beneficent animal and the impairment of its life-sustaining milk. When butter, yogurt, and ghee are made from the organic milk now being produced by many small dairies, they are our most nourishing and healing foods. Among them, ghee stands out as the elixir of excellent health.

Made from cow's milk, ghee is one of the most ancient, nourishing foods known. It has always been used as a healing food, and its very preparation is a life-enhancing *sadhana* that helps promote self-clarity. By following this graceful practice, *ojas*, *prana*, and *tejas* come into harmonic balance within the body. Making ghee is one of the simplest, most rewarding forms of meditation I know.

Sushruta, the ancient Ayurvedic seer, regarded ghee as an intelligence-building principle that fosters the body's confidence and virility when used internally. The sage Charaka praises its ability to promote memory and immunity. From the perspective of *sadhana*, ghee is associated with the vital-tissue element of love. Ghee is able to penetrate deep within the body's tissues, making it a perfect vehicle for conveying herbal powders, essences, and medicines into the body.

Ghee is made by boiling sweet butter, thereby ridding it of enzymes that encourage bacterial growth. The quality of the ghee depends on the quality of the butter, the means of making it, and how it is stored. If stored properly, the older the ghee, the more medicinal value it has. Used in small quantities, ghee is ideal for cooking, because it adds *ojas* to the food. It blends with food nutrients without losing its medicinal quality, so that it soothes and nourishes bodily constituents.

Ghee is good for all *doshas* and is specifically recommended for *pitta*. It requires no refrigeration, as the elements that cause butter to spoil have been removed. Easy to store, it does need to be refrigerated, kept covered, away from direct sunlight or heat, and free from water or any other contaminants.

### The Practice: Making Ghee

GHEE

*heavy stainless-steel saucepan*
*stainless-steel spoon*
*storage jar*
*1 pound organic sweet butter*

Sterilize the saucepan, spoon, and storage jar in advance by immersing them in boiling water. Melt the butter in the saucepan over a low flame. Continue to heat until it boils gently and a buff-colored foam rises to the surface. Do not stir the melted butter or remove the foam. Allow the ghee to cook gently until the foam thickens and settles to the bottom of the pan as sediment. When the ghee turns a golden color and begins to boil gently, with only a trace of tiny air bubbles on the surface, it is done.

Remove from heat. Once it is cool, pour the liquid into a clean glass jar, making sure that the sediment remains on the bottom of the pan. (The sediment is traditionally eaten as a snack by mixing with brown sugar.)

### The Practice: The Ceremony of Ghee

The ancient Vedic monks basked in the joyous ceremony of making ghee, practicing it as a means of meditation to awaken the true Self.

The seers frequently performed the ghee-making ceremony at *purnima*, during the full moon, to evoke inner tranquility. It is said in the Vedas that the cow is primarily guided by the energies of the moon, and that its milk reflects this luminous, calming energy. The guru would often instruct his disciples to "gather a herd of cows." This was a figurative expression meaning "go and gather, or strengthen, your resolve and commitment to a spiritual life." The making of ghee became one of the means by which the seers were able to acquire and practice these qualities. They gathered to prepare the ghee while observing profound silence, often minding its progress by closing their eyes and listening to its sounds as it matured through various phases of production.

In its earliest stage, the ghee is quiet. Then suddenly, as it begins to foam, it awakens with the gentle sound of raindrops falling on a tin roof. As the foam descends to the bottom of the pot, you may hear the sounds of a gurgling stream. Then it becomes quiet once again, filling the air with its rich, fragrant aroma. When the golden liquid of the ghee begins to bubble, it approximates the rhythmic sound of a water drum. Then each bubble disappears with an occasional *plop* and dissolves into a lasting silence.

You, too, can perform this ancient ceremony once a month to invite a more peaceful life. As the Vedic monks discovered, this *sadhana* can evoke a tranquil mind and bring forth healing energies. Observe your ghee-making *sadhana* in silence and remain mindful of the aromas, sounds, and presence of this delightful ceremony.

The food *sadhana* practices, when followed carefully, have unsurpassed healing effects on the mind, body, and spirit. I often "prescribe" spice grinding; the squatting postures; recipes for making ghee, *masalas*, and chutneys; and the re-creation of the kitchen as sacred space for people who have severe illnesses or are in the midst of a crisis. It took a brush with mortality for me to return to the Vedic lifeways and *sadhanas* that are my heritage. I hope that you will be motivated to incorporate the food *sadhanas* into your daily routine long before any disease or illness becomes manifest. These simple, ancient practices will sustain and nourish you as you reclaim your ancestral memories and revive your *buddhi*. Explore the recipes, use the postures, and celebrate your kitchen as you journey further along the path of practice.

# Appendix 1
## YOUR METABOLIC TYPE

The five elements congregate in each individual in patterns of energy known as *doshas*, which rule the functions of the body. The teachings of the *doshas* is the science of Ayurveda, the earth's oldest extant tradition of healing, healthful living, and longevity. Understanding the *doshas* helps us understand how to get and stay healthy.

Western medicine developed from investigating the microcosm, the physical world of matter and microbes. Ayurvedic medicine, however, sprang from a deep and penetrating inquiry into the macrocosm. A holistic system, Ayurveda cures by removing the source of disease, which can only happen after you identify the source of the disease—not just the symptoms. According to the Vedic seers, disease is caused by living in ways that transgress nature's laws and rhythms and by ignoring our own innate wisdom—dissonant use of the mind and senses, eating improperly, and ignoring our inner rhythms and the cycles of the seasons.

## THE DOSHAS

Knowing which *dosha* is dominant in your body helps you understand your physical rhythms. All Ayurvedic diagnosis begins with the *doshas*, a classic example of energy and matter in dynamic accord. The literal meaning of *dosha* in Sanskrit is "toxicity" or "impurity," since *doshas* become visible usually when they are in a state of imbalance. In a state of balance or health, we cannot detect the *doshas*. In a state of imbalance or disequilibrium, however, the *doshas* become visible as mucus, bile, wind, and all bodily discharges. If we ignore these early signs of disorder, imbalances can quickly become full-blown disease.

The three *doshas* coexist to varying degrees in all living organisms, and each is formed by a union of two elements in dynamic balance. Air and space, both ethereal elements, form the *vata dosha*. In *vata dosha*, air expresses its kinetic power of mobility which is *vata's* physio-psychological nature. *Dryness* is an attribute of motion and when excessive, it introduces *irregularity*, changeability into the body and mind. The element of fire forms the *dosha* known as *pitta*. In *pitta dosha*, fire expresses its transformational power, which is *pitta's* physio-psychological nature. *Heat* is an attribute of transformation and when in full force, it produces *irritability*, impatience of the body and mind. In *kapha dosha*, water expresses a stabilizing force. Heaviness is an attribute of *stability*, which is *kapha's* physio-psychological nature. Excessive *heaviness* introduces lethargy into the body and mind.

Each *dosha* also has a primary function in the body. *Vata* is the moving force, *pitta* is the force of assimilation, and *kapha* is the force of stability. Together they are an impressive example of seemingly adversarial forces coexisting in potential harmony. *Vata* is the most dominant *dosha* in the body, since air, its main element, is much more pervasive in the world than fire and water. *Vata* tends to go out of balance much more quickly than *pitta* and *kapha*. *Vata* governs bodily movement, the nervous system, and the life force. Without *vata's* mobility in the body, *pitta* and *kapha* would be rendered lame. It is most influenced by the *rajas* principle. *Rajas* is one of the three *gunas*, the primary constituents of nature, and it is the activity-oriented principle.

*Pitta* governs enzymatic and hormonal activities, and is responsible for digestion, pigmentation, body temperature, hunger, thirst, and sight. *Pitta* acts as a balancing force for *vata* and *kapha* and is most influenced by the *sattva* principle, which is the principle of peacefulness, and is the highest of all.

*Kapha* governs the body's structure and stability. It lubricates joints, provides moisture to the skin, heals wounds, and regulates *vata* and *pitta*. *Kapha* is most influenced by the principle of *tamas*, which is the principle of inertia.

*Vata, pitta,* and *kapha* pervade the entire body, but their primary domains are in the lower, middle, and upper body, respectively. *Vata* dominates the lower body, pelvic region, colon, bladder, urinary tract, thighs, legs, arms, bones, and nervous system. *Pitta* pervades the chest, umbilical area, lower stomach, small intestine, sweat and sebaceous glands, and blood. *Kapha* rules the head, neck, thorax, chest, upper stomach, fat tissues, lymph glands, and joints.

Apart from its main site, each *dosha* has four secondary sites located in different areas of the body. Together, these five sites are considered to be each *dosha*'s centers of operation, which include the various support systems through which the entire body functions.

The *doshas* interact continuously with the external elements to replenish their energy within the body. Each of the *dosha*'s five sites has a specific responsibility toward the maintenance of the organism. *Doshas* also exist in the more subtle aspects of the body and universe, such as the life force and the mind. Thus they are energetically much more influential in the maintenance of our overall health than their mere physiological expressions would suggest. In fact, as they manifest within the physical body, they continually need to be cleansed out of the body in order to maintain harmonious internal rhythms.

Each of the *dosha*'s sites is located within organs where its energy and function are manifested the most. The primary seat of *vata*, for example, is the large intestine. The air of the colon also affects the kidneys, bladder, bones, thighs, ears, and nervous system. *Vata*'s four remaining seats are the skin, lungs, throat, and stomach.

The stomach is *pitta*'s main seat in the body. The fire of the stomach affects the small intestine, duodenum, gall bladder, liver, spleen, pancreas, and sebaceous glands. Other seats for *pitta* are the blood, heart, eyes, and skin.

*Kapha*'s main seat is also the stomach; the water of the stomach affects the lymph glands and fat tissues. Other sites for *kapha* are the lungs, heart, tongue, joints, and head. The water of the head also affects the nose, throat, and sinuses.

Since each *dosha* is formed from two elements, it bears the qualities of both. *Vata* types, for example, influenced by the reigning elements of air and space, tend to be free-spirited and somewhat ungrounded. *Pitta* types are generally fast, fluid, and fiery, patterned as they are after fire and water. And those in whom *kapha* is dominant tend to be slow and methodical, since they are heavily affected by the characteristics of their main elements, water and earth. Every moment of every day, we are able to see the *doshas* in action through the elemental qualities we find in ourselves and the environment.

## ELEMENTAL SOURCE OF METABOLIC TYPES

1) *vata*      air/space
2) *pitta*     fire/water
3) *kapha*     water/earth

## QUALITIES OF THE METABOLIC TYPES

| *Vata* (like wind) | *pitta* (like fire) | *kapha* (like water) |
|---|---|---|
| dry | oily | oily |
| cold | hot | cool |
| light | light | heavy |
| mobile | intense | stable |
| | | dense |
| erratic | fluid | |
| rough | fetid | smooth |
| bitter | sour | sweet |
| astringent | pungent | salty |
| pungent | salty | sour |

## YOUR AYURVEDIC CONSTITUTION

The *dosha* that is dominant in you determines your metabolic type. Knowing what type you are provides you with helpful tools for maintaining a healthy life of balance. It also helps in diagnosing disease. Although disease has numerous causes, including genetic, environmental, and karmic factors, irritation of the *doshas* will always affect your health. The proportion to which *vata*, *pitta*, and *kapha* exist within you is what makes your constitution different from someone else's.

Your constitution is determined at birth by the states of balance or imbalance of your parents' rhythms during conception, as well as from the particular permutations of the five elements in the sperm and ovum at the time of conception. Once you are born, your constitution remains constant throughout your lifetime, but the condition of your *doshas* can change owing to disharmonious factors in your lifestyle and environment. The practices of *sadhana* can help bring the *doshas* back into a state of harmony and they certainly can help maintain your health.

In chapter 11, you were given a series of questions to help you figure out your metabolic type. There are other clues to help you determine your own or another's constitution. *Vata* types have hair that is thin and dry and often kinky or frizzy. Their skin has a grayish hue. They tend to be thin and angular, because they're formed by the wind, like a lean desert plant. Their eyes are usually brown, narrow, and uneven in shape, and their skin is always dry around the eyes. Likewise, they often have dry, cracked skin. *Vata* types have trouble putting on weight and often seem mentally distracted. Generally their physical problems are in the lower body—the large intestine and colon—because that's the seat of *vata*. They tend to have conditions such as constipation, insomnia, flatulence, arthritis, and osteoporosis.

Their greatest strength is their strong and sensitive spirit. They strive for inner freedom and are generally environmentally and spiritually attuned. They have deep faith and are generally flexible and adaptable to life's varying situations.

The *pitta* type will tend to have straight hair that is reddish in color. Does this mean that if you're of African descent you can't be *pitta*? Of course not. The Indian people who developed Ayurveda were people of color and of course *pitta* types can be dark-skinned and light-skinned. Even if you are dark-skinned and have essentially black hair, there may be a reddish tinge to the hair; it can be straight, but it will get prematurely gray. *Pitta* skin may have a reddish tone as well, and regardless of the underlying skin color, it will be oily and warm.

*Pitta* types tend to be shapelier and more athletic than *vata* or *kapha* types. Their body has the shape of an inverted triangle—broad-shouldered and slim-hipped. They tend to eat spicy, pungent foods, and sweat a lot. They can be moderate in weight. *Pittas* can have brown or hazel eyes, or greenish ones like tigers. They may be fiery or volatile or aggressive in temperament. Their physical problems are generally related to the stomach, liver, spleen and small intestine—hyperacidity, diarrhea, poor sight, skin rashes, liver, spleen, and blood disorders are some of the common complaints of *pitta* types. Their strengths are that of good physical stamina, strong intelligence, and mental focus. They also tend to be successful, courageous, and practical in their dealings.

*Kapha* types are the most voluptuous, with abundant, wavy hair. They have what I call a "moonlit" complexion, meaning that the hue is very fair regardless of color. Many dark people have translucent skin that looks as if the moon is reflected in it. Their eyelashes are long and curled, and the eyes themselves tend to be big pools. They have a cool and complacent temperament. They have moist skin that can be oily, but is always cool; their hands and feet are typically cool. The weak spot for *kapha* is in the upper body: lungs, throat, thyroid, and tonsils. They tend to be susceptible to conditions such as colds, coughs, allergies, tonsillitis, and bronchitis. Their strengths are those of physical and maternal endurance, calmness, and patience. Humility, nurturance, and fortitude are common *kapha* virtues.

I myself am a *vata-pitta* type. My skin tends to be dry. I have a strong spiritual temperament, with a deep love for my inner freedom, although I can be impatient. My lower body is my weakest part as it was also the site of my cancer condition.

My mother is also a *vata-pitta* type and I have inherited many of her qualities. My father is a *pitta-kapha* type and I have inherited his abundant, wavy *kapha* locks, his quick and alert mind, and his tendency to excel.

The box below summarizes the characteristics of the nine different body types—*vata*, *pitta*, and *kapha*—and the various combinations of the three *doshas*. You will also find examples of celebrities who are typical of each metabolic type.

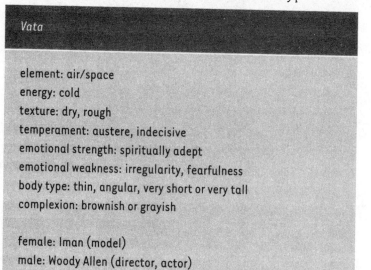

### Vata

element: air/space
energy: cold
texture: dry, rough
temperament: austere, indecisive
emotional strength: spiritually adept
emotional weakness: irregularity, fearfulness
body type: thin, angular, very short or very tall
complexion: brownish or grayish

female: Iman (model)
male: Woody Allen (director, actor)

### Pitta

element: fire/water
energy: hot
texture: oily, soft
temperament: fiery, vibrant
emotional strength: materially adept, visionary
emotional weakness: indulgent, aggressive

body type: athletic, well shaped
complexion: yellowish or reddish

female: Andrea McArdle (Broadway actress)
male: Mick Hucknall (lead singer of the band Simply Red)

## Kapha

element: water/earth
energy: cool
texture: smooth, dense
temperament: methodical, slow
emotional strength: maternal, nurturing
emotional weakness: attachment, greediness
body type: heavy, compact
complexion: pale, clear

female: Mama Cass Elliot (singer)
male: Jackie Gleason (actor, comedian)

## Vata-Pitta

element: dominant, air/space
           subordinate, fire/water
energy: cool
texture: sometimes dry, sometimes oily
temperament: sometimes indecisive and sometimes fiery
emotional strength: spiritually inclined, goal-oriented
emotional weakness: irregular, fearful, and sometimes aggressive
body type: thin, tall, or lanky
complexion: brownish or yellowish

female: Gwyneth Paltrow (actress)
male: John Malkovich (actor)

## Pitta-Vata

element: dominant, fire/water
subordinate, air/space
energy: warm
texture: oily, sometimes dry
temperament: cheerful, sometimes aggressive
emotional strength: materially adept, goal oriented
emotional weakness: ambitious, intolerant
body type: moderate to thin, well shaped
complexion: yellowish or tan

female: Sharon Stone (actress)
male: Tom Cruise (actor)

## Kapha-Vata

element: dominant, water/earth
subordinate, air/space
energy: cold
texture: smooth, dense, sometimes dry and rough
temperament: extreme tendencies, sometimes methodical and
sometimes indecisive
emotional strength: nurturing, spiritually inclined
emotional weakness: unmotivated, attached
body type: moderate to heavy (easy to gain weight)
complexion: pale, sometimes dark

female: Kathy Bates (actress)
male: William Conrad (actor)

## Vata-Kapha

element: dominant, air/space
                subordinate, water/earth
energy: cold
texture: dry, sometimes smooth
temperament: extreme tendencies, mercurial, irregular
emotional strength: spiritually adept, maternal
emotional weakness: isolated, fearful
body type: thin to moderate (easy to gain weight, easy to lose
   weight)
complexion: dark, sometimes pale

female: Whoopi Goldberg (actress, comedian)
male: Danny DeVito (actor)

## Pitta-Kapha

element: dominant, fire/water
                subordinate, water/earth
energy: warm
texture: soft, moist
temperament: decisive, patient
emotional strength: well balanced, materially adept
emotional weakness: possesive, indulgent
body type: well shaped, moderate to heavy
complexion: reddish, sometimes pale

female: Drew Barrymore (actress)
male: Leonardo DiCaprio (actor)

**Kapha-Pitta**

element: dominant, water/earth
           subordinate, fire/water
energy: cool, sometimes warm
texture: smooth, dense, moist
temperament: slow but methodical
emotional strength: excellent stamina, tenacious
emotional weakness: stubborn, lethargic
body type: solid, curvaceous, and heavy
complexion: pale, sometimes reddish

female: Rosie O'Donnell (comedian, actress)
male: John Candy (comedian, actor)

The *rishis* gave us wonderful symbols for the three types. *Vata* is represented by a six-pointed star, like the symbol of Sri Yantra or Star of David, *pitta* by an inverted triangle, and *kapha* by a square. Whatever our type, we can respect and rejoice in our own nature and the natures of those around us. In this beautiful universe we are able to coexist and complement each other because of our differences and vulnerabilities. From the standpoint of *sadhana*, our vulnerabilities can become our greatest strengths, because when we recognize that we have a soft spot, we can allow ourselves to grow to a deeper level of consciousness.

The Indian poet Kalidasa puts it this way: "In the birth of the Himalayas, the boundless jewel among mountains, only one fault exists, that of the snow. But like the immense splendor of the moon, whose luminous light drowns out its dots, coldness could never be the destroyer of her beauty." Like the snow, vulnerability cannot destroy the beauty of the boundless jewel of our anatomy. It is an intrinsic part of human nature. We tend to be self-conscious and try to hide our sensitivities, which actually can make them more entrenched and potentially harmful. When we can allow our tenderness to show, the universe sends its healing energies to nurture and support us.

## NURTURING EACH METABOLIC TYPE

The Ayurvedic principle of "like increases like" helps us nourish our individual rhythms and achieve balance in our lives. According to this principle, we are also nurtured by the elements and inclinations that are not innate to our metabolic type. Just as an individual who has a predominant quality of air in her nature has to work on building more stability, one who is extremely fiery should develop more moderation in his activities. We should avoid the intake of things that are like our own qualities, qualities that we already have, and increase the intake of things that are unlike our constitutional attributes. The chart below lists the properties that nurture each metabolic type.

| Vata: nurtured by fire, water, and earth | Pitta: nurtured by water, air, space, and earth | Kapha: nurtured by fire, air, and space |
|---|---|---|
| consistent | calm | stimulating |
| moist | cool | dry |
| heavy | substantial | warm |
| smooth | aromatic | light |
| hot | sweet | pungent |
| sweet | bitter | bitter |
| salty | astringent | astringent |
| sour | | |

# NURTURING YOUR
# PERSONAL RHYTHMS

These balancing principles are to be applied especially during your most vulnerable seasons. (See appendix 2 for more information about the six seasons of the Ayurvedic calendar.) Each *dosha* is increased in its own season. These are times of increased opportunity to gain a deeper understanding of our inner rhythms. The *vata* seasons are early fall and autumn. The *pitta* seasons are spring and summer. The *kapha* seasons are early and late winter. Follow the recommendations presented below that are most appropriate to your dominant metabolic type, as determined in the previous exercise. Depending on your imbalances and seasonal needs, you may choose to engage from time to time in the nourishing regimens of *doshas* other than yours, but once your most dominant *dosha* is brought into a state of balance, it will pull the secondary *doshas* into alignment.

*For Vata Type—Nourishing Quick and Irregular Rhythms*

Balancing Principle: Stability

• Maintain a steady routine around eating and sleeping habits
• Choose only the activities that create ease and allow yourself adequate time to complete them
• Take ample rest
• Eat wholesome, fresh, warm, moist, and nourishing foods
• Avoid bitter, cold, fermented, stale, and raw foods
• Buffer yourself against cold, damp, and wet environments
• Make an effort to embrace warmth, love, and healthy rituals and routines

*For* Pitta *Type—Nourishing Fast and Decisive Rhythms*

Balancing Principle: Moderation

- Rise with the sun and go to bed by ten P.M.
- Plan activities ahead to avoid time pressure
- Ease yourself out of all stressful activities and maintain only those projects that create ease
- Eat wholesome, moderately cool or warm, substantial, and calming foods
- Avoid hot, spicy, oily, salty, fermented, and stale foods, as well as the use of stimulants
- Shield yourself against hot, humid, and stressful environments
- Make an attempt to embrace serenity and calmness

*For* Kapha *Type—Nourishing Slow and Methodical Rhythms*

Balancing Principle: Stimulation

- Engage in stimulating physical exercise every day
- Open yourself to new and invigorating experiences
- Rise with the sun every day
- Eat wholesome, light, warm, pungent, and stimulating foods
- Avoid cold, oily, rich, and excessively sour or salty foods
- Buffer yourself against cold, damp, and wet environments
- Unburden yourself of all old loads and lighten your heart

If you like, you may make the appropriate principles into affirmations, for example, "I embrace serenity and calmness in my life," or "I eat only wholesome, substantial, calming, and moderately cool or warm foods." Commit the affirmations to memory or write them on a piece of paper, so that you can repeat them from time to time.

# THE WISE EARTH AYURVEDIC CALENDAR: THE SEASONS, JUNCTIONS, AND DAILY RHYTHMS

## RECLAIMING THE SEASONS

Our rhythms are directly connected to the seasons, because our metabolic nature, or *prakriti*, is derived from the penetrations of the five elements in the sperm and ovum that occur during conception. When we take in the earth's foods in harmony with its seasons, we strengthen our rhythms. By observing the provisions of the seasons, we can achieve our optimal state of health. In this sense, our well-being depends on an intuitive balancing of our being with nature.

The seasons evolve from the cosmic rhythms. They are the responses of the earth's yearly journey around the sun, divided into two distinct phases, the northerly and southerly. The northerly phase begins at the winter solstice in late December, the southerly phase at the summer solstice in late June. Throughout these two phases, the six seasons run their courses in a flowing, cyclical manner. The six seasons of the Ayurvedic calendar are as follows:

- Spring: March 15–May 15
- Summer: May 15–July 15
- Early fall: July 15–September 15

- Autumn: September 15–November 15
- Early winter: November 15–January 15
- Late winter: January 15–March 15

During the northerly phase (approximately December 20–June 20), the body is weakened because the sun absorbs moisture and humidity from the earth, and three tastes are dramatically enhanced: bitter, astringent, and pungent. Conversely, during the southerly phase, the sun's energy wanes, and the moon's energy gains strength. The moisture and cooling relief of the moon's influence helps to revive the human mind and body. During this phase, the remaining three tastes are dominant: sour, salty, and sweet. By decreasing the consumption of the tastes that are dominant during a specific season while increasing the others, we interact with the dynamic play of the seasons in a complementary way that keeps us healthy. By observing the seasonal influences on our food, we remain in harmony with nature. This is the easiest way to keep our *doshas* in a state of balance.

## THE SEVEN ANNUAL CYCLICAL JUNCTIONS

When the seasons change, we experience a sympathetic internal shift. All life-forms open themselves up to receive cosmic redirection from nature during these crucial seasonal transitions, so we are likely to be more vulnerable and unsettled. The Ayurvedic texts say that a disease can take root in the body only during the junctions between the seasons, when all nature is in flux. Because of the upheaval dominating these junctions, the body's natural immunity becomes virtually defenseless against impending disease.

Nevertheless, these seasonal junctions can become times

of glorious opportunity when we mindfully acknowledge and observe them. Because they invite us to empty the irrelevant and toxic from our organic being, we can cleanse and redirect our lives, provided we take time to abide consciously within ourselves. In accord with the universe's innate and pervasive cycles of seven, these seasonal junctions arrive seven times a year, at the onset of each season, even in tropical and semitropical climes where the transitions between the seasons are less dramatic. When the necessary precautions for cleansing, nourishing, and securing the body are taken, we are better able to cross over these vulnerable junctions. The seven seasonal junctions are as follows:

- Late winter to spring: March 21–April 7
- Spring to summer: May 21–June 7
- Northerly to southerly phase: June 8–June 21
- Summer to rainy season or early fall: July 21–August 7
- Rainy season to autumn: September 21–October 7
- Autumn to early winter: November 21–December 7
- Southerly to northerly: December 8–December 21
- Early winter to late winter: January 21–February 7

The dates provided may vary slightly depending on the seasons' natural irregularities and seasonal patterns in different parts of the world.

Special attention should be paid to the autumn-to-early-winter junction, when the earth changes its course from a southerly to northerly direction. This most crucial time of year, in terms of our health, is called *Yama Damstra*. In Vedic tradition Yama is the Lord of Death, who goes prowling for souls. Like police officers who have to fill a quota of traffic tickets by the end of the month, Lord Yama has to fill his own quota of souls for the underworld during this time of year. There is a restlessness in the atmosphere. Sensing

Yama's approach, all creatures are fearful. It is not a good time to be teetering on the brink of death, because he would certainly snatch you. *Sadhanas* such as fasting, meditation, and prayer help restore balance within the body and spirit at this juncture.

## DAILY RHYTHMS

The cyclical transitions of the days, seasons, lifetimes, and eons are all replicated in our personal rhythms. The six cosmic phases that make up each day, for instance, directly influence our breath and the emotions related to it. By allowing the daily rhythms to reveal themselves through our breath, we are able to reconcile and substantiate our profound meaning within nature.

These six phases expand and contract under the sun's influence. Just before dawn, for example, when the sun is about to rise, the *vata* (or airy) aspect of the universe dominates, bringing forth dryness, cold, and erratic mobility. We need warmth, moisture, and stillness at this time to maintain our balance with nature. That is why the ancients advised that the *sadhanas* of *pranayama* (breath control) and meditation be performed in the early morning. Both activities serve to enhance the breath, providing both warmth and comfort to the organism.

At daybreak, the *kapha* (or watery) aspect of the universe begins to flow out of the body as we are rising from a night's rest. The qualities of coolness, heaviness, and stagnancy pervade the body, so we need to briefly activate the solar breath (a simple procedure outlined on page 136) and do some form of movement or exercise to generate warmth and invigorate the organism.

At midday, when the sun is at its peak and tends to sap

the body's energy, the *pitta* (or fiery) aspect of the universe prevails, bringing forth hot, aggressive energies. At this time, we seek a cooling reprieve by briefly activating the lunar breath and reducing our physical activity so as to invite calm and coolness to the organism.

In the early afternoon, when the sun's energy begins to flag, the *vata* aspect of the universe returns. Once more, *pranayama* and meditation help to calm the breath and maintain stasis with nature.

At sunset, when the sun descends to the horizon, the *kapha* aspect of the universe begins to pour back into the body, inducing it to relinquish the tasks of the day. Once again, we increase our solar breath briefly and move about in wholesome ways to invigorate the body.

And at midnight, even though the sun is farthest away from the earth, the *pitta* aspect returns, increasing physical and emotional heat. The body's heat is at its peak once again, controlled by the vibrational heat waves of the sun. At midday and midnight, the *pitta* aspect of the universe is at its height. If we are awake at this time, we should rest from all mental and physical activities and briefly activate the lunar breath to induce cool tranquility within the system.

## Wise Earth Ayurvedic Chart of the Six Seasons

| Season | Junction | Taste | Energy |
|---|---|---|---|
| Spring<br>(March 15–May 15) | (May 21–June 7) | Astringent | Rebirth |
| Summer<br>(May 15–July 15) | (July 21–August 7) | Pungent | Play |
| Early Fall<br>(July 15–September 15) | (September 21–<br>October 7) | Sour | Celebration |
| Autumn<br>(September 15–<br>November 15) | (November 21–<br>December 7) | Salty | Surrender |
| Early Winter<br>(November 15–<br>January 15) | (January 21–<br>February 7) | Sweet | Gathering |
| Late Winter<br>(January 15–March 7) | (March 21–April 7) | Bitter | Reprieve |

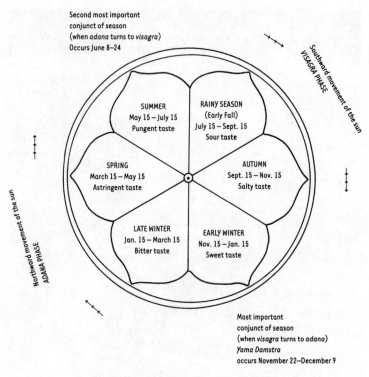

Second most important
conjunct of season
(when *adana* turns to *visagra*)
Occurs June 8–24

Southward movement of the sun
VISAGRA PHASE

Northward movement of the sun
ADANA PHASE

SUMMER
May 15 – July 15
Pungent taste

RAINY SEASON
(Early Fall)
July 15 – Sept. 15
Sour taste

SPRING
March 15 – May 15
Astringent taste

AUTUMN
Sept. 15 – Nov. 15
Salty taste

LATE WINTER
Jan. 15 – March 15
Bitter taste

EARLY WINTER
Nov. 15 – Jan. 15
Sweet taste

Most important
conjunct of season
(when *visagra* turns to *adana*)
*Yama Damstra*
occurs November 22–December 9

*Wise Earth Ayurvedic Mandala of the Six Seasons*

# SEASONAL MENUS
# AND RECIPES

Our ancestors, who lived off the land, worked according to the seasons, sowing and harvesting at the appropriate junctions of the year. While you should know your *dosha* and body type, so that you are aware of which types of foods to eat and which to avoid, it is even more important to eat foods that are appropriate to each particular season. When your diet consists of fresh, seasonally grown fruits and vegetables, your body's rhythms are in balance with nature. This is a crucial aspect to maintaining good health.

I have grouped the menus below according to the six seasons. I have also noted which *doshas* are most vulnerable during each season and which foods they should therefore avoid during that time, so that you can fine-tune the menus to your individual needs. Be flexible in terms of the *doshas* and make slight adjustments as necessary, so that you can plan menus that are suitable to everyone in your family.

Before you turn to the menus, here are some general points of information about how to promote healthy digestion.

## TIPS FOR DIGESTIVE HEALTH

As a general rule:

• The main meal should be eaten at lunchtime or as an early dinner (four to five P.M.). The quantity of food ingested should be no more than two *anjali* (two hands cupped together).

• The other two meals should be small, about one *anjali*.

• Fruits should be eaten alone, about one hour before or after a meal, because fruits tend to ferment in the digestive tract.

• Fruits should not be eaten with milk or other dairy products, because the acidity of the fruit in the stomach curdles the milk in the stomach.

• Sweet and sour tastes are a disharmonious combination. One counteracts the other and irritates digestion, so that the digestive fires becomes sluggish.

• Avoid complex food combinations, especially when dairy is involved, such as tacos or lasagna; also any combination of bread, cheese, and fruits.

• Drink ½ cup of warm water before each meal to activate *agni*, the digestive fire. Avoid drinking water or other fluids with the meal. The liquid douses the digestive fire and makes the process sluggish. Taking water or fluids directly after the meal has the same counterproductive effects and promotes lethargy and weight gain.

• Chew the meal thoroughly and joyfully to aid proper assimilation of nutrients and digestion, so that the vital tissues are well nourished, the body's hunger is fed, and emotional cravings are satisfied.

• Practice eating your meals in a spirit of harmony and gratitude to conserve the bodily juices for the massive task of digestion. When we attend to digestion, we attend to our health. Remember: All disease occurs as a result of poor digestion and assimilation in the body.

In chapter 11, I described which tastes are most beneficial to each of the *doshas*. Here is a quick summary of the relationship between doshas and tastes:

| Doshas and Their Natural Tastes | | |
| --- | --- | --- |
| *Vata* | *Pitta* | *Kapha* |
| Bitter | Sour | Sweet |
| Astringent | Salty | Sour |
| Pungent | Pungent | Salty |

| Beneficial Tastes for Each *Dosha* | | |
| --- | --- | --- |
| *Vata* | *Pitta* | *Kapha* |
| Salty | Bitter | Pungent |
| Sweet | Sweet | Bitter |
| Sour | Astringent | Astringent |

## MEASURING YOUR INGREDIENTS

The Vedas refer to the hands and feet as the "organs of action." When we use our organs of action, we engage in the moment-to-moment recollection of the five elements of our nature. Our hands are vital extensions that enable us to touch, and be in touch with, creation. The way of *sadhana* exhorts us to use our body as the ruler and measuring cup for all our needs. We are born with all the tools we need to exercise our gifts for practicing *sadhana*, including those needed to feel and measure foods as we prepare them.

In keeping with this principle, you will want to become comfortable with using your hands and eyes for measuring food quantities. This will help you to increase the joy and delight you bring to your everyday life and nourishment.

*Anjali*—the volume that can be held by your two hands cupped together—is a reliable way to estimate how much food you should eat. Two *anjali* of grain or vegetables is designed by nature to fill your own stomach. You can determine the amount of food you need when you are cooking for a group by measuring two *anjali* for each adult and one *anjali* for each child. You can gauge the necessary amount of spices or accents you need for a dish by your own pinch, i.e., what fits between your thumb and forefinger, because it is tailored to provide a suitable amount for your own personal body needs. *Angula* refers to the distance between the joints of each finger. This unit of measure was designed by nature to measure spices and herbs, such as cinnamon sticks and ginger.

## USING YOUR HANDS TO MEASURE FOOD

- Amount in your cupped hands (1 anjali) = equivalent of 1 cup
- Size of your pinch = equivalent of $1/8$ teaspoon
- Size of three-finger pinch = equivalent of $1/2$ teaspoon
- Size of five-finger pinch = equivalent of 1 teaspoon
- Size of your palm = equivalent of 1 tablespoon
- Length of your finger joint = equivalent of $3/4$ inch (1 *angula*)

Use only those tools that are absolutely needed. Practice cooking without measuring cups, spoons, and other unnecessary kitchen paraphernalia. These adjuncts are distracting and interrupt your direct energetic exchange with the food.

It may be difficult at first to take this conscious step, to trust the accuracy of your own physical-spiritual apparatus. Over time, however, you will become comfortable enough to return to the original and most natural system of measurement—using your own body.

## MANTRAS FOR THE SEASONS

As you practice the food *sadhanas*—while you are cutting fruits and vegetables, grinding the spices, cooking the foods, and when you sit down to your meal—you can bring positive energy to the experience by reciting mantras that are appropriate to the season that you are in. These simple affirmations remind us that the cyclical nature of our own biorhythms reflects the cyclical nature of the universe, and that we can use the seasons as a guide for our own spiritual transitions.

| Season | Mantra |
|---|---|
| spring | regenerate and transform |
| summer | celebrate and rejoice |
| early fall | reorganize and revitalize |
| autumn | harvest and simplify |
| early winter | gather and contain |
| late winter | rest and reflect |

## MENUS AND RECIPES

Here are just a few of the recipes and menus that I have developed and teach at the Wise Earth School. I hope that once you have sampled these dishes, you will be motivated to consult other recipe guides that honor the Ayurvedic tradition and, in time, create your own recipes, based on the principles of the food *sadhanas*.

## SPRING SEASON
## (MARCH 15 – MAY 15)

*Kapha* and *pitta* vulnerable time.
*Kapha:* Avoid excess sweet, sugars, refined carbohydrates, and fatty foods.
*Pitta:* Avoid excess sour, salty tastes; oily, fatty foods; and intoxicants.

### LUNCH:

> Ginger and Scallion Soup
> Soft Millet
> Almond Lime Squares
> Cinnamon-Mint Tea

### DINNER:

> Spinach Masala
> Steamed Asparagus
> Barley and Lotus Seeds
> Vedic Rose-Cherry Pudding

### GINGER AND SCALLION SOUP | Serves 4

*1¹/₄ gallons water*
*¹/₄ cup quinoa*
*¹/₂ cup oat bran*
*3 tablespoons fresh, minced ginger*
*1 clove of garlic, crushed*
*1 teaspoon white pepper, finely ground*
*1 tablespoon rock salt*
*6 scallions, chopped*
*1 tablespoon organic ghee*
*1 bunch watercress, for garnish*

Bring water to a boil in a large, heavy-bottomed soup pot. Add the quinoa, oat bran, ginger, garlic, pepper, and salt. Stir, cover, and simmer on medium-low heat for 25 minutes. Add scallions and ghee, and continue to simmer for 10 minutes. Garnish with sprigs of watercress and serve hot with two dollops of soft millet (millet recipe follows).

## SOFT MILLET | Serves 4

*2 cups millet*
*5 cups boiling water*
*1 pinch of sea salt*

Wash millet until water runs clear and add to boiling water. Add salt. Cover and simmer over medium-low heat for 25 minutes. Serve warm.

## ALMOND LIME SQUARES | Serves 4

*2 cups barley flour*
*1/4 cup unrefined brown sugar*
*2 tablespoons organic ghee*
*1/2 teaspoon rock salt*
*1/4 cup warm water*
*1/4 cup toasted almonds, finely crushed*
*juice of 2 limes*
*2 tablespoons grated lime zest*
*1 teaspoon baking powder*
*oil*

Preheat oven to 350 degrees. In a large bowl, combine the flour, sugar, ghee, and salt. Add the warm water, crushed almonds, lime juice, and zest, as well as the baking powder, and mix into a thick batter. Lightly oil a small square baking dish and pour batter into it. Bake for 20 minutes, or until a fork inserted comes out clean. Serve warm.

## CINNAMON-MINT TEA | Serves 4

*8 cups water*
*2 cinnamon sticks*
*12 fresh mint leaves*
*1 pinch cinnamon powder*
*1 tablespoon Sucanat*

Bring water to boil in a medium saucepan. Add cinnamon sticks, and allow to boil for 10 minutes. Remove from heat, add mint leaves, cinnamon powder, and Sucanat. Cover and let steep for 5 minutes before serving. Cinnamon sticks may be removed from tea before serving and retained for other use.

## SPINACH MASALA | Serves 4

*2 bunches spinach*
*1 tablespoon organic ghee*
*1 tablespoon Spring Masala (see recipe on page 317)*
*1 teaspoon tamarind paste*
*¹/₄ cup warm water*
*1 teaspoon unrefined brown sugar*
*1 teaspoon rock salt*

Wash the spinach, and trim the stems. Melt ghee in a large skillet, and roast the Spring *Masala* for 30 seconds, until the ghee starts to bubble. Add the wet spinach. Stir, cover, and let simmer for 3 minutes, until the leaves turn limp. Dilute the tamarind in the warm water, and add to the spinach mixture, along with the brown sugar and salt. Stir, cover, and simmer for 3 minutes more. Serve warm with Steamed Asparagus and Barley and Lotus Seeds.

## STEAMED ASPARAGUS | Serves 4

*24 asparagus spears*
*1 tablespoon organic ghee*
*¹/₂ fresh lime*

1 teaspoon black pepper, finely ground
1/2 teaspoon rock salt

Trim asparagus, and place in a steamer over boiling water. Steam for 3 to 4 minutes. Remove from steamer and place in a serving dish. Melt the ghee over asparagus; squeeze lime juice over it and sprinkle with black pepper and salt. Serve at once with cooked grain of your choice.

## BARLEY AND LOTUS SEEDS | Serves 4

3 1/2 cups water
2 cups pearl barley
1/4 cup dried lotus seeds
1 teaspoon sunflower oil
pinch of rock salt

Bring water to a boil in a medium-size saucepan. Wash the barley and lotus seeds and add to the boiling water. Add the oil and salt. Stir, cover, and simmer over medium-low heat for 20 minutes. Remove from heat and let stand for 10 minutes. Serve warm.

## VEDIC CHERRY-ROSE PUDDING | Serves 4

1 cup Cream of Wheat
1/2 cup spelt flour
1 cup cow's milk (organic)
1/2 cup rosewater
1/4 cup pitted dates
1/4 cup pitted fresh cherries
1/4 cup Sucanat
1 teaspoon cardamom powder
1/2 teaspoon ground nutmeg
1/2 teaspoon turmeric powder
1 handful fresh, organic rose petals for garnish

Preheat oven to 350 degrees. Oil a shallow baking dish and set aside.

Sift the flours into a mixing bowl and pour in milk and rosewater. Mix into a smooth batter. Cut dates and cherries into tiny pieces and add to batter. Stir in Sucanat and spice powders, and pour batter into prepared baking dish.

Bake for 15 minutes, until the pudding cake is barely set and the top is golden brown. Spoon out the pudding cake into dessert bowls, garnish with a few rose petals, and serve warm.

## SUMMER SEASON
## (MAY 15 – JULY 15)

*Pitta* vulnerable time.

Avoid excess pungent, hot peppers, garlic, oily or fatty foods, complex food combinations, intoxicants.

### LUNCH:

Cucumber Raita with Yogurt and Dill

Pea, Carrot, and Bulgur Salad
with Orange and Saffron Dressing

Melon and Mango Slices

### DINNER:

Lentil and Coconut *Dhal*

Dill and Scallion Chapati

Mango Chutney (see page 326)

Sweet *Lassi*

### CUCUMBER RAITA WITH YOGURT AND DILL | Serves 4

*2 cucumbers*

*¹/₂ cup organic plain yogurt*

*1 teaspoon fresh lemon juice*

*2 tablespoons fresh dill, minced*

*1 pinch of black pepper*
*1 pinch of rock salt*

Wash and peel the cucumbers and slice them lengthwise. Remove the seeds by running a teaspoon along the center of the cucumbers. Slice them cross-wise, very thinly. In a bowl, combine the yogurt, lemon juice, dill, black pepper, and salt. Add the cucumbers, toss, and serve immediately.

## PEA, CARROT, AND BULGUR SALAD WITH ORANGE AND SAFFRON DRESSING | Serves 4

*3 cups water*
*1 cup bulgur*
*1 cup fresh peas*
*1 cup carrots, diced*
*1 cup radicchio, finely chopped*
*1/4 cup cilantro, finely minced*
*1 teaspoon dried tarragon*
*1 tablespoon sunflower oil*
*1/2 orange, juiced*
*1 strand saffron*
*1/2 teaspoon rock salt*

Bring 3 cups of water to a boil. Add bulgur, cover, and cook over medium heat for 10 minutes, until bulgur is firmly cooked. Remove from heat and pour into a colander. Pour cold water over bulgur to keep the grains from sticking. Blanch the peas and carrots in the remaining water for 5 minutes. Strain and put in a large bowl. Fold in the bulgur, along with radicchio, cilantro, and tarragon. Combine oil, orange juice, saffron, and salt, pour over the mixture. Toss and serve at once.

## MELON AND MANGO SLICES | Serves 4

*1 small honeydew melon*
*1 large ripe mango*
*juice of 1 lemon*
*sprinkle of unrefined brown sugar*

Cut the melon in half; core and peel. Cut evenly into $1/2$-inch-thick slices, and set aside. Slice the mango in half, avoiding its large seed. Peel the halves and slice them. Arrange the melon and mango slices on a dessert platter, sprinkle with lemon juice and sugar, and serve.

## LENTIL AND COCONUT *DHAL* | Serves 4'

4 cups water
$3/4$ cup green lentils
4 bay leaves
$1/2$ teaspoon turmeric
$1/2$ teaspoon rock salt
1 teaspoon sunflower oil
$1/2$ teaspoon cumin seeds
$1/2$ clove garlic, grated
1 fresh green chili pepper
$1/4$ cup fresh coconut, shredded
1 small bunch fresh cilantro, chopped

Bring the water to boil in a medium-size saucepan. Wash and strain the lentils and add to the boiling water, along with the bay leaves, turmeric, and salt. Cover and simmer over medium heat for 15 minutes. Heat the oil in a small skillet and roast the cumin seeds and garlic for 1 minute, until the seeds turn golden brown. Add to the *dhal* by rinsing the skillet in the *dhal* water. Add the pepper and shredded coconut and continue to simmer for an additional 10 minutes. Toward the end of the 10 minutes, introduce the cilantro to the *dhal*. Remove from heat, cover, and allow *dhal* to sit for 5 minutes before serving with the Dill and Scallion Chapati and Mango Chutney.

## DILL AND SCALLION CHAPATI | Serves 4

2 cups spelt flour
2 tablespoons fresh dill, minced
1 scallion, chopped
$1/2$ teaspoon black pepper, finely ground

1 pinch of rock salt
3/4 cup warm water
1 teaspoon organic ghee

In a large bowl, combine the flour, dill, scallions, pepper, and salt. Introduce the water, a bit at a time, to knead into a pliable dough, for about 5 minutes. Allow to sit for 2 hours, covering the bowl with a thin, damp cotton towel. Set aside a small bowl of spelt flour to use for rolling the chapati (see Making Chapati on page 323).

Directly after cooking the chapati, daub one side with the ghee and serve immediately.

## SWEET LASSI | Serves 4

Lassi is a traditional North Indian spiced yogurt drink that is generally used as a digestive aid after meals.

1 pint organic yogurt
1 cup almond milk
2 cups warm water
1/4 cup unrefined brown sugar
1 teaspoon cardamom powder
1/2 teaspoon clove powder
1/2 teaspoon rock salt
fresh mint, for garnish

Blend all ingredients except mint in a large bowl, whisking with an eggbeater until the lassi becomes smooth and frothy. Garnish with mint and serve in large cups.

# EARLY FALL/RAINY SEASON (JULY 15 – SEPTEMBER 15)

*Vata, Pitta,* and *Kapha* vulnerable time.

*Vata:* Avoid astringent, bitter tastes and excess cold, dry foods.

*Pitta:* Avoid excess pungent, salty, oily, fatty foods, and intoxicants.

*Kapha:* Avoid excess sweet, salty, cold, oily, and fatty foods.

## LUNCH:

Red Lentils and Quinoa

Baby Carrots in Lemon Ghee

Cardamom and Ginger Tea

## DINNER:

Buckwheat *Biryani*

Early Fall Potato Curry

Pear Chutney

Berry Heaven Tart

## RED LENTILS AND QUINOA | Serves 4

*1 cup red lentils*

*4 cups water*

*2 dried bay leaves*

*1/2 teaspoon of rock salt*

*1 cup quinoa*

*1 teaspoon organic ghee*

*1 teaspoon cumin seeds*

*1/2 teaspoon fresh ginger, minced*

*1/2 teaspoon garlic, minced*

*1/4 cup fresh parsley, minced*

Thoroughly wash the lentils. Bring water to boil in a soup pot. Add the lentils, bay leaves, and salt, and simmer over medium heat for 10 minutes. Wash the quinoa in a fine sieve and add to the *dhal*. Continue to simmer for an additional 5 minutes. Heat the ghee in a small cast-iron skillet, and roast the cumin seeds, ginger, and garlic for a few minutes, until they turn golden brown. Remove from heat and immediately pour the ghee-roasted spices into the *dhal*, by rinsing the entire skillet in it. Cover and simmer for 3 more minutes. Garnish with parsley and serve warm.

## BABY CARROTS IN LEMON GHEE | Serves 4

*2 pounds baby carrots*
*1 tablespoon organic ghee*
*juice of 1/2 lemon*
*1 tablespoon corn oil*
*2 tablespoons minced fresh lemon thyme*
*1 teaspoon coriander powder*
*1 teaspoon rock salt*
*2 handfuls of dandelion leaves for garnish*

Wash the baby carrots and trim the stems. Blanch for 5 minutes in boiling water. Drain and put in a large bowl. Add the ghee and lemon juice to carrots. Heat the oil in a small skillet and sauté the lemon thyme for 30 seconds. Add coriander and salt. Remove from heat and add to carrots. Toss and serve over Red Lentils and Quinoa; garnish it with the dandelion leaves.

## CARDAMOM AND GINGER TEA | Serves 4

*8 cups water*
*1 teaspoon fresh ginger, peeled and grated*
*10 cardamom pods*
*1/2 teaspoon cardamom powder*
*1/2 fresh lemon, juiced*

Bring water to boil in medium saucepan. Add ginger and cardamom pods, cover, and simmer for 5 minutes. Strain the tea and reserve roughage to use in your bath water. Add cardamom powder and lemon juice to tea. Cover and steep for 5 minutes before serving.

## BUCKWHEAT *BIRYANI* | Serves 4

Biryani *is a traditional North Indian dish, generally made from rice, vegetables, nuts, and dried fruits.*

*1 cup cracked buckwheat*
*1½ cups water*
*1 tablespoon sunflower oil*
*1 teaspoon cumin seeds*
*1 teaspoon mustard seeds*
*1 teaspoon Early Fall Masala (see recipe on page 318)*
*1 teaspoon coriander powder*
*½ teaspoon rock salt*
*1 small russet potato, finely diced*
*1 cup cauliflower florets, finely chopped*
*½ red bell pepper, finely chopped*
*2 tablespoons cilantro, minced*
*1 teaspoon fresh ginger, minced*

Rinse buckwheat and drain. Bring water to boil in medium saucepan. Put in the buckwheat, cover securely and simmer on low heat for 10 minutes, until all water is absorbed. Heat oil in a large skillet or wok on medium heat and roast the cumin and mustard seeds for 1 minute, until the mustard seeds pop. Quickly add the *masala*, coriander powder, and salt, and lower heat and stir roasted spices for a few seconds. Add the potato, cauliflower, bell pepper, cilantro, and ginger, stirring frequently. Sprinkle in a palmful of water as you stir the mixture. Cover securely and continue to simmer on low heat for 5 minutes, until the potato is cooked. Gently fold in buckwheat and serve warm.

## EARLY FALL POTATO CURRY | Serves 4

12 early fall potatoes
1 tablespoon coriander seeds
1 tablespoon ajwain seeds
1 tablespoon sunflower oil
1 teaspoon turmeric powder
1 teaspoon cumin powder
1/2 teaspoon cardamom powder
2 dried red chilies
1 teaspoon rock salt
1/2 cup water
1/2 cup organic yogurt

Scrub the potatoes and cut into quarters. Dry-roast the coriander and ajwain seeds for 2 minutes in a large cast-iron skillet, until they are golden brown. Remove from heat and crush the seeds with a mortar and pestle. Heat the oil in the same skillet, and add the seeds, along with the potatoes. Add turmeric, cumin, and cardamom powders, along with the chilies and salt. Stir and simmer for 3 minutes, before adding the water. Cover and simmer on medium heat for 15 minutes, until the potatoes are very soft. Remove from heat and immediately fold in the yogurt. Serve at once over the Buckwheat *Biryani* with Pear Chutney.

## PEAR CHUTNEY | Serves 4

1 teaspoon black mustard seeds
1 tablespoon ghee
1/4 cup grated fresh ginger
1 cup peeled and thinly sliced firm Bartlett pears
1/4 cup currants

Sauté mustard seeds in ghee until they pop. Stir in ginger, pear slices, and currants. Stir gently and cook over medium heat for 3 minutes or so, until the currants swell.

## BERRY HEAVEN TART  |  Serves 4

2 cups fresh blackberries
1 cup fresh raspberries
$^1/_2$ cup unrefined brown sugar
2 tablespoons arrowroot starch
$^1/_8$ cup cold water
1 pinch rock salt

Prepare a sweet tart dough and place it in an oiled rectangular baking dish (see recipe for Sweet Tart Shell below). Preheat oven to 370 degrees.

Wash the berries and mash half of them into a pulp. Set aside the whole berries. Pour the mashed berries and sugar into a medium-size saucepan and bring to a boil on medium heat. Dilute the starch in cold water and pour into fruit mixture, along with the salt. Reduce heat, stir frequently until mixture thickens, then remove from heat and set aside.

Arrange the whole berries in the unbaked tart shell and pour the fruit mixture over them. Bake for 30 minutes, until the edges of the shell turn golden brown. Serve warm.

## SWEET TART SHELL

1 cup unbleached whole wheat flour
1 tablespoon unrefined brown sugar
1 pinch of rock salt
2 tablespoons sunflower oil
$^1/_4$ cup warm water

To make the tart shell, combine flour, sugar, and salt, gradually adding the oil. Use sufficient water to knead the dough into a firm ball. Roll out the dough into a circle, large enough to cover an 8-inch tart pan. Chill until the shell is stiff. If filling and crust are to be baked together, dough is now ready to be used. For a prebaked pastry shell, continue with the following directions.

Preheat oven to 350 degrees and bake the shell for 15 minutes, until the edges are lightly brown. Cool on a rack.

# AUTUMN
# (SEPTEMBER 15–NOVEMBER 15)

*Vata* vulnerable time.
Avoid excess cold, dry, astringent, bitter foods.

## LUNCH:

Russet Potatoes with Ghee and Dill
Mesclun Salad
Fruit-and-Nut Compote

## DINNER:

Basmati *Kichadi*
Blossoms of Broccoli with Garlic
Ganesha's Pudding

## RUSSET POTATOES WITH GHEE AND DILL | Serves 4

*2 handfuls small russet potatoes*
*1 tablespoon organic ghee*
*2 tablespoons fresh dill, coarsely chopped*
*1/2 teaspoon fresh, white peppercorns*
*1/2 teaspoon nutmeg, freshly grated*
*1/2 teaspoon rock salt*
*1/4 cup water*

Scrub russet potatoes and cut into halves. In a large cast-iron skillet, melt the ghee over medium heat. Lay the potatoes facedown in the skillet for a few minutes, until they are browned. Stir in fresh dill, pepper, nutmeg, and salt. Add water, cover, and simmer over low heat for 20 minutes. Pour the potato mixture in the center and serve with mesclun salad.

## MESCLUN SALAD | Serves 4

*Mesclun is a Provençal term for a salad mixture of greens and young, tender lettuces. Recently, mesclun mix has become very popular in the big chain supermarkets and health-food stores.*

*1 small head oak leaf lettuce*
*2 curly endives*
*2 tablespoons sunflower oil*
*1 lemon, juiced*
*1/2 teaspoon freshly ground black peppercorns*

Wash and towel-dry the lettuces. Tear them into small pieces and place in a large salad bowl. Pour oil and juice, along with the pepper, into a jar. Cover with a tight-fitting lid and shake to mix the dressing. Toss the salad with just enough dressing to coat the greens.

## FRUIT-AND-NUT COMPOTE | Serves 4

*2 cups water*
*1/4 cup apricots, halved and pitted*
*1/4 cup dried figs, thinly sliced*
*1/4 cup raisins*
*2 cinnamon sticks*
*6 cardamom pods*
*1 tablespoon unrefined brown sugar*
*1/4 cup pecans, coarsely chopped*

Bring the water to boil in a heavy-bottomed saucepan. Add all other ingredients except for the pecans, cover, and simmer on low heat for 30 minutes, until all the fruits are tender. Garnish with pecans and serve warm.

## BASMATI *KICHADI* | Serves 4

*3 1/2 cups water*
*2 cups basmati white rice*
*1/4 cup split yellow mung beans*

1 teaspoon rock salt
1 teaspoon sesame oil
1 teaspoon cumin seeds
red oak lettuce, for garnish

Bring water to a boil in a medium-size saucepan. Wash rice and mung beans and add to the water, along with the salt. Cover and simmer on medium-low heat for 12 minutes, or until the *kichadi* turns fluffy. Remove from heat, and set aside. Heat the oil in a small skillet. Roast the cumin seeds for a few minutes until they are golden brown. Gently stir the roasted seeds into *kichadi*. Serve at once, over whole lettuce leaves.

## BLOSSOMS OF BROCCOLI WITH GARLIC | Serves 4

1 bunch green sprouting broccoli, with leaves
1 bunch purple sprouting broccoli, with leaves
1 bunch rapini
1 teaspoon olive oil
4 cloves garlic, finely minced
1/4 cup water

Wash the bunches of broccoli and rapini thoroughly, separating leaves from sprouts. Heat oil in a large skillet and brown the minced garlic for 2 minutes. Add the leaves and sprouts. Pour water, stir, cover, and simmer for 3 minutes. Serve hot over mixture of cooked Basmati *Kichadi*.

## GANESHA'S PUDDING | Serves 4

2 cups chick pea flour
1/4 cup almond oil
1/4 cup warm water
1 tablespoon organic ghee
1/4 cup unrefined brown sugar
1/2 teaspoon natural almond essence
1/2 teaspoon cardamom powder

Mix all the ingredients together in a large bowl. Heat a large cast-iron skillet and pour in the batter. Cook on medium heat for 15 minutes, until the batter is slightly browned. Remove from heat, and let stand for 5 minutes before serving.

## EARLY WINTER
## (NOVEMBER 15–JANUARY 15)

*Kapha* vulnerable time.
Avoid excess sweet, cold, oily, or fatty foods.

### LUNCH:

Red Pepper Loaf with Melted Ghee
Mizuna and Lemon Salad

### DINNER:

Red Cabbage and Onion Soup
Millet Supreme
Walnut and Pear Cake

### RED PEPPER LOAF WITH MELTED GHEE | Serves 4 (2 loaves)

*2 red bell peppers*
*2 cups warm water*
*1 teaspoon dried tarragon*
*1/2 teaspoon cayenne powder*
*1 tablespoon natural yeast*
*1 teaspoon rock salt*
*4 cups barley flour*
*1 teaspoon sunflower oil*

Spear the whole peppers with a fork and char over open flame, until the skin turns black. Run cold water over them and peel off the skin. Remove core and seeds and cut into 1/2-inch-thick strips. Set aside.

Combine water, tarragon, cayenne, yeast, and salt. Stir until the yeast dissolves. Add flour gradually, along with most of the peppers, setting aside a few pieces for garnishing. Knead into a sticky dough and transfer into a large oiled bowl. Cover securely and let rise in a warm place for 40 minutes. Punch down the dough, cover, and let rise again for 40 minutes. Divide the dough into two equal pieces and put on oiled baking pan. Brush tops of loaves with oil, garnish with reserved pepper slices, and bake at 425 degrees for 10 minutes. Reduce heat to 350 degrees and bake for 20 minutes more. Remove from oven, allow to sit for 15 minutes. Slice and serve with melted ghee.

## MIZUNA AND LEMON SALAD | Serves 4

1 fresh lemon
2 teaspoons rock salt
1 large bunch mizuna leaves

Wash lemon and cut in very thin slices, retaining the skin. Season the lemon slices with salt. Arrange the seasoned lemon slices on top of the mizuna greens and serve.

## RED CABBAGE AND ONION SOUP | Serves 4

$1/2$ gallon water
1 small red cabbage, shredded
2 red onions, chopped
1 tablespoon coriander powder
$1/2$ teaspoon cayenne powder
1 tablespoon dried dill
1 tablespoon dried parsley
2 cloves garlic
1 tablespoon rock salt
$1/4$ cup cashew butter
1 red onion, thin half-moon slices

Bring water to a boil in a large soup pot. Add the cabbage and onions, along with coriander and cayenne powders, dried dill, parsley, and salt. Lightly crush the garlic cloves with a hand stone and remove the skin. Add the lightly crushed cloves of garlic to the soup mixture. Cover and simmer on medium heat for 35 minutes, until onions are practically dissolved. Add cashew butter and stir the soup until it dissolves. Garnish the hot soup with thinly sliced red onions. Remove from heat, cover, and let sit for 5 minutes. Serve hot with a heaping dollop of Millet Supreme.

## MILLET SUPREME | Serves 4

3 1/2 cups water
2 cups millet
1/4 cup fresh peas
1/2 teaspoon turmeric
1/2 teaspoon cumin powder
1/2 teaspoon ajwain seeds
1 teaspoon rock salt
1 tablespoon sunflower oil
1/4 cup currants
1/4 cup roasted almonds, slivered
juice of 1/2 lemon

Bring water to a boil in a medium-size saucepan. Thoroughly wash the millet and add to boiling water, along with the peas, turmeric, cumin powder, ajwain seeds, and salt. Cover and simmer on medium heat for 20 minutes. Heat the oil in a small skillet, and add the currants and almonds. Stir for a few minutes until the currants begin to swell. Add the lemon juice. Add to the millet, and continue cooking for 10 minutes more. Serve warm.

## WALNUT AND PEAR CAKE | Serves 4

oil and flour to prepare pan
2 tablespoons organic ghee
1/4 cup unrefined brown sugar
1/2 teaspoon natural vanilla essence
1 teaspoon cinnamon powder

$1/2$ teaspoon ginger powder

$1/2$ teaspoon ground nutmeg

$1/2$ teaspoon rock salt

$1/2$ cup water

$1/2$ cup spelt flour

$1/2$ cup crushed walnuts

$1/2$ cup dried pear slices

Preheat oven to 350 degrees. Oil and flour a baking pan. Set aside.

Combine the ghee, sugar, vanilla essence, spice powders, and salt in a bowl. Add a palmful of water and whisk the mixture until smooth. Gradually fold in the flour, adding the remaining water. Mix in the walnuts and dried pear slices. Pour the batter into the prepared pan and bake for 30 minutes at 350 degrees.

# WINTER
# (JANUARY 15 – MARCH 15)

*Kapha* and *Vata* vulnerable time.

*Kapha:* Avoid refined sweets and excess cold, unctuous, salty, fatty foods.

*Vata:* Avoid excess cold, dry, bitter foods.

## LUNCH:

Creamy Butternut Squash Soup

Seven-Grain Bread

## DINNER:

Caraway Brown Rice

Whole Mung *Dhal*

Sauteed Golden Beets with Late Winter *Masala*

Apple Date Torte

## CREAMY BUTTERNUT SQUASH SOUP | Serves 4

$1/2$ gallon water
1 small butternut squash, peeled and cut into 1" cubes
$1/2$ cup rolled oats
1 tablespoon dried cilantro
1 tablespoon cumin powder
1 teaspoon coriander powder
$1/2$ teaspoon turmeric powder
$1/2$ teaspoon black pepper, finely ground
1 tablespoon fresh ginger, grated
juice of 1 fresh lemon
1 tablespoon rock salt
1 tablespoon soya oil
2 scallions, chopped
parsley
landcress

Bring water to boil in a large pot. Add squash, oats, cilantro, spice powders, black pepper, fresh ginger, lemon juice, and salt. Cover and simmer on medium heat for 35 minutes. Use a flat-bottomed ladle to puree the squash. Heat oil in a small skillet and sauté scallions for about 2 minutes, then add to the creamed soup. Cover and simmer 5 minutes. Serve hot and garnish with fresh parsley and landcress.

## SEVEN-GRAIN BREAD | Serves 4 (4 rolls)

1 tablespoon natural yeast
$1/2$ cup warm water
2 tablespoons sesame butter
$1/2$ cup spelt flour
$1/2$ cup unbleached whole wheat flour
$1/2$ cup soya flour
$1/2$ cup millet flour
$1/2$ cup oat bran

$^{1}/_{2}$ cup rolled oats
$^{1}/_{2}$ cup cracked wheat
1 tablespoon Sucanat
$^{1}/_{2}$ teaspoon rock salt
$1^{1}/_{2}$ cups warm water

Dissolve the yeast in warm water, then dilute the sesame butter in the yeast solution. Combine the flours, bran, rolled oats, cracked wheat, Sucanat, salt, and remaining water together, then add to the yeast–sesame butter mixture.

Knead into a sticky dough. Transfer dough to a large oiled bowl. Cover securely and let rise in a warm place for 40 minutes. Punch down the dough, cover, and let rise again for 40 minutes, until it doubles in size.

Form dough into four rolls and place on oiled baking trays. Bake at 350 degrees for 25 minutes.

## CARAWAY BROWN RICE | Serves 4

2 cups long-grain brown rice
$3^{1}/_{2}$ cups boiling water
1 pinch of sea salt
2 teaspoons caraway seeds

Wash rice until water runs clear and add to boiling water. Add salt. Cover and simmer over medium-low heat for 25 minutes. Dry-roast caraway seeds in a small cast-iron pan until golden. Add to rice mixture and cook an additional 5 minutes. Serve warm.

## WHOLE MUNG DHAL | Serves 4

1 cup whole mung dhal
$2^{1}/_{4}$ cups water
$^{1}/_{4}$ teaspoon turmeric
1 pinch of sea salt
1 tablespoon ghee
1 minced green chili pepper
$^{1}/_{2}$ teaspoon grated ginger

*1 tablespoon Late Winter* Masala *(see recipe on page 318)*
*1 teaspoon fresh lemon juice*

Wash mung dhal until water runs clear. Soak in 3 cups of cold water overnight. Drain. Boil 2 cups of water and add dhal, turmeric, and salt. Cover and simmer over medium heat for 50 minutes.

In a small skillet, heat ghee and green chili pepper and ginger for a few minutes. Add the Late Winter *Masala* toward end of browning. Add to dhal with lemon juice and remaining water. Cover and continue to simmer for an additional 30 minutes over low heat.

## SAUTEED GOLDEN BEETS WITH LATE WINTER *MASALA* | Serves 4

*4 golden beets*
*1 tablespoon sunflower oil*
*1 tablespoon Late Winter* Masala *(see recipe on page 318)*
*2 yellow onions or shallots, half-moon slices*
*1 teaspoon rock salt*
*1 tablespoon minced fresh parsley*

Scrub the beets and cut into bite-size pieces. Heat cast-iron skillet with sunflower oil. Stir in Late Winter *Masala* until slightly browned. Add shallots, beets, and salt. Stir and add two tablespoons of water. Cover and allow to cook on medium heat for 5 minutes. Remove from heat, garnish with fresh parsley, and serve hot.

## APPLE DATE TORTE | Serves 4

*2 cooking apples*
*$1/4$ cup dates*
*$1/2$ teaspoon cardamom powder*
*$1/2$ teaspoon ground nutmeg*
*1 pinch of rock salt*
*1 cup whole wheat pastry flour*
*$1/2$ teaspoon baking powder*
*2 tablespoons walnut oil*

*¹/8 cup maple syrup*
*¹/8 cup applesauce*

Preheat oven to 350 degrees. Wash and core the apples, slice thin, and set aside. Remove seeds from dates, and cut into thin strips. Combine apples, dates, cardamom, nutmeg, and salt in a mixing bowl, then set aside.

Combine flour and baking powder, then sift into a separate bowl. Add the oil and maple syrup to flour mixture, along with the applesauce. Mix into a batter and pour into an oiled baking dish. Layer fruit mixture on top of batter. Bake for 45 minutes, until a fork inserted in center of torte comes out clean. Serve warm.

# GLOSSARY OF
# SANSKRIT TERMS

**Aditi.** "vast, abundant space"; cosmic womb of creation; the Source, Aditi is sometimes depicted as the Cow of Plenty; one who feeds the celestials, humans and spirit; the Perfumed One

*advaita.* the doctrine of monism, according to which reality is ultimately nondual, comprised of One Whole; the vision of Vedanta

*agni.* "fire"; one of the fire elements; god of the element fire, invoked through Vedic ritual

*ahamkara.* ego; the "I" notion; cosmic memory recorder

*ahara rasa.* ingested nutrients, before they are digested

*ahimsa.* "nonharming"; abstinence from harmful thought, action, or word; a significant moral discipline in Vedic life, Buddhism, and Jainism

*ajna.* limitless power; name of sixth chakra

**Alvar.** "one who rules the Divine through devotion"; a group of renowned poet-saints of South India who worship the god Vishnu

*anahata.* fearless, unafflicted; nature of the black antelope; symbol and name of fourth chakra

*ananda, anandam.* essence of reality; pure joy; the mind-transcending experience of the Ultimate Reality, or Self

*annam.* literally, "that which grows on the earth"; food

*apana.* fourth air of the cosmos; keeper of the void or empty space within; preserves spirit of nonattachment (also, one of five bodily airs; air controlling ejection of bodily wastes)

**apsaras.** celestial beings

**arogya.** "health"; the opposite of disease (*vyadhi*); excellent state of well-being; true nature of the Self

**Atharva Veda.** "Atharvan's knowledge"; one of four Vedic hymn collections that deals with magical spells, rituals, and yoga (see also *Rig Veda, Sama Veda,* and *Yajur Veda*)

**Atman.** Indwelling Spirit; soul within body; conscious self

**avidya.** ignorance of our essentially infinite nature

**Ayurveda.** "science of life"; Mother of Medicine; a holistic system of medicine and health which comes from the *Atharva* and *Rig Vedas*; ancient authorities on Ayurveda are Charaka, Sushruta, and Vagbhata; Ayurveda covers many areas of medicine, including general, surgery, physiology, gynecology, psychology, pediatrics, diseases of the head, pharmacology, veterinary science, herbology, tonics and rejuvenation, sexual rejuvenation, science of the subtle body, demonology; Ayurveda is a nature-based system of health and healing which springs from the native wisdom of the sages and their uncompromised adherence to the cosmic rhythms; the aim of Ayurveda is longevity and health achieved by balancing energies (especially the *doshas*, or bodily humors) at all levels of being, subtle and gross, through innumerable methods and therapies selected in accord with the individual's constitution, lifeways, and nature; Ayurveda, as a holistic form of medicine, is kin to all native medicine traditions, such as Chinese, African, Amerindian, Native American, and South American; among the first surgeons was Sushruta (600 B.C.E.), whose *Sushruta Samhita* is studied to this day (Hippocrates, the Greek father of medicine, lived two centuries later.)

**Bhagavan.** "one who possesses sixfold virtue"; a god of the *Rig Veda*, lord of wealth, fame, power, knowledge, happiness, compassion.

**bhakti.** faith, devotion

**bhramari.** a bee; a traditional breath practice in which the practitioner imitates the bee and vibrates the entire nervous system, brain and body, by buzzing the vocal cords

**bija.** "seed"; as in *bija* mantra; a karmic imprint on the subconscious

**bija mantra.** "seed syllable"; a primordial sound, such as *ham, rang, hrim*

**bindu.** "drop"; the dot placed above the Sanskrit letter M in syllabic word or mantra; the nasalized sound itself; also, an energy center of consciousness in the head directly above *ajna* chakra

**brahmacharini.** one whose life is devoted to Self-Knowledge; one whose conduct is *Brahman*, pure consciousness; spiritual aspirant in Vedic monastic lineage, who observes rigorous spiritual disciplines

**Brahmacharya.** one of the foundational practices of yoga, renunciation of the material world and devotion to scriptural study; the observance of chastity in thought, word, or action

**Brahman.** Absolute Consciousness, which is distinct from Brahma, the Creator

**brahmana.** Brahmin; "evolved or mature soul"; the mature soul, which is exemplary of wisdom, tolerance, and humility; from Brahman, "growth, evolution, swelling of the spirit"; also, a member of the priestly class of Vedic society

**brahma shabda.** cosmic sound

**brahmavidya.** literally "knowledge of Brahman"; knowledge of the self as one with consciousness

**buddhi.** cognition; faculty of personal wisdom; intuitive faculty; resolve of the mind; the intellect; *buddhi* is characterized by discrimination (*viveka*), voluntary restraint (*vairagya*), cultivation of inner quietude (*shanti*), contentment (*santosha*), and forgiveness (*kshama*). Also, Buddhi-Mercury, son of Shiva; deity who rules Wednesday

**causal body.** *karana sarira,* the inmost body; the soul form

**chai.** Indian tea mixed with milk and sugar

**chakra.** "wheel"; the energy centers of consciousness located within the human being's subtle body. (There are fourteen major chakras in all; seven primary chakras can be seen psychically as multipetaled lotuses. These are situated along the spinal column from the base to the cranial chamber. Additionally, there are seven chakras, barely visible, that exist below the spine. These are the centers of karmic consciousness, the seat of all negative emotions.)

***chandra-mauli.*** "moon-crested"; a particular blood vessel in the vulva which acts as a magnetic lodestone, drawing the energy of the moon to revitalize the womb

***chandra-mukha.*** "moon-faced"; a Sanskrit name for the vagina

**chapati.** thin Vedic flatbread baked on a skillet and allowed to balloon over an open fire

***chit.*** pure awareness; transcendent consciousness, beyond all thought

***chitta.*** "mind"; "consciousness"; the psyche or consciousness that depends on the play of attention, as opposed to *chit*

**Dakshinamurti.** "south-facing form"; the god Shiva depicted sitting under a *pipala* tree, silently transmitting Jnanam, the knowledge of Self to four *rishis* at his feet

***damaru.*** "drum"; a small double-headed, hourglass-shaped drum used in Vedic rituals and meditation practices (the sound of this drum is associated with the element of space)

***darshana.*** "vision"; "sight"; seeing the Divine; seeing with inner or outer vision (The eyes are the locus through which energy is exchanged. Gods, goddesses, and gurus are said to "give" *darshana* and disciples and devotees to "receive" *darshana*. Also, *darshana* is receiving the grace and blessing of the deity, holy person, or place. This direct infusion of energy and blessing from the venerated being is a long-standing tradition and sought-after experience of Hindu faith.)

***deva.*** "shining one"; "god"; refers to one of the many Vedic deities; *devas* are seen as powerful beings in the subtle realms of existence

**Devabhasa.** communication of the gods; original name of the Sanskrit language

**Devi.** "the shining one"; name for the Divine Mother

***dhal.*** traditional Indian bean soup

**Dhara Devi.** "support"; a name of the Earth Goddess

***dharana.*** "sustaining"; concentration; prolonged focus of attention on a single mental object and leading to meditation

**dharma.** from *dhri*, "to sustain, carry, or hold"; Divine law; law of being; right action according to the laws of nature; also, the path of righteousness, virtue, justice, and truth (Dharma is the inherent nature of the human and its fulfillment is the profound aim of human destiny.)

*dhup.* pine kindling used in Vedic fire rituals

*dhyana.* "meditation"; meditative contemplation or absorption; the seventh limb of Patanjali's eightfold yoga

*dosha.* literally, "fault," "flaw," or "defect"; one of the three forces which springs from the five elements within the body, *vata* (air/space), *pitta* (fire/water), and *kapha* (water/ earth); also, *dosha* refers to the five flaws of human nature: lust, anger, greed, fear, and delusion

**Durga.** one who is difficult to attain; the eight-armed Vedic Warrior Goddess who rides a lion and drums the world into being with her *damaru* (drum); a name for Shiva's consort, who symbolizes Self-knowledge

*dvani.* dynamic, audible sound

**Gaja.** "elephant"; elephant symbol of the fifth chakra, *vishuddha*

*gandarva.* "fragrant"; the name of the celestial musicians

**Gayatri.** the celebrated mantra of the *Rig Veda* imparted to the Brahmanas at the time of their initiation into *Brahmacharya* at the age of eight (The Gayatri mantra is considered the greatest among Vedic hymns. It is addressed to the sun-god as a form of the divine light. Gayatri is also called the Mother of the Vedas, and protects those who recite it.)

**ghee.** purified butter, prepared by simmering unsalted butter on low heat until all the water content of the butter boils off and the milk solids remain. Ghee is considered a primary elixir of good health.

*gopi.* cowherdess; the name of god Krishna's devotees said to be the incarnations of the *rishis*

*guna.* quality, nature, or virtue; three primary constituents of nature (i.e., *sattra, rajas, tamas*)

*ha.* Sanskrit syllable representing the solar energy

*hamsa.* "gander"; generally translated as "swan," the breath, or life force *(prana)*; a type of wandering ascetic

**hatha yoga.** "yoga of force"; the yoga of physical and mental discipline developed by the seers as a means of physical, emotional, and spiritual revitalization (This practice has been used as preparation for meditation and integration of lunar and solar energies. Hatha yoga consists of postures *[asanas]*, internal cleansing practices *[dhanti or shodana]*, breath control *[pranayama]*, locks *[bandha]*, and sacred hand gestures *[mudra]*, all of which regulate and energize the flow of prana and purify body, mind, and spirit.)

**ida-nadi.** "soothing conduit"; the lunar, feminine current flowing along the left channel of the spine

**jnana, jnanam.** liberating knowledge; according to the *rishis*, *jnana* is the last of the four successive stages *(padas)* of spiritual unfoldment

**jnani.** a wise person; awakened one; according to the Vedas, it is possible to gain enlightenment even while still embodied—the Self-realized sage who is thus liberated is known as a *jnani* or *jiva-mukti*

**kala.** "time"; an integral aspect of the finite world; nutritional membrane for tissues; "body crystal"

**Kali.** "darkness"; "time"; Vedic goddess Kali, who destroys illusions, is honored in India as an aspect of the Divine Mother from whom all are born and to whom all must return. (According to Vedic cosmology, we are living in the age of Kali. Kali energy is what moves through us in times of stupendous change and transformation.)

**Kali yuga.** "yoke of Kali"; the fourth and final phase of universal existence, the age of cosmic dissolution that is said to precede the dawn of a golden era (This period is traditionally held to have commenced in 3102 B.C.E.)

**kama.** "desire"; a deity, the Vedic Cupid; also, excessive desire or lust, one of the obstacles on the spiritual path

**Kameshvara.** a name for Shiva; Lord of Desire (*kama*=pleasure, desire; *Isvara*=Supreme Personal God)

**Kameshvari.** a name for Shakti; Goddess of Desire, consort of Kameshvara (*kama*=pleasure, desire; *Isvari*=Supreme or Personal Goddess)

**kapalabhati.** "skull-luster"; comprised of three practices to clear passages of breath, remove phlegm, and give beauty and vitality

**kapha.** biological water humor; the principle of potential energy, which controls body stability and lubrication

**karma yoga.** "yoga of action"; the necessary performance of actions that are in harmony with one's innermost purpose, nature, and being *(sva-bhava)*; a primary life practice in yoga

**kosha.** "sheath"; Vedic term for a bodily casing, of which there are five: the food-body, breath-body, mind-body, cognitive-body, and infinite-body or Infinite Self

**kundal.** "coiled"; referring to the serpentine force of kundalini

**kundalini.** the primordial cosmic force embedded in the root chakra; primal energy of manifestation symbolized by a coiled serpent at the coccyx of the spine (the kundalini's ascent to the crown chakra creates a temporary state of transcendence into the Absolute Reality)

**linga, lingam.** the phallus as both creative aspect and supreme consciousness of the Divine; "Mark of Shiva"; sign

**Maha-kala.** "great time"; "dissolver of time"; one of the names and forms for Shiva, Maha-kala devours time and with it all forms and, by so doing, helps the soul to transcend all dualities

**Mahashakti.** "Great Mother"; the feminine power aspect of the Divine

**mala.** traditional Vedic prayer beads, generally consisting of 108 beads; garland of flowers

**manas.** "mind"; "understanding"; the lower, or empirical, mind; seat of desire and governor of the sensory and motor organs *(Manas* is characterized by desire and willpower.)

**mandala.** circular, mystical diagram; a circular diagram without beginning or end which symbolizes the infinite; a picture or group of syllables or words used in meditation to access the infinite inner realm

**mandir.** Hindu temple

**manipura.** "city of gems"; third chakra; psychic center at the solar plexus which governs willpower

**mantra.** "mystic sound"; a sound, syllable, word, or phrase imbued with significant power, drawn from Sanskrit (Mantras are recited to invoke the energy of the deities and to enforce an energetic field of protection. When chanted, mantras help to quiet the mind, harmonize the body's inner rhythms, and evoke our deep spiritual qualities. Traditionally, to be effective, mantras must be given by the preceptor through initiation.)

**mantra yoga.** the yoga of mystic sound and recital of the Vedic chants

*marma.* Ayurveda's vast tapestry of the anatomical reflex points of the body; junctions of *pranic* energy; vital junctures where muscles, tendons, joints, and ligaments intersect; somewhat synonymous with acupuncture points

*masala.* a traditional mixture of Indian spices

**maya.** "measure"; the creative, divisive force of the Divine; the mirage that hides the Ultimate Reality; relative reality; the principle of manifestation; the cosmic creative force of creation, preservation, and dissolution

**Maya Shakti.** Mother Nature; the primordial force behind creation

*mithya.* interdependent; that which has its basis in something else (for example, the whole manifestation has its source in the Absolute Reality)

*moksha.* "liberation"; "release"; liberation from the cycles of rebirth (according to Vedanta, the highest of four possible human pursuits or goals); final liberation or self-realization

**mudra.** "seal"; a sacred hand gesture which expresses specific powers or energies. (Mudra practice helps to conduct consciousness in the body; mudras are a vital, integral aspect of Vedic ritual, worship, prayer, dance, and yoga.)

*muladhara.* "foundation"; "supported"; first chakra; four-petaled psychic center, located at the base of the spine; it is here that the serpent power *(kundalini-shakti)* lies dormant.

*muni.* an ascetic, or forest-dwelling sage, who has kinship with all creatures; also, one who practices *mauna*, silence

*nada.* manifested sound

*nadi.* "conduit"; "channel"; according to Ayurveda, the human anatomy consists of a network of 72,000 subtle conduits or nerve channels, along which flows *prana*, the life force (of these channels, three are most significant—they are *ida*, *pingala*, and *sushumna*)

**Nataraja.** "King of Dance"; God Shiva is the cosmic dancer, and his dance is the dance of the entire cosmos, depicting spirituality and creativity in perfect unison (Through the cosmic dance, Shiva demonstrates that which is created is inseparable from its creator. Nataraja represents the Primal Soul [Paramesvara], power, energy, and life of all that exists. This cosmic dance symbolizes stillness and motion merging into One Consciousness.)

**Navaratri.** Hindu festival celebrating the Divine Mother in her three primary forms: Saraswati, Lakshmi, and Durga

**ojas.** "glow of health"; primeval energy held in the body and which may appear as one's aura; energy produced through disciplined yogic practice, especially the practice of chastity

**pada.** the foot; section, stage, or path; according to *Shaiva Siddhanta*, there are four *padas* or stages for the soul to move through

**Parashakti.** one of two primordial aspects of creation; Goddess Shakti as the basis of creation; beyond time, space, and form

**Parashiva.** one of two primordial aspects of creation; God Shiva as the pillar of consciousness; Absolute Reality

**Pashupati.** "Lord of Souls"; Shiva as Lord of the Creatures

**Patanjali.** Traditionally regarded as the author of the yoga sutras and of the *Brahma-Sutra of Badarayana*, one of the foundational works of the Vedanta tradition. Patanjali lived in 200 C.E. Also the name of the Sanskrit grammarian who lived in 150 C.E.

**pingala-nadi.** "tawny conduit"; the solar, masculine current flowing along the right channel of the spine

**pitri.** "forebear"; "ancestor" (the ancestor plays a significant role in the daily life of the Vedic people)

**Pitri Paksha.** a specific time of year when the ancestors' spirits are remembered and nourished with rites, rituals, and prayers

**pitta.** biological fire humor; the principle which controls digestion and the enzymatic and endocrine systems

**prakriti.** "primary matter or nature"; potentiality of physical cosmos; gross energy from which all the elements are formed; the three qualities of *sattva*, *rajas*, and *tamas* are the intrinsic energies of *prakriti*; active principle of manifestation; synonymous with *maya* *prajna.* "wisdom"; liberating wisdom; that which gives way to the Transcendental Reality

*prajna-paradha.* "crimes against wisdom"; going against the grain of the cosmic intelligence; perverting the mind to engage in activities known to be unwholesome

*prana.* life force; vital air; from the root *pran* (to breathe); principal form of the five airs of the body; called "ki" or "chi" in Oriental medicine; the five *pranas* are *prana, apana, smana, udana,* and *vyana*; one of the three primordial conditions of the cosmos (*ojas, tejas,* and *prana*)

*pranayama.* "breath control"; the regulation or expansion of the breath, which is an integral limb of Patanjali's eightfold yoga.

*puja.* Vedic ritual or ceremony

*pujari.* Hindu priest; pundit

*Purana.* "ancient lore"; a popular religious body of work on Vedic cosmology and theology

*Purusha Sukta.* a hymn from the *Rig Veda* composed by the sage Narayana (Purusha is the cosmic person, having a thousand heads, a thousand eyes, a thousand feet, and encompassing the earth, spreading in all directions into animate and inanimate things.)

*rajas.* cosmic force of activity; one of the three *gunas* (*sattva, rajas,* and *tamas*); excess *rajas* causes the mind to become overactive, unstable

*rasa.* taste; lymph or plasma; the first of the seven vital tissues; also, aesthetic or refined beauty

*Rig Veda.* "knowledge of praise"; the oldest collection of Vedic hymns; the most sacred Vedic scripture (See also *Atharva Veda, Sama Veda,* and *Yajur Veda.*)

*rishi.* "seer"; a term for an enlightened being, a wise and psychic visionary (In the Vedic age, *rishis* lived in forest or mountain retreats, either alone or with disciples. The *rishis* were the greatest visionaries, who were the inspired conveyors of the Vedas and who infused their creative force of vision of the Ultimate Reality into the wellspring of Vedic tradition. Sage Narayana, considered to be the first *rishi* to "see" and articulate Vedic vision, came to be known as Adi

Rishi, "the first seer." The knowledge he shares is in the six-teen mantras known as *Parusha Sukta*. This was the earth's first information on the cosmic anatomy and ecology.)

*rita.* cosmic rhythm; sacred order of the universe

**Rudra.** "wielder of stupendous powers"; "red, shining one"; the name of Shiva as the universal force of dissolution and re-absorption (Rudra-Shiva is revered as the "terrifying One" and the "Lord of Tears.")

*sadhaka.* one who practices *sadhana*; a spiritual aspirant

*sadhana.* wholesome, everyday practices observed in accor-dance with the cyclical rhythms of nature; spiritual prac-tice that awakens the power of awareness; healthy, joyful response to life

*sadhu.* "virtuous one, unerring and pure"; a holy person dedi-cated to the search for consciousness

*sahasrara.* "a thousand petals"; the seventh chakra, situated in the crown of the head

*samadhi.* "sameness"; "standing within one's Self"; state of cos-mic union with the Divine; state of true yoga, in which the meditator and the object of meditation are one; *samadhi* has two levels: *savikalpa samadhi* (identification or oneness with the essence of an object) and *nirvikalpa samadhi* (iden-tification with the Self, in which all modes of conscious-ness are transcended and Absolute Reality—beyond time, space, and form—is experienced

*samana.* third of five airs of the body; keeper of balance

**Sama Veda.** "knowledge of chants"; the Vedic hymns contain-ing the chants used in ceremonies and rituals (See also *Atharva Veda, Rig Veda,* and *Yajur Veda*.)

*samsara.* misery created by misperceiving the Self as separate from the Whole

*sat, satyam.* "truth"; "existence"; "being"; that which is the Ulti-mate Reality; the cosmic truth

*satsanga.* "in the company of the real"; the traditional Vedic practice of sitting in the beneficent presence of saints, sages, and enlightened beings who communicate or trans-mit the cosmic truth

*sattva.* cosmic force of equilibrium; naturally peaceful and balanced state of a healthy body and mind; one of the three *gunas* (*sattva, rajas*, and *tamas*)

**Shakta Upanishad.** text disclosing the teachings related to Shakti, the feminine aspect of the Divine

**shakti.** cosmic feminine force; power, energy; power of consciousness

**shanti mudra.** the sacred hand gesture of cosmic peace

**siddhi.** "perfection"; "accomplishment"; spiritual perfection that results from complete identification with the Ultimate Reality

**sitali.** the cooling breath; a specific *pranayama* practice wherein the breath is inhaled through the mouth by curving the tongue to form a channel

**smriti.** "memory"; "remembered knowledge"; the tradition of the *rishis* which gave way to revelation, *sruti*

**sruti.** what is heard; cosmic revelation as heard, seen, and articulated by the Vedic seers

**sukhasana.** posture of ease or comfort

**sukshma-prana.** subtle life force

**Surya.** Vedic sun-god

**sushumna.** "she who is most gracious"; central and main channel within spinal column (This channel extends from the root chakra at the base of the spine to the crown chakra of the head, and it is along this central pathway that the aroused kundalini must ascend.)

**svadhisthana.** "one's own base"; sacred chakra situated directly below the navel

**tamas.** cosmic force of inertia; natural state of the body during rest or of the universe during dissolution; one of the three *gunas* (*sattva, rajas*, and *tamas*)

**tanmatra.** energy quanta; a measure of energy

**Tantra.** "loom"; a body of sacred scripture originated in the early centuries of the Common Era, pertaining to Tantrism and primarily dealing with ritual practices centering on the feminine divine principle *shakti*

**tapas, tapasya.** "heat"; "glow"; asceticism; observance of austerities and yogic disciplines to induce inner luminosity and vitality; intense disciplines imbibed by the sages, seers, and yogis

**tejas.** effulgent, brilliant energy; the light of pure consciousness within the body; subtle fire; one of the three primordial conditions in creation (*ojas*, *tejas*, and *prana*)

**tha.** Sanskrit syllable representing the lunar energy

**udana.** second of five breaths of the body; rising air; universal keeper of memory and personal sound

**Upanishad.** "sitting near"; Vedic scriptures composed from what was seen and articulated by the celestials and *rishis* (The Upanishads expound the metaphysics of Oneness, the Whole, nondualism [*Advaita Vedanta*]. Over two hundred Upanishads exist, although Vedic traditionalists recognize only 108 of them. These Upanishads are organized in eight distinct groups. Originally, Vedic texts were not written, but memorized and transmitted from teacher to pupil by word of mouth.)

**Ushas.** "dawn"; Daughter of Heaven, the light of dawn that illuminates the world; consort of the sun-god, Surya; Vedic cow goddess

**Vac.** "speech"; a feminine deity, as the Mother of the Vedas (She is said to have four *padas*, or aspects, human speech being one of the four *padas* that is known to humans.)

**vajra.** "unyielding"; a thunderbolt (the weapon of Indra, Lord of the Firmament)

**varnas.** pure vibration; profound silence; unmanifest sound

**vasana.** "trait" or "characteristic"; desire or longing; in Patanjali yoga, the subtle subliminal imprints in the mind, stamped there as a result of our actions and volitions

**vata.** biological air humor; the principle of kinetic energy in the body, mainly concerned with the nervous system and which controls all body movement

**vikriti.** state of imbalance and disease in the body, generally caused by disharmonious habits and lifeways; disharmonious habits

**vina.** an ancient Indian stringed instrument (Goddess Saraswati is depicted as playing the vina.)

**vishuddha.** "purity"; the fifth chakra, situated in the throat; center of divine love

**Vriksha-Natha.** a name for Shiva, Protector of the Vegetation

**vyana.** fifth air of the cosmos; air of circulation

*yajna.* "sacrifice"; the ritual sacrifices fundamental to Hinduism (In the Vedic era, external sacrificial ritual was internalized in the form of deep meditation.)

**Yama.** "Lord of Death"; one who receives the souls of the deceased

**Yama Damstra.** period of time between November 22 and December 9, when the earth begins its northward rotation around the sun (According to the Vedas, Lord Yama actively scours the earth for souls during this time. This time holds within it an innate structure of fear and mental disturbance for human beings.)

**yoga.** from the root *yuj* (to join or unite); spiritual discipline or mystical practice to merge body, mind, and spirit, or inner and outer universe; one of six classical schools of thought presented by Patanjali in his *Yoga-Sutra*

**yoni.** the womb; source of creation

**yoni mudra.** "womb-seal"; a sealing hand posture or gesture wherein the fingers are intertwined and the aspirant's attention is directed within to find the source of his/her being

**yuga.** "yoke"; according to Vedic cosmology, there are four *yugas*, or stages of existence in the world, each consisting of several thousand years

# VEDIC RESOURCES

## Vedic Studies

Wise Earth School of Ayurveda
(Bri. Maya Tiwari)
90 Davis Creek Road
Candler, NC 28715
(828) 258-9999
www.wisearth.org
e-mail: health@wisearth.org

Mother Om Mission
(Bri. Maya Tiwari)
Guyana, South America
www.motherom.org
e-mail: health@wisearth.org

Arsha Vidya Gurukulum
(H. H. Swami Dayananda Saraswati)
P.O. Box 1059
Saylorsburg, PA 18353
(570) 992-2339
e-mail: avp@epix.net

## Ayurvedic Studies

Wise Earth School of Ayurveda
(Bri. Maya Tiwari)
90 Davis Creek Road
Candler, NC 28715
(828) 258-9999
www.wisearth.org
e-mail: health@wisearth.org

\* \* \* \*

American Institute of Vedic Studies
(Dr. David Frawley)
P.O. Box 8357
Santa Fe, NM 87501
(505) 983-9385

Ayurvedic Healing Arts Center
16508 Pine Knoll Road
Grass Valley, CA 95945
(916) 274-9000

Ayurvedic Institute & Wellness Center
(Dr. Vasant Lad)
P.O. Box 23445
Albuquerque, NM 87192-1445
(505) 291-9698

The Chopra Center for Well-Being
7630 Fay Avenue
La Jolla, CA 92037
(858) 551-7788
Fax: (858) 551-9570

Himalayan Institute
RR1, Box 400
Honesdale, PA 18431
(800) 822-4547

Institute for Wholistic Education
33719 116th Street, Box SH
Twin Lakes, WI 53181
(414) 889-8501

Lotus Ayurvedic Center
4145 Clares Street, Suite D
Capitola, CA 95010
(408) 479-1667

New England School of Ayurvedic Medicine
1815 Massachusetts Avenue
Cambridge, MA 02140
(617) 876-2401


## Vedic Music and Dance

Rajkumari Cultural Center
84-25 118th Street #1F
Kew Gardens, NY 11415
(718) 805-8068
e-mail: goraj@juno.com

Yogi Hari's Ashram
2216 NW 8th Terrace

Ft. Lauderdale, FL 33311
(800) 964-2553
www.yogihari.com

## Suppliers of Ayurvedic Herbal Products

Auroma International
P.O. Box 1008, Dept. ABC
Silver Lake, WI 53170
(414) 889-8569

Ayurveda Center of Santa Fe
1807 Second Street, Suite 20
Santa Fe, NM 87505
(505) 983-8898

Ayurvedic Concept
6950 Portwest Drive, Suite 170
Houston, TX 77024
(713) 863-1622

Ayurvedic Institute & Wellness Center
11311 Menaul N.E., Suite A
Albuquerque, NM 87112
(505) 291-9698

Ayurveda Yoga Institute
263 Teaneck Road
Ridgefield Park, NJ 07660
(201) 440-3106

Ayush Herbs, Inc.
10025 N.E. 4th Street
Bellevue, WA 98004
(800) 925-1371

Banyan Trading Co.
P.O. Box 13002
Albuquerque, NM 87192-3002
(505) 275-2469
www.banyantrading.com

Bazaar of India Imports, Inc.
1810 University Avenue
Berkeley, CA 94703
(800) 261-7662

Herbal Vedic Products
Ayur Herbal Corporation
P.O. Box 6054
Santa Fe, NM 87502
(414) 889-8569

Lotus Herbs
1505 42nd Avenue, Suite 19
Capitola, CA 95010
(408) 479-1667

Maharishi Ayurveda Products
International Inc.
417 Bolton Road
P.O. Box 541
Lancaster, MA 01523
(800) 255-8332

Sushakti
1840 Iron Street, Suite C
Bellingham, WA 98225
(888) 774-2584
e-mail: info@ayurveda-sushakti.com

Tej Ayurvedic Skin Care, Inc.
162 West 56th Street, Room 204
New York, NY 10019
(800) 310-0179


## Vedic Bookstores

Arsha Vidya Bookstore
P.O. Box 1059
Saylorsburg, PA 18353
(570) 992-2339
e-mail: avp@epix.net

South Asia Books
P.O. Box 502
Columbia, MO 65205
(314) 474-0166

## Vedic Musical Instruments and Sacred Items

Jai Vishwa Gifts
2353 County Road P
Malmo, NE 68040
(402) 642-9238
Fax: (402) 642-5240
e-mail: peace2u@tvsonline.net
(*dholak* drums, harmonium, Himalayan singing bowls, Vedic hand cymbals, prayer beads, Vedic idols, statues, and posters, and sacred items for Vedic rituals and ceremonies)

# BIBLIOGRAPHY

*Ancient Indian Historical Tradition.* F. E. Pargiter. Delhi: Motilal Banarsidass, repr. 1972. First published 1922.

*Antal and Her Path of Love: Poems of a Woman Saint from South India.* Vidy Dehejia. Albany, NY: S.U.N.Y. Press, 1990.

*Arsha Vidya (The Vision of the Rishis).* Swami Dayananda Saraswati. Saylorsburg, PA: Arsha Vidya Gurukulam, 1990.

*Atma Bodha of Sankaracarya.* 2d ed. Vidyaratna T. N. Menon. Palghat, India: The Educational Supplies Depot, 1964.

*Autobiography of a Yogi.* Paramahansa Yogananda. Los Angeles, CA: Self-Realization Fellowship, 1987. First publ. 1946.

*Ayurvedic Medicine, Past and Present.* Pandit Shiv Sharma. Calcutta, India: Dabur Publications, 1975.

*Caraka Samhita.* P. V. Sharma. Delhi, India: Chaukhambha Orientalia, 1981.

*A Celtic Anthology.* Little Grace Rhys. New York, NY: Thomas Y. Crowell Co., 1927

*Celtic Myths & Magick: Harnessing the Power of the Gods and Goddesses.* Edian McCoy. St. Paul, MN: Llewellyn Publications, 1995.

*Dancing with Siva: Hinduism's Contemporary Catechism.* Satguru Sivaya Subramuniyaswami. Concord, CA: Himalayan Academy, 1993.

*The Death of Nature.* Carolyn Merchant. New York, NY: Harper & Row, 1980.

*The Doctrine of Vibration: An Analysis of the Doctrines and Practices of Kashmir Saivism.* Mark S. G. Dyczkowski. Albany, NY: S.U.N.Y. Press, 1987.

*Doctrines of Pathology in Ayurveda.* Vidyavilas Ayurveda Series, #3, Prof. K. R. Srikantha Murthy. Varanasi, India: Chaukhambha Orientalia, 1987.

*The Edited Works of Ramana Maharshi.* Edited by Arthur Osborne. London: Rider, 1986.

*Essays on the Gita.* Sri. Aurobindo. Pondicherry, India: Sri Auribindo Ashram, 1949.

*The Ever-Present Origin.* Jean Gebser. Athens, OH: Ohio University Press, 1985.

*Faith in a Seed: The Dispersion of Seeds and Other Late Natural History Writings.* ed. Bradley P. Dean. Washington, DC: Island Press, 1993.

*Gitanjali.* Rabindranath Tagore. New York: Collier Press, 1971.

*The Goddesses and Gods of Old Europe.* Marija Gimbutas. Berkeley, CA: University of California Press, 1974.

*Gorakhnath and the Kanphata Yogis.* George W. Briggs. Delhi: Motilal Banarsidass, repr. 1973.

*Great Systems of Yoga.* Ernest Wood. New York: Citadel Press, 1968.

*A Handbook of Ayurveda.* Vaidya Bhagwan Dash and Acarya Manfred M. Junius. New Delhi, India: Concept Publishing Co, 1983.

*The Heart of the Goddess.* Halle Iglehart Austen. Berkeley, CA: Wingbow Press, 1990.

*The Heart of Yoga: Developing a Personal Practice.* T. K. V. Desikachar. Rochester, VT: Inner Traditions International, 1995.

*Hindu Mysticism.* Surendranath Dasgupta. Delhi: Motilal Banarsidass, 1927.

*Inspired Talks.* 3d ed. Swami Vivekananda. Madras, India: Sri Ramakrishna Math, 1921.

*Japa: Mantra Meditation.* Swami Dayananda Saraswati. Saylorsburg, PA: Arsha Vidya Gurukulam, 1990.

*Kali: The Feminine Force.* Ajit Mookerjee. New York: Destiny Books, 1988.

*Loving Ganesha: Hinduism's Endearing Elephant-Faced God.* Satguru Sivaya Subramuniyaswami. Concord, CA: Himalayan Academy, 1996.

*Madhava Nidanam (Roga Viniscaya) of Madhavakara: A Treatise on Ayurveda.* Jaikrishnadas Ayurveda Series, #69. Prof. K. R. Srikanta Murthy. New Delhi, India: Chaukhambha Orientalia, 1987.

*Mantra Kirtana, Yantra and Tantra.* Swami Mayananda Jyoti. Bombay, India: D. B. Taraporevala Sons & Co, 1991.

*Mantra-Yoga-Samhita.* Ram Kumar Rai. Varansi, India: Chaukhambha Orientalia, 1982.

*Mystic Saints of India: Shankaracharya.* Prem Lata. Delhi, India: Sumit Publications, 1982.

*Nada Brahma: The World Is Sound.* Joachim-Ernst Berendt. Rochester, VT: Destiny Books, 1987.

*Path to Bliss: A Practical Guide to Stages of Meditation.* Dalai Lama. Translated by Geshe Thubten Jinpa and edited by Christine Cox. Ithaca, NY: Snow Lion, 1991.

*The Power of Myth.* Joseph Campbell. New York, NY: Doubleday, 1988.

*The Ramayana of Valmiki.* New Delhi, India: Chaukhambha Orientalia, 1984.

*The Sadhana and the Sadhya.* Swami Dayananda. Purani Jhadi, Rishikesh, India: Sri. Gangadhareswar Trust, 1984.

*Saundarya Lahari (Inundation of Divine Splendour).* (Based on Swami Tapasyananda's translation.) Sri. Sankaracarya. Madras, India: Sri Ramakrishna Math, 1991.

*The Serpent Power, Being the Satcakranirupana and the Padukapanchaka.* 10th ed. Arthur Avalon [see also John Woodroffe]. Madras, India: Ganesh & Co., 1974. First published 1913.

*Shiva: An Introduction.* Devdutt Pattanaik. Mumbai, India: Vakils, Feffer and Simons, 1997.

*Srimad Bhagavad Gita: Bhasya of Sri Sankaracarya.* Sri Ramakrishna Math (Sanskrit edition) Madras, India: Mylapore, 1983.

*Sushruta Samhita.* Translated by K. L. Bhishagratna (Sanskrit series.) Varanasi, India: Chaukhambha Orientalia, 1981.

*A Tagore Reader.* Amiya Chakravarty. Boston, MA: Beacon Press, 1961.

*Tantra of the Great Liberation (Mahanirvana Tantra).* Translated by Arthur Avalon. New York: Dover, 1972.

*The Tantric Tradition.* Agehananda Bharati. London: Rider and Co., 1965; New York: Samuel Weiser, rev. ed., 1975.

*Tattwa Shuddhi: The Tantric Practice of Inner Purification.* Swami Satyasangananda Saraswati. Munger, India: Bihar School of Yoga, 1984.

*Teaching Tradition of Advaita Vedanta.* Swami Dayananda Saraswati. Saylorsburg, PA: Arsha Vidya Gurukulam, 1990.

*Tools for Tantra.* Harish Johari. Rochester, VT: Destiny Books, 1986.

*Turning Point: Science, Society, and the Rising Culture.* Fritjof Capra. New York, NY: Bantam, 1983.

*Upadesha Sahasri of Sri Sankaracarya.* Sri Ramakrishna Math. (Sanskrit/English edition.) Madras, India: Mylapore, 1984.

*Upanishad Bhasyam,* Vol. 1. (Sri Shankara Bhagavatpada's version, Sanskrit edition.) Varanasi, India: Mahesh Research Institute, 1949.

*The Upanishads.* Translated by Eknath Easwaran. Tomales, CA: Nilgiri Press, 1996.

*The Upanishads and Self Knowledge.* Swami Dayananda Saraswati. Saylorsburg, PA: Arsha Vidya Gurukulam, 1990.

*The Vedas: Harmony, Meditation and Fulfillment.* Jeanine Miller. London: Rider, 1974.

*Viveka Chudamani of Sri Sankaracarya.* Swami Madhavananda. Calcutta, India: Aovaita Ashram, 1982.

*Viveka Chudamani of Sri Sankaracarya.* Swami Turiyananda. Madras, India: Sri Ramakrishna Math, 1998.

*When the Drummers Were Women.* Layne Redmond. New York: Three Rivers Press, 1997.

*Yoga: The Method of Re-Integration.* Alain Danielou. London: Christopher Johnson, 1949.

*Yoga Philosophy of Patanjali.* rev. ed. Hariharananda Aranya. Translated by P. N. Mukerji. Albany, NY: S.U.N.Y. Press, 1983.

## SELECT PERIODICALS

*Hinduism Today.* A bimonthly magazine for Hindus and students of Hinduism published by the Himalayan Academy and founded by H. H. Satguru Sivaya Subramuniyaswami.

Address: *Hinduism Today,* 107 Kaholalele Road, Kapaa, HI 96746-9304. Editorial tel.: (808) 822-7032. Subscription tel.: (808) 823-9620 or (800) 850-1008.

*Yoga & Health.* A monthly magazine published by Yoga Today Ltd. and edited by Jane Sill.

Address: *Yoga & Health,* 21 Caburn Crescent, Lewes, East Sussex BN7 1NR, England.

*Yoga Journal.* A bimonthly magazine published by the California Yoga Teachers Association and edited by Kathryn Arnold.

Editorial offices: 2054 University Avenue, Berkeley, CA 94704.

Subscription address: *Yoga Journal,* P.O. Box 469018, Escondido, CA 92046-9018. Tel.: (510) 841-9200.

# INDEX

Bri. Maya grew up and was educated in British Guiana (now Guyana). Born of Eastern Indian parents, whose great-grandparents had emigrated to the Indies as indentured laborers, at fifteen she moved to New York City to become a successful fashion designer. At twenty-three, forced by ovarian cancer to redirect her life, Bri. Maya left a highly successful career and returned to her ancestral India to study the ancient Indian spiritual tradition of Vedanta and Ayurvedic medicine. She is now an internationally renowned teacher and practitioner of Ayurveda and is the founder of the Wise Earth School, an Ayurvedic, nature-based facility for healing in Asheville, North Carolina, where she lives. Bri. Maya is also the founder of the Mother Om Mission (M.O.M.), headquartered in Guyana, South America, with a base in Queens, New York, a charitable organization the goal of which is to provide Ayurvedic health care to at-risk communities throughout the world. Bri. Maya gives numerous lectures at major conferences, where she has taught thousands of attendees, and as a spiritual teacher conducts *satsangas*—the traditional Vedic forum for the spiritual master to share wisdom and spirituality—throughout the world to give solace to the grieving and afflicted. Also a traditional guru and spiritual mother to hundreds, Bri. Maya is called Maya Ma (Mother Maya) by her devotees. She has been featured on the cover of *Yoga Journal,* has made radio and television appearances, and writes a regular column for *Hinduism Today,* an international Hindu newspaper that has over a million readers. Bri. Maya returns to India annually for a three-month silent meditation retreat. She is the author of *Ayurveda: Secrets of Healing* (Lotus Light) and *Ayurveda: A Life of Balance* (Healing Arts Press).